Ten Years of Viewing from Within
The Legacy of Francisco Varela

Edited by

Claire Petitmengin

imprint-academic.com

Copyright © Imprint Academic, 2009

No part of this publication may be reproduced in any form
without permission, except for the quotation of brief passages
in criticism and discussion.

Published in the UK by Imprint Academic
PO Box 200, Exeter EX5 5YX, UK

Published in the USA by Imprint Academic
Philosophy Documentation Center
PO Box 7147, Charlottesville, VA 22906-7147, USA

ISBN 978 184540174 0

A CIP catalogue record for this book is available from the
British Library and US Library of Congress

Contents

About Authors	4
Editorial Introduction, *Claire Petitmengin*	7
Describing the Practice of Introspection, *Pierre Vermersch*	20
The Explicitation Interview, *Maryse Maurel*	58
The 'Failing' of Meaning, *Natalie Depraz*	90
On the Cultivation of Presence in Buddhist Meditation, *Charles Genoud*	117
Experiencing Level, *Marion Hendricks*	129
Iteratively Apprehending Pristine Experience, *Russell T. Hurlburt*	156
Exploring Moments of Knowing, *Jane Mathison & Paul Tosey*	189
Aligning Perceptual Positions, *Connirae Andreas & Tamara Andreas*	217
Sensory Awareness, *Russell T. Hurlburt, Christopher L. Heavey & Arva Bensaheb*	231
Listening from Within, *Claire Petitmengin et alii*	252
Mindfulness Based Psychological Interventions, *Pierre Philippot & Zindel Segal*	285
Pre-Reflexive Experience and its Passage to Reflexive Experience, *Daniel N. Stern*	307
What First & Third Person Processes Really Are, *Eugene Gendlin*	332
The Validity of First-Person Descriptions as Authenticity and Coherence, *Claire Petitmengin & Michel Bitbol*	363

ABOUT AUTHORS

Claire Petitmengin is a senior lecturer at Télécom et Management SudParis and member of the Centre de Recherche en Epistémologie Appliquée in Paris. Since her doctoral thesis of 1998 (under the direction of Franciso Varela), her research has focused on pre-reflective lived experience, the methods enabling us to become aware of it and describe it, and to detect experiential generic structures. Her research evaluates the reliability of these methods, and their educational and therapeutic applications. She is also interested in the process of mutual guidance and refinement of first person and third person analyses in the context of 'neuro-phenomenological' projects.

Connirae Andreas has a MA in Clinical Psychology from the University of Colorado, and a PhD from NCU in Psychotherapy. She co-founded NLP Comprehensive (with Steve Andreas), teaching and developing new material since 1977, and has co-authored and edited numerous books and articles including *Heart of the Mind*, *Core Transformation*, and the Core Transformation Trainer Packet.

Tamara Andreas has a MM (Masters in Music) from Ohio State University and offers trainings in a range of NLP methods, including Aligning Perceptual Positions and Core Transformation. She is co-author of *Core Transformation* and is the presenting trainer for the DVD training, 'Core Transformation: the Full 3-day Workshop', which includes a complete teaching on Aligning Perceptual Positions.

Michel Bitbol was trained in Paris (France) as a medical doctor, as a physicist and as a philosopher. He is presently Director of research in philosophy at the Centre de Recherche en Epistémologie Appliquée, and he teaches Epistemology at the University Panthéon-Sorbonne. He worked as a research scientist in biophysics 1978–1990, then turned to philosophy of physics, developing a neo-Kantian approach to quantum mechanics. Later on, he focused on the relations between the philosophy of physics and the philosophy of mind and consciousness, working in close collaboration with the late Francisco Varela.

Natalie Depraz lectures in philosophy at the University of Paris IV, and is attached to the ENS (École Normale Supérieure) and CNRS (Centre National de la Recherche Scientifique). She specialises in phenomenological philosophy, has published numerous books and articles on Husserl, and is a founding editor of the journal *Alter*.

Charles Genoud has been a practitioner of Tibetan Buddhism since 1970. A student of the Venerable Geshe Rabten, Dilgo Khyentse

Rinpoche, and other teachers in the Tibetan tradition, he has also practiced *Vipassana* meditation in Burma and India. He has studied the practice of Sensory Awareness with Michael Tophoff and Charlotte Selver. Co-founder of the Vimalakirti Center for Meditation in Geneva, Switzerland, Charles Genoud conducts meditation retreats in the United States, Europe, Brazil, and the Middle East. He is the author of the book *Gesture of Awareness*.

Christopher Heavey received his PhD in clinical psychology from UC Los Angeles and is Associate Professor of Psychology at the University of Nevada at Las Vegas, where he explores inner experience using the Descriptive Experience Sampling method.

Marion Hendricks is the Director of The Focusing Institute, an International not-for-profit organization, giving workshops and lectures on Focusing-Oriented Psychotherapy world wide. She graduated from and received her client-centred training at the University of Chicago. She interned at the Post-Graduate Center for Mental Health in New York City, and then worked as a psychologist-trainer in the New York State Hospital system. She was a core faculty member at the Illinois School of Professional Psychology in Chicago for ten years, establishing and teaching the Experiential/Client-Centred specialization.

Russell T. Hurlburt is Professor of Psychology at the University of Nevada at Las Vegas. He explores inner experience — thoughts, feelings, sensations — using the Descriptive Experience Sampling method, which he originated, using random beepers and intensive interviews to provide qualitative descriptions of inner experience.

Jane Mathison originally trained as a biologist and taught Vertebrate Zoology and History and Philosophy of Science at a London Polytechnic. She trained in NLP (Neuro-Linguistic Programming) in 1988, and became interested in its potential for gaining insights into the various layers of conscious experience, completing the first doctoral thesis in NLP in 2003 under Paul Tosey. She has since worked at the School of Management, University of Surrey, where she is currently a Research Fellow, investigating learning, and developing NLP and Explicitation as tools for phenomenological research.

Maryse Maurel is a retired mathematics professor. In addition to her teaching activities, she has contributed to mathematics education research (Institut de Recherche sur l'Enseignement des Mathématiques and Institut Universitaire de Formation des Maîtres, Nice), and development, training and research work on explicitation (Groupe de Recherche sur l'Explicitation). She has thus been able to incorporate the results of pedagogical research in mathematics, and the use of the explicitation interview, into her teaching methods.

Pierre Philippot is Professor of Psychology at the Louvain University where he presides over the Psychological Science Institute. His teaching and research cover cognitive regulation of emotion and autobiographical memories, respiratory feedback in emotion, and emotional facial expression recognition, and emotion-focused psychotherapy. He founded and directs a psychology clinical centre specializing in the treatment of emotional disorders in his home university.

Zindel Segal is Head of the Cognitive Behaviour Therapy Unit at the CAMH, Clarke Divsion and Professor of Psychiatry and Psychology at the University of Toronto. He is also the Head of Psychotherapy Research. He received his undergraduate training in Psychology at McGill University and completed his graduate work at Queen's University. Dr. Segal is an associate editor for *Cognitive Therapy and Research* and serves on the editorial boards of a number of other journals. He has published over 70 scientific papers and 7 books.

Daniel N. Stern trained at Harvard University; Albert Einstein College of Medicine,1960; Bellvue Hospital, NY,The National Institute of Health, and Columbia University. He holds posts at Université de Genève, the Department of Psychiatry at Cornell, and the Columbia University Center for Psychoanalysis. He has worked over thirty years at the interface between research and practice; developmental psychology and psychodynamic psychotherapy; infant observation/experimentation and the clinical reconstruction of early experience; and the interpersonal and intrapsychic perspectives. He has published six books and several hundred journal articles and chapters.

Paul Tosey joined Surrey University in 1991, where he is Senior Lecturer in Management. He previously lectured at Edinburgh University, where he became a teaching Fellow in 2007, and has trained to Master Practitioner level in NLP. He has published widely on transformative learning, on Gregory Bateson's work, and on NLP. In 2008 he chaired the world's first International Research Conference on NLP.

Pierre Vermersch, born in 1944, studied psychology at the University of Aix en Provence before joining CNRS in Paris in 1971, where his research focused on Piaget's theory for understanding adult cognition. Since 1988 he has developed the 'explicitation interview', an interview technique designed to produce a detailed verbalization of lived experience, and leaded the GREX Research Group on Explicitation.

Claire Petitmengin

Editorial Introduction

This special issue commemorates the tenth anniversary of the publication of *The View from Within* (Varela & Shear, 1999), where Francisco Varela in collaboration with Jonathan Shear designed the foundations of a research program on lived experienced.

In the Editors' Introduction: 'First-person methodologies: What, Why, How?' (Varela & Shear, 1999a), they demonstrated that it was essential to lift the ban which had until then excluded lived experience from the field of scientific research, and to design rigorous methods enabling researchers to collect 'first person' descriptions of the 'lived experience associated with cognitive and mental events' (p. 1), that is descriptions provided by the subject living them. They also introduced the idea that the process which enables us to become reflectively conscious of one's experience and to describe it has a specific structure, and that it is possible and important to study it.

The objective of this commemorative issue is to examine and refine this research program on first person methods, through contributions based on empirical research. We have tried to keep close to the spirit of the original by gathering contributions of researchers who do not only propose first person descriptions, but who also try to describe the very process of description, in order to make this process reproducible — a necessary condition for any scientific understanding.

The 'Pre-Reflective' and Implicit Character of Lived Experience

But why should we need methods to study our lived experience? Our lived experience being the most immediate and intimate thing about us, is it not directly accessible? However it is a fact that the individuals who genuinely and concretely tried to describe their lived experience, as well as the researchers who tried to collect such descriptions, met serious difficulties and usually only gathered rather poor descriptions.

Who amongst us would be able to describe spontaneously and precisely the lived experience associated with his recollection, decision, reading or emotional processes? Very fortunately, all of us are used to living the experiences of remembering, taking a decision, reading, and feeling emotions. But usually, we have only a very partial awareness of the way we proceed. And when we have to describe these experiences, it is much easier for us to express what we know, what we have heard or read about them, than the way we have really lived them. This is clearly shown by the well-known experimentations of Nisbett and Wilson (1977), which are amongst the most quoted in the domain of consciousness studies.

Moreover, strangely, we are not aware of this deficit of awareness. Usually, we do not imagine that a particular process is necessary to enable us to become aware of our lived experience, which is the first and main obstacle to individual awareness as well as to the development of a science of lived experience: why, as an individual, should I set myself the task of acquiring an awareness which I am not aware that I lack? Why, as a researcher, should I give myself the project of designing methods enabling the development of such an awareness?

The main reason for our lack of awareness seems to be our usual absorption in the content, the object, the 'what' of our activity, to the detriment of the 'how'. We are a little like a blind person exploring objects with the tip of his cane, whose attention is entirely directed toward the object, and who ignores the contact and variations of pressure of the cane in the palm of his hand. Like the blind person, we use this information in action, but usually it remains largely unnoticed. This unnoticed character concerns even our most ordinary perceptive activities. For example, if we look at a landscape, or a painting, we immediately recognize elements on which our attention focuses and in which it becomes absorbed. At the same time, it is as if our gaze directed itself, projected itself toward the object, over there. Our attention is absorbed into the object, we lose contact with the immediate visual sensation. 'In seeing, I attend to features of what there is to see. But I can also attend to how seeing feels, to what the activity of seeing is like for me, and to the ways it feels different from freely imagining and from remembering. In attending to experience in this way, I can become aware of features I do not normally notice (attend to), precisely because they usually remain implicit and pre-reflective' (Thompson, 2007, p. 286). Whether we are touching, seeing, listening, imagining, remembering, understanding or deciding, whether we are performing a concrete or an abstract activity, a large part of our experience, although 'lived through' subjectively, is not immediately accessible to reflective consciousness and verbal description. We experience it, but in a 'pre-reflective'[1] way. While the term 'implicit' emphasizes its unformulated character, the term 'pre-reflective' thus emphasizes its unnoticed character.

By 'reflective' experience we mean an experience which is lived while being fully aware of itself or self-aware. By 'pre-reflective' experience, we mean an experience (for example of pain) which is lived without being fully aware of itself or self-aware. We use the word 'pre-reflective' with the meaning 'which does not recognize itself'. However, the underlying metaphor of the mirror implies a distancing which is not relevant here, and some authors of this issue prefer to use the term 'pre-reflexive' only to emphasize the absence of auto-reference. It is also important to note that in our view, reflective experience does not imply a particular mental state which would take the initial experience (of pain) as its object; neither does it involve a self, an ego, an 'I' or a subject, while pre-reflective experience would be I-less or ego-less.

However in this introduction and in this whole issue, the aim is not to give a definitive and conceptually completely satisfying definition of the term 'pre-reflective'. We do not even claim that 'pre-reflective' is the right word to designate this aspect of our experience, not only because of the connotations mentioned above, but also because the 'pre' seems to imply that pre-reflective experience should always be followed by reflective experience. Our lack of awareness of what is most intimate to us — our own experience — is a great mystery, which consciousness studies are only just beginning to investigate. Our goal is only to pinpoint this little-explored dimension, and ideally to induce the reader to refer to it and recognize it in his or her own experience. We also wish to suggest that it constitutes an immense potential research field, which could usefully be explored in detail. 'Exploring the pre-reflexive represents a rich and largely unexplored source of information and data with dramatic consequences' (Varela and Shear, 1999a, p. 4).

Now we would like to propose a map of the different dimensions of this exploration, which will then enable us to present the organization of the different articles of this issue.

---

[1] To use the vocabulary of Husserl (1913), later adopted by Sartre (1936 and 1938) and Ricœur (1950). Piaget (1974) speaks of 'consciousness in action'. 'Pre-reflective' translates the French word 'pré-réfléchi' and sometimes 'pré-réflexif'.

The Process of Becoming Aware

All the articles in this issue indeed show that a specific process may enable us to become reflectively aware of the pre-reflective part of our experience. 'There are numerous instances where we perceive phenomena pre-reflexively without being consciously aware of them, but where a "gesture" or method of examination will clarify or even bring these pre-reflexive phenomena to the fore' (Varela and Shear, 1999a, p. 4). For example, specific gestures may enable us to learn how to stabilize our attention, which is usually extremely capricious, on the particular experience that we are exploring; or to identify and abandon ('bracket') the beliefs and representations which surreptitiously substitute for the description of the experience itself; or to redirect our attention from the content of the experience, the 'what', which usually entirely occupies us, towards the modes of appearance of this content, the 'how'; or to produce a verbal description of this 'how' and evaluate the relevance of this description.

This process of becoming aware and describing may unfold at two different levels: *the level of experience, and the level of the experience of becoming aware of one's experience*. Let me take an example. While writing the present article, my attention is completely absorbed in the ideas that I am trying to express. On the one hand, thanks to specific gestures, I may become aware of the pre-reflective part of this experience: the rapid succession of inner images, inner comments, slight emotions, that usually accompanies my activity of writing in a pre-reflective way. On the other hand, this very process of becoming aware and describing is also an experience, which is usually performed in a pre-reflective way. And for this particular experience, I can also turn my attention from the 'what' or content of this experience (i.e. the rapid succession of inner images, inner comments, slight emotions I am becoming aware of), towards the 'how', the gestures which enable me to become aware of this content. How do I proceed in order to stabilize my attention on the experience to be described (i.e. my experience of writing)? How do I proceed in order to pass from the verbalization of my representations, commentaries and beliefs about this experience, towards the description of the experience itself? How do I reorient my attention from the 'what' to the 'how' of my experience of writing?

These *gestures* enabling us to become aware and describe our experience must in turn be clearly distinguished from the (mostly linguistic) *devices* enabling an interviewer or a therapist to induce them in the context of a research or therapeutic session.

The Structured Character of Experience

The articles in this issue also converge towards the conclusion that our experience is not just a 'draft', but has a precise *structure*. Analysing and comparing descriptions of the same type of experience has enabled the authors to detect features presenting a striking regularity from one experience to another and from one subject to another. On the basis of these recurrent characteristics, each author (or group of authors) has identified generic experiential categories which are independent of the experiential content, in other words the structure of the corresponding experiences.

Amongst the experiential structures which are in the process of being explored, one is particularly interesting for us as researchers in the domain of consciousness studies: the structure of the very process of becoming aware of our experience and describing it. What the contributors to this volume seem to be discovering, while describing this process, is that it is composed of a definite succession of precise acts and stances. This finding confirms the possibility of 'a unified description of the structural dynamics of the act of becoming aware in its procedural dimension' (Depraz *et al.*, 2003), which had been hypothesized by Varela and his colleagues. Becoming aware of one's lived experience is not a random event, but the result of precise acts, of which a first 'sketch of a common structure' (Varela and Shear, 1999a, p. 7) is emerging. This structure shows two specially striking features. First, the process of becoming aware of one's pre-reflective experience does not seem to be a process of distancing and objectification, or to entail 'a kind of doubling or fracture or self- fission' (Zahavi, 2008, p. 90) between an observer and an observed, a reflecting and a reflected subject. On the contrary, this process seems to consist of coming into closer contact with one's experience. Second, the gestures involved in this process do not consist of accumulating new knowledge, but rather of striping ourselves of the knowledge that prevents us from entering into contact with our experience. They are gestures of letting go and reduction rather than accumulation and enrichment.

The very existence of this structure has two important epistemological consequences. The first is that it makes the description of lived experience *reproducible*. Reproducibility is the foundation of any scientific validation. To be considered as scientifically valid, an observation must be verifiable or falsifiable, at least potentially, by any other researcher. And in order to be verifiable or falsifiable, it must be reproducible, that is it must be accompanied by a generic description of its very process of production.[2] In the domain of consciousness studies, this requirement of reproducibility means that a first person description should not only be the result of a definite process of becoming aware and describing, but also be accompanied by a precise generic description of this very process. And it is the structured character of this process that makes it possible to provide a generic description enabling its reproduction, and therefore a disciplined and rigorous study of lived experience.

The second consequence of the structured character of lived experience — one however which will not be developed further in this special issue which focuses on first person methodologies — is that it enables a mastered and explicit 'circulation' between first and third person analyses (Varela and Shear, 1999a, p. 2). Experiential categories may indeed be used as criteria for neuro-physiological analyses, enabling the detection of unnoticed structures on this level, and the ascription of meaning to them. Conversely, the detection of new neuro-physiological structures may help us to refine the reflective consciousness of the corresponding experience and to discover new structures on the experiential level. The detection of experiential structures is thus the kingpin of the neuro-phenomenological project initiated by Francisco Varela (1996).

Viewing From Within?

A refinement of the methods for studying pre-reflective experience would probably entail a renewal of the main issues of consciousness studies. For example these methods highlight the importance of the 'felt' and intermodal dimension of experience, termed 'felt senses' by Eugene Gendlin and 'dynamic forms of vitality' by Daniel Stern, two researchers whom Francisco Varela considered as pioneers. These subtle rhythms and movements, although usually unnoticed, seem to play a fundamental role in the constitution of a 'self' and in our interpersonal relationships as well in the process of emergence, understanding and expression of meaning.

The exploration of the pre-reflective micro-dynamics of lived experience also enables us to access a dimension where the separation which is usually felt between the objects, the other people, which are over there 'outside', and my own perceptions, emotions and thoughts which seem to be localised 'inside', is less rigid than in the experience which we are usually reflectively aware of. Strangely, the more

---

[2] The description of the very process of production seems to be a necessary condition of reproducibility, however we do not pretend that it is a sufficient one.

attention is detached from its absorption in objects to enter into contact with experience, the more reduced becomes the corresponding distinction between and 'exterior' and 'interior'. Far from presupposing this distinction and considering it as 'given', our exploration of pre-reflective experience instead leads us to be interested in the way it is constituted. Therefore we do not consider ourselves as 'introspectionists', in the sense that we turn our gaze exclusively 'inwards'. We have nevertheless chosen to keep the expression 'from within' in the title of this issue, not only to pay homage to Francisco Varela, but also to refer to a particular mode of relationship with one's experience, consisting in coming into close contact with it or 'dwelling in' it.

Content of this Issue

For this special issue, I chose to invite researchers who use a concrete and disciplined practical method for becoming aware of and describing lived experience, while also trying to describe their method. But instead of classifying the articles according to their methods, I found it more insightful to articulate them around the different axes of exploration of lived experience that we have just defined.

The first group of articles focuses on the structure of the very process of becoming aware of one's lived experience and describing it, and (for some of them) on the devices enabling interviewers to induce this process and overcome its difficulties.

In the opening article, **Pierre Vermersch** draws on his practice of the *explicitation*[3] interview method to provide a description of the very process of introspecting. He focuses on two aspects of the introspective practice: introspection as becoming reflectively aware and introspection as recollecting, by throwing fresh light on them based on Husserlian theories of consciousness modes and of retention. He also describes the use of generic experiential categories as a guide for a skilled practice of introspection in research.

Thanks to excerpts from interviews, **Maryse Maurel** illustrates some of the techniques used by the explicitation interview method to guide a subject from a pre-reflective to a reflective consciousness of his experience. She also provides a brief insight into the applications of the explicitation interview, notably in the fields of sport, health, training and artistic creation.

---

[3] The French word 'explicitation' means 'to make explicit'. In this introduction, I chose to use this French word instead of 'elicitation', whose meaning is more ambiguous in English.

The article by **Natalie Depraz** is an original work of self-explicitation of a singular personal experience of emergence of meaning into consciousness — or more exactly an experience of loss of meaning. After a brief account of the methodological devices used for achieving this work of explicitation, the author disentangles and unfolds three interwoven chronological threads: the successive moments of the explicitation process which enabled her to become aware of more and more deeply pre-reflective dimensions of the initial experience; the various difficulties, resistances and emotional shocks faced during this process, the awareness of which followed its own dynamics; and as a result of this explicitation process, the chronology of the initial experience.

In the following article, **Charles Genoud** deals with the cultivation of presence in *vipassana* meditation. He describes the redirection of the mind which is required to be present to experience, which means to be conscious of being conscious of something, instead of being absorbed into the object that is being perceived or thought of. He examines a few of the concepts that we usually impose upon our experiences when we are absorbed in the exploration of objects: inner character, temporality, intentionality, personality, duality of a subject facing an object, whereas being present means suspending these concepts.

Relying on her practice of the 'Focusing' method, **Mary Hendricks** highlights a generic experiential category termed 'Experiencing Level', which does not concern the content of experience but the manner in which what a person says relates to felt experience. This experiential category is a variable whose specificity is that it can be evaluated according to precise linguistic and somatic — i.e. 'third person' — criteria. Through transcript material taken from psychotherapy sessions, Mary Hendricks illustrates low, middle and high experiencing levels, and how the subject's experiencing level can be increased or hindered by the therapist's prompts. She also shows that having defined this variable in terms of observable indicators makes it possible to formulate exact steps for teaching high experiencing.

In the next article, **Russ Hurlburt** focuses on the learning process enabling someone to apprehend their experience and especially to 'bracket presuppositions', highlighting its iterative structure. Through the transcription of a single first interview with the Descriptive Experience Sampling method (DES), he shows the difficulties of this process, its different stages and the devices which may enable the interviewer to facilitate it.

As it has both methodological and substantive purposes, the article by **Jane Mathison** and **Paul Tosey** provides a transition between the first and the second group of articles. In the first part, they illustrate through excerpts from two explicitation interviews the tools provided by neuro-linguistic programming (NLP) for collecting first person accounts. In the second part, they show the application of these tools to the explicitation of two insights or 'moments of knowing', while highlighting the common features of these moments.

The second group of articles gives examples of generic experiential structures identified from samples of first person descriptions, and provides some insights into the process of identifying these structures. All of them focus on the structure of perception.

Connirae Andreas and **Tamara Andreas** describe and refine a generic experiential structure of perception termed 'perceptual position' in neuro-linguistic programming (NLP). Through a concrete example of an interview, they show that this structure does not only concern visual perceptions, but also auditory and kinaesthetic perceptions. They further show that our visual, auditory and kinaesthetic perceptions may be split in different perceptual positions at the same time, or on the contrary be 'aligned'. Through perceptual positions, the article also gives a striking example of the pre-reflective dimension of lived experience, and illustrates the explicitation techniques used in NLP.

The analysis of hundreds of interviews led **Russ Hurlburt** and **Chris Heavey** to identify a specific mode of sensory or perceptual experiencing, which they subsume under the experiential category 'sensory awareness'. This phenomenon involves the subject being immersed in the experience of a particular sensory aspect of his or her external or internal environment without particular regard for the instrumental aim or perceptually complete-objectness. Although highly frequent in all the sensorial modalities, this phenomenon is usually unnoticed and particularly difficult to recognize.

Claire Petitmengin and her colleagues focus on the specific experience associated with listening to a sound. On the basis of a set of descriptions of this experience, they identify a threefold generic structure depending on whether the attention of the subject is directed towards the event which is at the source of the sound, the sound in itself, considered independently from its source, or the felt sound — three dimensions which are increasingly pre-reflective and difficult to detect. The authors describe this structure, as well as the method they used to gather descriptions of auditory experience and identify experiential categories from these descriptions.

The articles of the third group throw a fresh light on the issue of the transition from pre-reflective to reflective consciousness from developmental and psychotherapeutic perspectives, or use descriptions of this transition to draw epistemological consequences from them.

The article by **Pierre Philippot** and **Zindel Segal** presents and discusses the psychological interventions based on the development of mindful awareness as a psychotherapeutic tool, in particular mindfulness based stress reduction (MBSR) and mindfulness based cognitive therapy (MBCT). They examine their effectiveness in improving psychological and physical well-being, and speculate about the cognitive processes that might account for these effects, notably emotion regulation and self-awareness. They also examine how using first person methods to collect descriptions of the experience associated with these therapies might refine this understanding. Through this presentation, the authors deal with the important question of the effects of the process of becoming aware, in other words: what does reflective consciousness do to experience?

The article by **Daniel Stern** (who prefers to use the term 'pre-reflexive') deals with the question of the passage from non verbal pre-reflexive experience to verbal reflexive experience from a developmental perspective. After a description of the structure of pre-reflexive experience, where the 'dynamic forms of vitality' play an essential role, the article focuses on the following questions: is there an intermediary stage of non verbal reflexive consciousness between non verbal reflexive and verbal reflexive experience? In other words, can reflexive experience be non verbal? And what is special about the passage into the verbal reflexive domain?

Eugene Gendlin concentrates on the 'explication' process through which new concepts form from implicit and bodily felt understanding. In the first part of the article, he uses a description of this bodily knowledge, which is body–environment interaction, to question the usual distinction between 'third person' and 'first person' or 'from outside' and 'from within' perspectives, and to understand how this distinction originates. In the second part, Gendlin shows that although implicit understanding is used by everyone all the time, referring directly to it and speaking directly from it is a skill which can be learned. He gives us elements of his method (Thinking at the Edge) designed to facilitate the explication process and the emergence of new concepts, notably in the research field. He also explains how the explication model affects the theory of language.

Claire Petitmengin and **Michel Bitbol**, after an inventory of the criticisms of introspection, answer them by providing a description of the introspective process, description which is grounded in their practice of the explicitation interview technique as well as *vipassana* meditation. Far from consisting in observing one's experience, this process consists in coming into contact with one's experience, in becoming fully present to it. This description of introspection leads the authors towards a new conception of the validity of introspective reports, conceived as authenticity and performative consistency instead of correspondence, a conception which turns out to be the same as that which underlies the experimental sciences.

Conclusion

After ten years of viewing from within, our objective in this issue is to show that the very conditions of possibility of a 'first person' discipline are in the process of being established. A discipline requires methods:

'(1) providing a clear *procedure* for accessing some phenomenal domain,

'(2) providing a clear means for an *expression and validation* within a community of observers who have familiarity with procedures as in (1)' (Varela and Shear, 1999a, p. 6).

We have a specific domain of study: human lived experience. Increasingly refined and disciplined methods for studying this domain, associated with an increasingly precise language, become available. These methods and language give any researcher — provided that he has reached a sufficient level of mastery, as it is the case in any other discipline — the means of verifying the findings of another. They enable a research community to be progressively strengthened.

To develop this emerging research program and community, we do not require expensive machines. However we need financial, human and institutional resources (1) to compare and refine our different methodologies and harmonize their vocabulary, not on a conceptual basis but on the basis of a common lived referential; (2) to train other researchers who want to use these methods, notably young researchers; (3) to design and carry out projects to explore the different dimensions of human lived experience, whether it is identifying experiential structures or articulating experiential and neuro-physiological structures.

The potential applications are innumerable and sometimes urgent. In the pedagogical domain, could not a better understanding of the pre-reflective micro-dynamics of the process of emergence and understanding of meaning enable us to refine our teaching methods and 're-enchant' school? In the technological domain, could not a finer understanding of our cognitive processes make it possible to improve the design and evaluation of technologies supporting these processes? Could not this understanding enable a better knowledge of the way these technologies transform our lived experience, in order to accompany this evolution in a relevant way, and identify the possible risks? In the medical domain, do we not lack a better understanding of the lived experience associated with pain, with the different stages of illnesses, and with pharmacological and surgical treatments? Could not the prevention, diagnostic and treatment of pathologies be facilitated by a better knowledge of this experience? Could not such a bodily consciousness be learned?

Finally, is not the loss of contact with our experiencing the chief malaise of our society? 'In the years to come', wrote Francisco Varela, 'the taking into account of human experience and of its potential of transformation will become not only necessary, but really essential' (2000, p. 122). Rediscovering the contact with our lived experience could transform considerably not only our understanding of what consciousness is, but also our lives. We want to pay homage to Francisco Varela for the clear insight he had of this crucial issue and for having initiated this research programme.

Call for Responses

Other researchers are invited to participate in this debate by commenting on the articles in this issue. If a substantial number of responses are proposed, they will be published with replies from the authors — as was the case in *The View from Within* — in a special issue of *JCS* early in 2011. If only a few responses are received, they will be published individually in regular issues of *JCS*. In all cases publication will be at the editors' discretion; longer commentaries may themselves be subject to external review. Comments may target one article in the issue, or a theme which is referred to in several articles. We ask commentators to inform Claire Petitmengin or Anthony Freeman of their intention to contribute, if possible naming the article(s) they intend to target, before March 31st 2010 and to submit the full text of their proposed commentary by June 30th 2010.

Acknowledgments

I would like to thank Jack Petranker and Michel Bitbol for their help in editing this issue.

References

Depraz, N., Varela, F. & Vermersch, P. (2003), *On Becoming Aware: The Pragmatics of Experiencing* (Amsterdam: John Benjamin).

Husserl, E. (1913/1990), *Ideas Pertaining to a Pure Phenomenology and to a Phenomenological Philosophy* (Boston. MA: Kluwer Academic Publishers).

Nisbett, R.E. & Wilson, T.D. (1977), 'Telling more than we know: Verbal reports on mental processes', *Psychological Review*, **84**, pp. 231–59

Piaget, J. (1974), *La prise de conscience* (Paris: Presses Universitaires de France).

Ricœur P. (1950), *Philosophie de la volonté* (Paris: Aubier).

Sartre J.P. (1936), *L'imagination* (Paris: Presses Universitaires de France).

Sartre J.P. (1938), *Esquisse d'une théorie des émotions* (Paris: Hermann).

Thompson E. (2007), *Mind in Life: Biology, Phenomenology, and the Sciences of Mind* (Cambridge, MA: The Belknap Press of Harvard University Press)

Varela, F.J. (1996), 'Neurophenomenology: A methodological remedy for the hard problem', *Journal of Consciousness Studies*, **3**, pp. 330–35.

Varela, F.J. (2000), 'Le corps et l'expérience vécue', in *Les chemins du corps*, ed. Tardan-Masquellier (Paris: Albin Michel).

Varela F. J. & Shear J. (ed. 1999), *The View from Within: First-person Approaches to the Study of Consciousness*; A special issue of *The Journal of Consciousness Studies* (Exeter: Imprint Academic).

Varela F.J. & Shear J. (1999a), 'First-person methodologies: What, Why, How?', in Varela and Shear (1999), pp. 1–14.

Zahavi, D. (2008), *Subjectivity and Selfhood: Investigating the First-Person Perspective* (Cambridge, MA: MIT Press).

Pierre Vermersch

Describing the Practice of Introspection

Abstract: *The main objective of this article is to capitalise on many years of research, and of practice, relating to the use of introspection in a research context, and thus to provide an initial outline description of introspection, while developing an introspection of introspection. After a description of the context of this research, I define the institutional conditions which would enable the renewal of introspection as a research methodology. Then I describe three aspects of introspective practice: 1) introspection as a process of becoming aware, theorized through Husserl's model of consciousness modes; 2) introspection as recollection, through the model of retention and awakening in Husserl's theory of memory; 3) the use of universal descriptive categories for the description of all lived experiences, as a guide for skilled practice of introspection in research. Finally I examine the question of the validation of introspective data, suggesting a strong distinction between the ethical criterion and the epistemic criterion of truth.*

Keywords
Consciousness, descriptive categories, explicitation interview, Husserl, introspection, lived experience, phenomenology, pre-reflective.

Initial Questions, Primary Motivations

The main objective of this article is to capitalise on many years of research, and of practice, relating to the use of introspection in a research context, and thus to provide an initial outline description of introspection, while developing an introspection of introspection.

Let us take as a preliminary supposition that you have reached the conclusion that there is no point in carrying out research into consciousness, or into any other subject of study based on consciousness, without trying to gather information about what the subject is conscious of, in his own view. Because if not, we could find ourselves in the absurd situation of trying to say what someone else is conscious of! Why not ask him? If he is conscious, then he is conscious! And if he is, why could he not tell us about it? So is he conscious or not? To answer this question, it is necessary to be able to gather information about this matter. I can of course say, for the other person, in his stead, what affects him, that is what has an effect on him, whether he is conscious of this or not, by means of recordings of physiological indicators, but on the one hand I will not have the corresponding semantics, and on the other hand I will not know if the subject is reflectively conscious of this. That in fact is the question, and he is the only one who can enable us to establish this point. Sooner or later, the complement of all research on the living subject must also be able to say what he is living, what he is experiencing, in short everything of which he is already or can become reflectively conscious.

Let us suppose however that *you*, the person reading this article, have reached this conclusion, namely that you need to gather information about the experience of the subject (according to him), and thus about what he can be conscious of, or become conscious of. You have a new and meaningful research aim: to document the subjective dimension, to gather information from the subject about what he has experienced. You know that you must abandon the idea of *only* using indirect information, such as behavioural, physiological and neurophysiological traces, or video recordings, as this would inevitably mean you would have to use an interpretation strategy in your discourse about what the subject is conscious of, about what happened for him, in your view.

To achieve this new objective, you must practice — and thus know, and become competent and indeed expert in — a new data gathering methodology. Fundamentally, you have no other choice than to practice, and to have others practice, a form of *introspection*, that is to obtain descriptive verbalisations based on acts of introspection relating to a past lived experience (in the recent or more distant past).[1] Attempting to consider the resulting verbalisations alone, without taking into account the acts which give rise to them is a puerile strategy,

---

[1] In this introduction I have left out the question of current introspection and/or simultaneous verbalisation (Vermersch, 2008b) in order to consider only retrospective introspection.

which involves hiding from oneself the fact that one is requesting an act of introspection by asking questions to the other person (Fraisse & Piaget, 1963), and the damaging consequence is that you do nothing to guide the act of introspection as you did not know (or recognise) it. You harbour, as many others have done before, the illusion that you merely elicit verbalisations, and nothing more. You place yourself in the situation of not knowing how you obtain your data, how you informer generates them. You obtain answers and you go off to process them. If you do not obtain the answers, or if the spontaneous verbalisations are too poor in content, or non- existent, you immediately reach one of the following conclusions: (1) That the subject is unconscious and thus has nothing to say (see for example the work on implicit knowledge [Reber, 1993; Reder, 1996; Underwood, 1996]); (2) That he does not remember and thus will not remember, exit; (3) That in any case he has no access to the information, because there is no introspection, that it is a myth (see for example Nisbett & Wilson, 1977; (Nisbett & Bellows, 1977; Smith & Miller, 1978; White, 1980); (4) That there is in fact no experiential content, and thus nothing whatever to say (Lyons, 1986)! Whereas our interpretation of what these authors say suggests: (1) That the subject should first become conscious, i.e. reflectively conscious of what he may say, and that we know how to help the subject to carry out this transition; (2) That it is possible the subject may say that he does not remember, but that he can be helped to transcend this first impression and guided into mobilising a specific autobiographic memory; (3) That if the questions of the researcher relate to the causality of the situation ('Why did you do such and such a thing? Why have you changed criteria?'), it is understandable that the subject: (a) should not describe, but comment, or justify, as that is what he is asked to do, and that this is not introspection, but reasoning; (b) should express his spontaneous, or even naïve, theories, as he is not asked to describe what happened, and that as a result it is quite understandable that another subject, who has been introduced by the researcher in the position of a hidden observer, expresses the same thing as the subject who is directly involved in the experiment; (4) And finally that when there is apparently nothing to describe, it is perhaps necessary to consider the lack of introspective competence of the person making this affirmation, and the necessity of taking into account the technical nature of introspection and the obligation of being trained in these practices, so that they can be used intelligently and effectively.

Taking a radically first-person viewpoint (Vermersch, 2000), it is the researcher who for a time takes up the position of informer, with regard to his lived experience, and himself produces an introspection by a work of reiterated written expression, by taking advantage of his expertise as a researcher in the field he wishes to study. Taking a second-person viewpoint, the researcher invites one other person (or several other people) to act as informer(s), and must then guide the introspection process of the person (or persons) without thereby inducing the content of the description. This is usually termed 'conducting a research interview', and I have developed a specific interview technique: the explicitation interview (Vermersch, 1994; 2008) (see also the article by Maryse Maurel in this issue). In what I write, I thus assimilate the explicitation interview to retrospective introspection (Vermersch, 2008b), more exactly the explicitation interview is a form of guided retrospective introspection. The descriptive expertise which is the heart of introspection is not innate in any way, it is provided by the interviewer in the form of non-inductive guidance of the formulation of the experience. Auto-explicitation is a guided self-introspection (Vermersch, 2007b). The person who practices this is the one who has the introspective expertise.

Whatever the case considered, we therefore conclude that it is necessary to use introspection as a method for gathering research data about subjectivity.

The posture of my discourse: from introspective practice to its theorisation.

To explain what I am going to develop in this article, I think it is necessary to specify the type of research approach from which this information has been drawn, by briefly retracing the genesis of the explicitation interview technique. My approach is a little unusual in that it was not originally based on a research programme established on the basis of a theoretical framework and hypotheses which would determine specific means of collecting data. After initially focusing on the use of traces and observables, and particularly of video recordings, it became clear that what I used to call 'normal unconscious cognitive functioning', could not be documented solely by a viewpoint external to the subject, even though the use of experimental situations which are spontaneously rich in observables made it possible to go quite a long way by inference. I thus transcended the prejudices of the period, which had been inculcated into me at university, which suggested that verbalisation data were unreliable, uninteresting, reconstructed after the fact, and only reflected naïve prejudices and theories about people. The use of an interview technique had the practical purpose of transcending the limitations of behavioural data, and the gathering of verbalisation was only a means to an end. I thus obtained information that I did not think I would be able to obtain using the theoretical knowledge I had mastered. Not only did the conventional limitations of recollection memory seem to be easily transcended, but also if one had experience of the 'fragmentation of the description' and of looking for the 'useful level of detail', as was the case in the psychology of work, we thus obtained an abundance of precise details which the subject himself was amazed to discover in his past experience. Recognising his experience, accepting that it is his, and at the same time discovering with surprise that it is contained in his lived experience! There was here the prefiguration of a theoretical reflection on the nature of consciousness (direct or pre-reflective consciousness) and on the type of recollection memory which made it possible to allow this kind of autobiographical information to emerge. The description of the practice, and then the systematisation of the techniques used to question, to guide towards embodied memory, to fragment the description, etc., gave rise to an original interview technique which I have termed the 'Explicitation interview' (Vermersch, 1994; 2008). The education of researchers, students, human relations professionals, and philosophers, led quite naturally to the methodical construction of this interview and of the modes of its transmission in the form of one-week seminars. But, despite its effectiveness in research and in intervention modes such as the analysis of errors in education, or the analysis of practice of professionals, it was difficult for me to understand why this approach worked. What were the theoretical bases which could have introduced intelligibility, a modelling of what was at work?

What I will set out in this article, after having published it in stages over the last fifteen years or so, mainly in France in the review *Expliciter* (www.expliciter.fr), describes this modelling. It has involved looking back at the history of introspection, to understand why there were so many criticisms, and so many rejections and taboos, about the first-person viewpoint. This is what I had outlined in my article in *JCS* ten years ago (Vermersch, 1999) and in the book written jointly with N. Depraz and F. Varela (Depraz *et al.*, 2003), showing that there were serious questions amongst all these criticisms, and others which were purely ideological and specific to a cultural and historic setting, but none of them represented an insurmountable criticism. Furthermore, the few authors who have taken a second look at introspection — (Burloud, 1927b; Humphrey,

1951; Mandler & Mandler, 1964) — have not understood why it was so virulently attacked on such an ill-founded basis.

This article thus consists of theorisations which are mainly inspired by the phenomenology of Husserl,[2] proposing a model of intelligibility of what we know how to do in practice. And I will outline[3] in a complementary way the various techniques used to apply these theories. Initially I will present the conditions which must be met to enable introspection to become a subject of research, both from the viewpoint of the authorisation a researcher or institution can give himself or itself to transcend the taboos attached to introspection, and which have gone through the 20th century completely unchanged, and from the viewpoint of the technical conditions to be met so as to enable the documentation of the introspection of introspection. I will then turn to the main theoretical points enabling an understanding of the possibility of introspection, and of how it can be related to practices assisting introspection.

Part One: Conditions Enabling the Study of Introspection

1. Social conditions for taking an interest in introspection

Why begin by looking again a data which are more social and more contingent, because they are historic, rather than phenomenological? We now know that sociological, institutional, ideological and sectarian conditions play an important role in the genesis, disappearance and refusal of research programmes. It would be easy to show this in

---

[2] Depending on viewpoints, one may designate the same act of seizing lived experiences 'into view', introspection (which is of course not the case of Husserl), 'immanent perception' by opposition to acts based on the mobilisation of the perceptive organs, 'apperception' to make use of the same opposition, and finally 'reflection', if we follow the translators of Husserl , to designate not an act of reflection in the sense of reflecting about an object of understanding, of reasoning, but an act mobilising a 'reflective activity', of carrying out the reflection, or if we take the term of Piaget of carrying out the 'réfléchissement' of the lived experience (Piaget & Coll, 1977). I must here clear up a possible misunderstanding about the relationship between phenomenology and introspection. The concept of introspection is radically rejected by Husserl, in that this involves for him a form of naturalisation, or an absence of the Husserlian founding gesture: 'the transcendental reduction'. But if one suspends this viewpoint, it may be observed that the act of Husserlian 'reflection', the cognitive movement by which I turn towards what is appearing, is nothing but an introspection carried out under a horizon of specific presuppositions about the status of what is focused on. In this sense, as far as the actual practice of gathering information about one's own experience is concerned, there are no major differences in acts between phenomenological 'reflection' and psycho-phenomenological introspection.

[3] Just a brief outline, in that these techniques have been thoroughly described elsewhere in my publications. The article by M. Maurel in this issue provides some examples with a commentary.

terms of the fate of each programme which focused on introspection at the start of the 20th century. But this would be the subject of another article. My intention here is to set out some institutional conditions which mean that an interest for introspection and, even more, interest for a description of introspection, have been combined.

1.1 Overcoming the first difficulties

The entire history of scientific introspection, since the start of the 20th century, has been littered with passionate and sectarian reactions, and by absolute prohibitions which although ill-founded prevented the practice of introspection. Initially, the idea of mobilising introspection as one of the essential methods for constructing scientific psychology was presented as obvious, from James onwards (James, 1901; 1890), up to the enthusiasm shown for the 'systematic experimental introspection' of Binet (Binet, 1922), the researchers of the Würzburg school (see Mandler & Mandler, 1964) and Titchener (Titchener, 1912; 1913). So the first obstacle to be overcome when one takes an interest in introspection is these taboos, to stop believing such absurd ideas as 'one cannot at once be in the street and on the balcony'. Or quite simply it is a matter of finding a research director, a laboratory or a university which agrees to take on board a research programme which includes the word 'introspection'. Taking an interest in introspection means that taboos which are still powerful must be overcome.

But if this is to be done, there must first be a clear epistemic motivation. I began my article with a similar argument. The strongest support for paying attention to what the subject may be reflectively conscious of currently comes — paradoxically — from the neurosciences. Because as neurological data have become increasingly precise, the question has arisen as to how they can be given a semantic, and how can they be clearly linked to subjective experience. And how could this be done other than by the expression of the subject himself, which can only be based on an introspective act.

However, even once we have gone this far, a final difficulty has to be overcome, i.e. the failure of the first attempts. This was the result of a failure to understand that the ordered practice of introspection is no easy matter; it is rather like considering that one can draw a portrait simply because one has eyes with which to see. As F. Varela stressed, introspection is technical, and calls for a learning process and expert guidance. Having cognition, and having a capacity for reflective activity do not make you into a researcher who is competent in the use of introspection. I hope that my article will throw light on to these points, by setting out the places in which the expertise is applied, bearing in mind that its acquisition will necessarily require practice.

1.2 Institutional conditions: the importance of the social and historic context.

To go beyond a naïve and uneducated use of introspection, and thus to enable it to become a research methodology, it seems to me that the minimum condition is first that it should be *effectively practised* by a community of researchers. This should take place over at least ten years or so, so that two or three successive research cycles (theses, publications, books) can begin to have cumulative effects, with each researcher having his own experience of introspection, and of guiding in an interview the introspection of other people. It must form part of research programmes, which must necessarily be accompanied by theoretical, methodological and epistemological courses about introspection, and also practical courses to acquire and perfect knowhow. All my arguments are in favour of the necessity of developing a genuine familiarity of use, so that progressively its function as a tool becomes a source of questioning, and can be detached until it becomes a subject of research. I do not believe that a single researcher on his own is capable of creating the conditions required for the development of this methodology, unless a research team is created. Historically, one might think that the great period of the conception of introspection as a means of research at the start of the 20th century should have provided an example of what I am suggesting. In fact, the three early 20th century research teams (the school of Würzburg in Germany, the Titchener laboratory in the United States, and Binet and his students in France), who set up a research programme founded on introspection, did not have the time before the disappearance of their programme, and before the effects of the First World War (1914–18) on academic life, to go far enough in the constitution of an expert community to develop a research programme on the introspection of introspection. All that emerged around the end of this period (1911) were remarks about the practice of guiding introspection. Several conditions were combined: researchers who were becoming expert practitioners, a widened international research community, several cycles of research realised (theses and publications), successively raising new questions, variations in practice, reflections on failures, etc. At this point in time, history intervened, and the two world wars consigned all this preparatory work to oblivion. Furthermore there was the debate on 'thought with or without images', which was raised before researchers had the means to answer this question. The data gathered were too powerful for the period in question. I have surveyed the few survivors who published a little, between the two wars or much later in the 1950s, manuscripts which were prepared in the 1930s. But these were only isolated individuals, the social fabric of research needed to be entirely reconstructed, and introspection had a bad press at the time, to say the least! The Grex (Groupe de recherche sur l'explicitation) was probably one of the few places[4] in Europe in which an expert community has been built up since 1988 (Maurel, 2008), and which after around 15 years of practice has turned towards the explicitation of explicitation. But it has only been able to do this, and overcome the taboos, by financing itself, in a sort of academic marginality, by accepting and valorising exploratory postures, even though several theses have been defended in their own specific university disciplinary framework (see also the article by M. Maurel in this issue).

2. Preliminary: how to gather information about introspection: V1, V2, V3.

To study introspection, it is necessary to first carry it out in practice, but also to practice it sufficiently to overcome the initial naïve mistakes, the first failures, and gradually to acquire expertise. Why should it be any different than for any profession, any activity in games, sport, music, etc. When this is the case, we therefore have a basic structure: a lived experience V1 which is taken as a reference and will form the subject of an introspective description after the fact. This time of introspection is therefore another lived experience, distinct from the first one, and which we will denote as V2. This is not a current introspection, but an introspection based on evocation, or the 'secondary remembrance'[5] of V1. These two initial phases enable the description and study of V1. This is the purpose of the use of an

---

[4] Mention may also be made of the work in France of De La Garanderie — a student of Burloud, familiar with Binet — but who has above all developed teaching applications, and who has not carried out or supervised research work. See De la Garanderie (1989) for example.

[5] Husserl uses the term 'secondary remembrance' to designate a clear intuitive donation of past lived experience. Intuitive is the opposite of signitive, and designates a donation as almost-relived, which I have referred to myself as 'evocation'. Husserl clearly distinguished between a 'signitive' mode (conceptual, based on knowledge and on discourse) and an 'intuitive' mode based on a perceptive donation, a donation of something relived for the memory, of imagination, in short all the modes of accessing an object as direct immediacy. I can 'know' the route which I took to come to the office, this is the signitive mode of recollection; or I can 'relive' or rediscover the sensoriality of the route of the

introspective method, to bring about the description of a reference lived experience which has been invoked or provoked, and which is the research subject.

> For example, I want to study the memorisation of scores by professional pianists. I ask a pianist to evoke a moment when he was involved in the activity of memorisation. The reference lived experience V1 is the moment when he learns a score by heart. In a second stage, V2, I carry out an explicitation interview, and I question him about how he went about memorising his score. I therefore propose that he should describe this past lived experience, that is introspect himself.

There are thus two separate stages: V1 the reference lived experience which is the experience studied, and V2, a lived experience whose main activity is to carry out a 'secondary remembrance' of V1 and its introspective description. If we only have these two stages, the introspection implemented in V2 has the status of an instrument. The researcher's attention is not concentrated on the instrument, but on what the instrument focused on and produces. As this is done, over the years, we gradually accumulate information about the difficulties in implementing the 'introspection' instrument. The researcher is also a practitioner; he becomes expert in his practices, and like any practitioner, he gathers information from his practice. This is something one can note in the methodological remarks of the successive research projects of the Würzburg school, which multiply as the research programme is developed; the same is true in the successive publications of Titchener and its PhD students. By effective practice, we thus begin to create sediments of observations, remarks about the use of introspection, the variety of types of introspection, facilities, difficulties encountered by different subjects, the favourable or unfavourable effects of the various formats of questions. As time goes by, we obtain an 'enlightened practice', researchers who become expert practitioners of research interviews, all of which feeds into the conception of the teaching courses for students, and the guidance of their data collections for theses and papers.

The following stage took simple commitment to this expert practice further, to detach introspection from its use, and make it into a subject of reflection, and then a subject of research in its own right. One may have various research strategies, but one which seems essential is to gather information in first and second person about the practice of introspection, and thus to practice an *introspection of introspection*, a

---

morning, it is then a recollection based on the 'intuitive' mode. Intuitive does not therefore mean fuzzy, inspired, approximate, without explanation, but rather immediate, sensorially founded, alive.

description of acts of introspection. This theoretical possibility was clearly seen by Husserl (Husserl, 1989) (see §77, 78), but he did not consider the difficulties of implementing it. If one wishes to take as a research subject acts of introspection — how the subject experiences introspection when he practices it — thanks to introspection, it is necessary to study a new reference lived experience characterised by the fact that the practice of introspection is mobilised in it, as this is the subject of study. This is the case with lived experience V2. V2 thus becomes the reference lived experience of a new time of introspection, and thus of a new lived experience which we will denote as V3. V3 is a new lived experience, which is dedicated to the practice of introspection on the previous introspective lived experience V2.

To study introspection, we therefore have an initial level of research complication. It is necessary to first create a situation in which introspection is used, and then with the same subject create a second situation, a second stage distinct from the first one, in which the previous situation is focused on. The differences between V1, V2, and V3 are shown in the table below.

Table 1.

The different lived experiences V1, V2, V3. The first column describes the meaning of each of these lived experiences, the second the dominant activity of each of these lived experiences, and the third the type of purpose associated with them.

The different lived experiences	*The dominant activity of each person in these lived experiences*	*Purposes associated with these lived experiences*
V1, reference lived experience	The subject works on a piece of piano music on a particular occasion.	Purpose of musical education. No psycho-phenomenological research purposes.
V2 explicitation lived experience, in the context of an interview situation or self-explicitation situation.	Descriptive introspection of reference lived experience V1.	*Research purpose* on musical education (it is the content of V1 which is the subject of study).
V3 explicitation lived experience of *acts* mobilised in V2 (the content of V2, which is V1, is not longer what is focused on).	Introspection of mental acts implemented in the practice of introspection during V2.	*Research purpose* on introspective acts (it is the V2 acts which are the subjects of study). Psycho-phenomenological purposes.

The principle is apparently simple, and it would seem that it just needed to be put into practice. But great difficulties then arise, which we had not anticipated, and which typically produce pragmatic knowledge derived from actual practice. In our first 'introspection of introspection' attempts (for example, we tried to describe the act of evocation by which we access the past using a specific recollection mode), we were simply unable to achieve our aim. It took several attempts, with varying degrees of success, to enable an understanding of the difficulties encountered and define ways of overcoming them. It is in fact quite delicate for several reasons. The first and most immediate is continuing to question V1. This is because the introspective activity developed in V2 is based on a strong presentification by evocation of V1, and so as soon as we draw the attention of the subject to the time V2 when he was introspecting, what is given first in the remembrance of V2 and is imposed with force, is the *content* of his activity: and thus the remembrance of V1. As a result, immediately the subject starts to re-describe V1, rather than the lived experience V2 and particularly *the acts* which he has used to focus on V1, to seize it, to hold it in place, to describe it. These acts do not belong to lived experience V1; they are acts of lived experience V2 which characterise the practice of introspection (Vermersch, 2006c). This leads to the second difficulty: it is necessary to discriminate in the focusing and in the descriptive expression the content of the reference lived experience V1 and the mobilised acts. We come up here against the fundamental distinction made by Husserl between noemata (phenomena) and noesis (act of consciousness). It is a matter of describing the noeses, the acts, and this is only accessible via the phenomenological reduction of the noematic content. Once a clear distinction has been drawn between these two aspects, it is also necessary in practice that the questions should skilfully lead towards a description of the noeses and towards stage V2; it is very easy to slide towards V1 and the content. But I will not go into detail here about the questioning techniques.

Numerous aspects of introspection can then be studied; there is an immense research programme to be devised and implemented in the framework of a research community. In the following, I will focus on a certain number of points which are in my view essential for an understanding of the implementation of retrospective introspection for research purposes.

Part Two: Theoretical and Methodological Elements Characterising Introspection

This part of my article is intended to set out in detail the theoretical and methodological bases which have emerged from all our observations resulting from the practice of introspection in the context of the explicitation interview, and more recently of self-explicitation. This overview presentation has been devised a posteriori in order to give it conceptual legibility.[6] The description of introspective access to the past lived experience has been conceived gradually not as a memory performance, but first of all as a question of becoming conscious and of perceptive activity. I intend to deal with this second part from three different and complementary viewpoints: based on Husserl, the phenomenological theories of modes of consciousness (1) and passive memory (2), which are intended to account for behaviour which is deliberately solicited in the mobilisation of introspection for research; the systematisation of universal categories of description of all lived experience (3) to enable an understanding of how one can deliberately organise perception activities in secondary remembrance.

I will now provide a brief description of these three points, before looking at them again in detail.

- The first viewpoint is based on a theory of modes of consciousness inspired by Husserl's phenomenology and characterises introspection first of all as a question of becoming conscious, i.e. as based on the necessity of a transition from a pre-reflective consciousness of the lived experience to a reflective consciousness of the same lived experience. This transition is an operation of 'reflection'. This reflection is both a conscientisation and a recollection. Taking into account the necessity of prior reflection provides many practical indications about the techniques it is necessary to mobilise in order to *facilitate* the act of introspection as well as *not to prevent it*, as many techniques aim to stop the subject from performing acts which effectively block authentic introspection or divert him away from authentic introspection.

- The second viewpoint is also based on a phenomenological theoretical framework, that of the specific memory of the lived

---

[6] I would specify at this point that it is not written in the order of the genesis, but in the order of intelligibility, which turns out to be quite different, if only because I was completely unaware of Husserl, at the same time as I was producing a systematisation of the explicitation interview technique.

experience as a field of information which is normally partly available *unbeknownst to the subject*. I am borrowing from Husserl his conception of 'passive memory' (Husserl, 1925/2001), which is based on the fact that unbeknownst to me and continuously many items of information are memorised inside me, which he terms 'retention'. And that in a complementary way — in line with theories of involontary memory or concrete memory (Gusdorf, 1951) — these retentions do not disappear, and can be awakened, either involuntarily by an associative shock, or deliberately by an 'awakening intention'. The hypothesis of passive memory and its awakening is opens up the possibility of obtaining an extraordinary quantity of details in recollections, particularly when the person is skilfully interviewed.

- The third is based on a methodology of description of lived experience, and with this aim amplifies introspection as a perceptive activity (or 'shifting of ones' view inside the past lived experience' as Husserl writes) stressing the practical importance of mastering descriptive categories which are generic for all lived experience, and the knowledge of technical aspects of the description of lived experience.

For the purposes of this article I will leave aside the very precise techniques developed for conducting an interview, which are essential if it is to be successful, such as: (1) taking into account the various facets of creating, maintaining and ensuring vigilance about the ethical and relational dimension (cf. the concept of 'communication contract' in the sense specific to the explicitation interview) (Vermersch, 1994; 2008, chap 6), and (2) mastering the prompts by clarifying the perlocutory effects sought by the interviewer — concerning which some indications are provided in this issue in the articles by Maryse Maurel for the explicitation interview, and by Jane Mathison and Paul Tosey for NLP.[7]

1. Introspection as becoming aware of prereflective lived experience.

If introspection was only a question of memory, just the fact of remembering what one experienced which was conscious, there would be no research question. Spontaneous practice shows that it

---

[7] In addition to the book 'L'entretien d'explicitation', the following may also be consulted: (Vermersch, 2006a; Vermersch, 2007a; Vermersch et al., 2003).

does not function so simply, and that the immediate recollection of one's own lived experience is poor, anecdotal, and soon exhausted. What I am aiming for first of all is to show that there is a fundamental gap between what the subject believes he knows about his lived experience and what he could in fact produce, particularly when he is guided by introspection/explicitation aid techniques. Phenomenologically, this question comes from the basic empirical observation, repeated in all reasonably thorough explicitation interviews, that often the informer finds more past information than he expects, and that he is often amazed to discover things (acts, taking of information, states, details) that he recognises having experienced, but surprise him because they only come back to him after the fact. It is as though, at the moment when he was experiencing them, he did not know them, and that at the moment he was about to talk about them, he did not know in advance that he would have something to say about these particular points, and that as a result he seems to be discovering it as he names it, while recognising it without hesitation as his own lived experience!

To make this empirical observation intelligible, the theory of modes of consciousness developed by Husserl struck me as very useful. Instead of the dichotomy — which is habitual in cognitive psychology — of one conscious mode and one unconscious mode, if one follows Husserl one must take a trichotomy into account. A distinction is thus drawn between the following three modes:

(a) An active unconscious mode (predonation field or phenomenological unconscious), whose existence does not presuppose a censorship mechanism, which could be termed the 'normal' or 'usual' unconscious, and which can only be studied by inference through a third-person viewpoint;

(b) A lived consciousness mode, which could be termed direct consciousness, consciousness in action, or to mark its difference with the following level, pre-reflective, irreflective or non-reflective consciousness;[8]

---

[8] The terms of 'consciousness in action' or 'direct consciousness' come primarily from the work of Piaget (Piaget, 1974). He showed in the study of the ontogenesis of intelligence, a stage when the child takes into account a property in his actions, but does not know how to name it; there is thus consciousness in action, which will change at the next stage. I have also used the concept of 'direct consciousness' as an equivalent. The terms: unreflective, pre-reflective and non-reflective come from phenomenology; they are all characterised by a private denomination focusing on the fact that this consciousness is not, or is not yet reflected. I will treat them as synonymous.

(c) A reflective consciousness mode — see the detailed presentation of Husserl's texts in Vermersch (2000}.

Table 2.

Modes of consciousness and transition between modes based on the work of Husserl.

(1) Phenomenological unconscious	Predonation field. Before any intentional seizing, a place of sedimentation of retentions.
Transition I	*Intentional seizing*, transition to direct consciousness. Donation.
(2) Consciousness in action	Direct, pre-reflective consciousness.
Transition II	*Reflection*, first reflective seizing, transition to reflective consciousness.
(3) Reflective consciousness	Product of 'reflection' in the Husserlian sense: 'to take into view'
Transition(s) III	'Phenomenological' seizing of consciousness.

In this article I will not attempt to repeat the detailed analysis made by Husserl, which can be found clearly set out for example in (Husserl, 1989, § 77 and 78). I would like to draw conclusions for the concept of pre-reflective consciousness. There is the simple and very enlightening idea that lived experiences are largely simply lived, without at the same time being 'viewed'. Husserl establishes this for current lived experiences, i.e. while I am thinking of something, I can direct my 'view' (pay attention, apprehend, perceive) for example towards my internal state and become aware of the fact that I am happy. I become aware that I am currently happy, but also, that I *was happy before* I turned towards my emotional state, and this is true for many things which happen in my lived experience. He also establishes it for lived experiences which are just over, seized in the primary recollection or retention, and also for lived experiences which are given later in the recollection memory which he calls 'secondary remembrance'. This constitutes one of the foundations of the phenomenological method, and indeed is a prerequisite for its possibility, that 'reflection' (which I may just as well term introspection) enables the perception of lived experiences, and particularly of lived experiences which were not 'viewed', and which can viewed after the fact. In other words, there normally exists a large proportion of aspects of our lived experience which are lived in the mode of non-reflective consciousness. In fact this does not mean that I am 'unconscious' of what I am doing or perceiving, but that I am fully conscious of it without at the same time being conscious of the way in which I do it. I perceive or I do x, without necessarily keeping in the view of my consciousness the way in which I organise my perceptive activity. Husserl establishes this point by simply inviting the reader to experience for himself, and to discover the lived evidence of the fact that I am not reflectively conscious of everything which happened in my lived experiences, and that I can by modifying my attitude turn towards a particular aspect of my lived experience and discover that it is present, that it was already there. This is proof that previously I was not present in it, I did not have reflective consciousness of it. As far as the practice of introspection is concerned, there are here many difficulties which must be clarified and overcome in practice. The first is that what relates to pre-reflective lived experience is normally invisible to me, and the second is that what is invisible to me (of which I am not reflectively conscious) I think I cannot recall and therefore that I am unable to recall (cf. the example of 'Claire and her keys' in the article by M. Maurel in this issue).

The absence of spontaneous phenomenality in the pre-reflective mode of consciousness and its consequences.

Pre-reflective consciousness by definition is normally invisible in the present moment, as if it were visible it would not be pre-reflective; being visible, being 'taken into view' as Husserl writes repeatedly and metaphorically, is a matter of reflective consciousness. Reflective consciousness appears through the modification which takes place when I take now into my view something which was not yet in my view, but was already in my lived experience. Husserl clearly makes a difference between 'living x' (consciousness in action, prereflected consciousness) and 'viewing x' (reflective consciousness). Pre-reflective lived experience can only be seized a posteriori in a form of memory, either just afterwards, or in a form of recollection which Husserl calls 'secondary remembrance', which is a contact with the past lived experience, in other words a form of relived experience emphasising an intuitive donation (a matter of immanent perception and not of knowledge) and which I for my part have termed 'evocation'. This is the most serious problem with the practice of introspection: practising introspection is going into myself to find information which is largely invisible until I have brought it into reflective consciousness. The pre-reflective dimension of lived experiences *only appears*, as Husserl stresses, *by contrast with the modification of consciousness which consists of directing one's view towards the lived experience itself*, and thus to 'become conscious' of it or bring it into 'reflective consciousness'. In this transition the unreflective character of lived experience clearly emerges, and by contrast the modification which consists of the transition into the reflective consciousness mode. This seizing into view already supposes a learning process, an exit from the natural attitude, it requires the construction of a new attitude: that of the phenomenological witness.

Reflection and recollection in secondary remembrance.

Another difficulty of retrospective introspection stems from a risk of misinterpretation. Not only is the pre-reflected dimension not spontaneously apparent, but moreover its non-appearance *may be wrongly attributed* to a memory problem. This confusion will be interpreted as the fact that the memory is defective, since what first appears to me is the fact that I cannot remember or can remember only a little about my lived experience. For when I am in recollection mode, what is given back most easily and immediately is mainly that which in the past lived experience was already reflectively conscious. But if pre-reflective consciousness does exist, its characteristic for me is that I do not know that it was existing, since it was pre-reflective, and as a consequence I do not know what I was directly conscious of in the pre-reflective mode. In other words, 'I do not know what I do however know'. But everything suggests to me that what I cannot remember, I do not remember and that it is lost. There is a discouraging confusion for the informer (even if he is trained) between the lack of an immediate recollection, 'I can no longer remember' and the lack of 'reflection'. For there to be recollection, it is necessary to carry out the reflection of the lived experience which has not yet been reflected. But this can be thought just as well in reverse: for there to be a transition to reflective consciousness, one of the ways is to 'view' the past lived experience. Intuitive seizing, authentic contact with the lived experience - whether it is in the immediate or later past - then becomes the privileged act producing the transition to reflective consciousness, it is by this means that is carried out the reflection of what has been lived in the mode of consciousness in action. And this is what makes the quality of authenticity of this contact so important for the production of faithful introspection. Of course, globally we remain in the setting of a recollection. Wherever a fundamental differentiation is to be made, it is in the recollection mode which is sought, i.e. a form of recollection which brings back the lived experience in its sensitive, intuitive dimension, in other words the affective or concrete memory as it was called at the start of the 20th century (Gusdorf, 1951). It is essential to re-establish contact with the lived experience, not as knowledge of the lived experience, but as an intuitive donation of the lived experience, in which reflection can then be carried out in a way which is commensurate with what has been memorised.

Two confusions are therefore possible: to believe that a lived experience was unconscious when in fact it was only pre-reflective, and to believe that there are no recollections when in fact there is only a temporary absence of reflection.

It is useful to point out some practical consequences about ways of questioning, so that we achieve coherence with the pre-reflective consciousness model and with accessing it through secondary remembrance. What is important is to elicit secondary remembrance to produce a transition to reflective consciousness and thus the possibility of a verbalisation. Each prompt has perlocutory effects (Vermersch, 2007; 2008a; Vermersch *et al.*, 2003) which modify the cognitive acts of the subject and his directions of attention. Thus all the questions in which the subject is asked to *explain* what he has done, or to give the *reasons* for it, will have the effect of preventing him from contacting his lived experience intuitively, while making him seize his lived experience as past *knowledge*, as an object for reasoning. *In fact reflection and reasoning are two mutually incompatible acts, in that it is very difficult to mobilise them both at the same time!* The practice of retrospective introspection is not so much a question of memory as primarily a question of presence to the past, a stance which gives primacy to the process of becoming aware of the pre-reflective dimension of the past. It is the authenticity of the intuitive contact with the past lived experience which will enable the 'letting come' of the information contained in this past, which I do not have the reflective consciousness to possess. This model thus gives primacy to a mode of relation to the past which I have named 'evocation' in the context of the explicitation interview, and to a mode of describing which sets out from this quality of relationship to the past, which I have termed 'an embodied discourse position'.

To sum up the first point, the consequences of the model of consciousness modes throw light on the mine of potential information opened up by accessing the pre-reflective dimension of lived experience. In the practice of introspection, this means giving special importance to the act of secondary remembrance as the way which enables reflection. Secondary remembrance does not consist in an effort of memory, but in letting something emerge during the evocation of a singular past lived experience. As a result, one of the major difficulties is created by the fact that the subject makes 'efforts' to remember, while one of the technical bases is to solicit an effortless memory, a letting come. What is at stake is authenticity, clarity, and fidelity to the intuitive donation of the past lived experience.

Epistemic coherence: the only lived experience is in one lived moment.

To access a lived experience, even a past one, and thus to create the fundamental condition for an authentic introspection of an intuitive donation of the lived experience, it is essential to focus on a specified situation and moment, as no lived experience exists in general. Relating to a 'lived experience in general' is not having a lived experience but having a thought about a class of lived experiences. It is undeniable that one can easily identify classes of lived experiences, which are the repetitions of the same action in the same circumstances, such as making coffee in the morning, taking the same route, carrying out the same professional gestures, etc. But relating to a class of lived experiences, to a generality, or to a time period which is too large and exceeds the unfolding of an action, does not mean giving oneself intuitively a lived experience, but having a thought relating to this class of lived experiences. Instead of a contact, we have an overview of a generality. Without an intuitive donation it becomes impossible to access the pre-reflective content inscribed in each lived moment; without this donation the subject will produce a 'signitive' discourse about generalities, invariants common to these actions. This opens the door for the expression of his naïve theories, i.e. what the subject believes he must do. It is more of a position consisting of giving a lesson or a lecture, and thus enunciating what one knows (or thinks one knows) already about what one does. This will not produce introspective information about what the informer does really when he is in action, and particularly what he does in the pre-reflective consciousness mode, which is always more than what he thinks he knows about what he does! This requirement is thus based on epistemic coherence; describing one's lived experience is describing a lived moment, a singular moment which is circumscribed and real (which I have in fact lived), because if not it is not a description of a lived experience. If the informer is not in authentic contact with a lived moment, he can say things, and even things which will interest all the disciplines which focus on the study of representations for example, but he does not inform us and does not inform himself about what he has experienced and of which he is not reflectively conscious.

The epistemic coherence of the practice of guided introspection is to lead the informer into the mode in which he can apprehend his lived experience, and describe it as a lived moment, with what was already reflected in the moment, and what comes to 'reflection' in secondary remembrance.

2. Theory of 'passivity'

In my view the idea of pre-reflective consciousness is in itself revolutionary for the cognitive sciences; taking account of pre-reflective lived experience greatly broadens the field of information available for research, and clarifies the format of prompts appropriate for introspective explicitation. It emphasizes a specific act: intuitive donation, the fact of taking into view that which had only been experienced, for the past lived experience it is then a matter of evocation or recollection. This is a theory which couples together consciousness and memory from the viewpoint of the transition to reflective consciousness. But the theories of memory of Husserl (Husserl, 1925/2001) and Vermersch (Vermersch, 2004; 2006b) offer on the one hand another extension in what it is possible to recollect through his theory of permanent 'passive memory' or retention, and on the other hand hypotheses relating to the possibility of deliberately awakening these retentions by 'awakening intentions'.

Passive memorisation or retention

Another apparently simple phenomenological idea is that of permanent passive memorisation of the lived experience: what Husserl calls 'retention' or 'primary recollection'. The psychology of memory has lately come to study implicit memory or incidental learning, or in another paradigm autobiographical memory, but it has taken little interest in the obvious fact that at each moment of our lives we 'memorise' many elements of our lived experience without having any intention of doing so. Alzheimer's disease shows us what happens when this is not the case.

> Tomorrow I will still remember the place in which I sat down in the room, people who were next to me or opposite me, what I was wearing, or what the weather was like, without me at any moment getting down to the task consisting of learning about the place where I sat down, etc. However, this is information which will remain available, without me knowing that I have it inside me, that it has been memorised inside me.

The whole of our life is surrounded by information which is acquired continuously in an involuntary, passive way. This information remains available depending on its usefulness, or if not it disappears from consciousness, but not from memory. We have here several ideas: the first is that of retention, as a permanent passive memorisation of elements of my lived experience; the second is that as the content of my lived experience is to some extent pre-reflective, and this is of course the case of retentions which are continuously acquired, I will only know it when I recognise it by its reflection. Its memorisation, if it has taken place, is in a way doubly unknown to me! I do not know it in the sense of not having reflective consciousness of it, but furthermore I do not know what has been memorised inside me. One can thus understand one of the main difficulties of retrospective introspection, which is quite discouraging for anyone attempting it alone: not only do I have the impression that I do not remember, but in any case, it appears to me with near-certainty (a false near-certainty) that nothing is available to be recollected. The resulting conclusion is that it does not work, and that it is impossible to carry out research by this method! When in fact one has 'simply' to create the conditions which enable the reflection of the lived experience.

What we have here is a powerful theory about the fact that what is available to recollection is far more important than what the subject believes he knows, because of passive memorisation and its pre-reflective nature. A second complementary hypothesis is that all these retentions are linked, interwoven and connected by resonances over distances, and associations of all kinds. And that each moment recalled in the evocation mode takes into view everything that is linked to it and can be seized provided that the view is shifted inside what is given. For this intuitive donation elicited by evocation will open up possibilities provided by the continuous interweaving of all the components of the lived experience. This means that each recollected lived element can give rise to and/or be the object of the placing into relationships with everything which is linked to it, by simply contiguity or by remote resonance. These possibilities of attachment are based on all the relational modes between elements belonging to the same lived moment, and they are innumerable; furthermore, they do not need to be memorised separately to open up the possibility of 'looking at them' in secondary remembrance. The practical question is then no longer recollecting, but discerning in what has already been recollected everything which is attached to it, and whose description may be relevant.

The field of what can come back into the memory is infinitely larger and more detailed than has been shown by the paradigms of memory study since Ebbinghaus. Wanting to check what is recognised or recollected out of a defined mnemonic material is ignoring everything that the subject can remember of the lived experience of having been exposed to this material. Of course in doing so, one cannot control in advance the span of what can be recalled, as what could form the object of a recollection can only be determined a posteriori. (Ancillotti & Morel, 1994).

Technically, this leads to questions which modify the direction of attention of the subject on the basis of what he has already grasped in the evocation, for example by prompts such as: 'and what happens just before' and 'what else are you paying attention to at this moment', etc.

Awakening of retentions: Empty focusing. Awakening intention.

In his theory of retention, Husserl conceives that retention 'gradually subsides', i.e. that it becomes less and less active, until it reaches the 'degree zero of activity'. This degree zero *is not a disappearance*, but a 'non-activity', just as immobility is not death, but the degree zero of movement. What is important is that their non-disappearance is accompanied by the possibility of being reawakened, and thus gaining access to reflective consciousness, and thus to the possibility of being verbalised. We know that these retentions will come back involuntarily through sensorial association, or resonance, as in the effect of Proust's famous 'madeleine dipped in tea'. The drawback is that in this case, they will only be awakened by chance and are thus not available at will. But the sensorial association effect may be deliberately sought, as well shown by the techniques of the Actor's studio (Strasberg, 1969) based on concrete memory. Husserl calls the medium of awakening 'a bridge to the past', an impression which awakens retention and gives back intuitive contact with the corresponding lived experience.

There then arises the technical question of possible aid, deliberate solicitation of the awakening of retentions linked to a singular lived moment. At least three techniques can be used to elicit this awakening of retentions which are relevant to the scope of the introspection:

- The first consists of simply guiding the person towards focusing on a singular lived experience rather than remaining on a general discourse, which is a necessary condition for evoking lived experience, as we saw earlier;

DESCRIBING THE PRACTICE OF INTROSPECTION   43

- The second deliberately uses an indirect perlocutory effect by inducing the evocation act thanks to a request which cannot be answered without relating intuitively to the past lived experience.
- The third mobilises an 'empty focusing' supported by an awakening intention, and thus an act projected towards something one is certain exists (I have experienced it), but which is not apparent to me, as though I did not remember it.

The first technique consists of guiding the informer towards a thematic focusing circumscribed by a singular moment of his lived experience. This means hearing in his discourse whether he is talking in a general way, and after a reformulation of what he has expressed, proposing to him, with his agreement, to let come back a moment in which what he wants to talk about actually took place. And if there are several, he should be tactfully encouraged to choose one of the lived experiences, and even more specifically 'one moment' in this singular lived experience, for example: 'by what he began with', 'the moment which particularly interests him', 'an important moment for him', etc. It should be understood that, in response to a generalising discourse, the mere fact of requesting 'an example', 'an occasion when that happened', or 'the last time it happened', already has the effect of channelling the attentional theme towards a focused field, and thus encouraging intuitive contact with the past lived experience. At the same time, the researcher observes the verbal and non-verbal apparition of the signs demonstrating the presence of an intuitive contact and thus the mobilisation of the act of secondary remembrance. If he does not identify them, he intervenes by using other techniques.

In fact, the second technique is a response to the fact that the researcher detects that the informer is not performing the act of secondary remembrance. Can one intervene? Can one help him perform the act thanks to appropriate prompts? The difficulty is that mobilising secondary remembrance is basically involuntary until one has become well practised, it cannot therefore be simply directly 'ordered' as such. On the other hand, it is possible to induce it by formulating questions that the subject can only answer by moving into the evocation position, and thus secondary remembrance. This can be done relatively easily if one asks a question such that 1/ the subject does not immediately know the answer, and 2/ to provide the answer, if he agrees to, he cannot base his answer on acquired conceptual knowledge, but must inform himself at the source, i.e. in his own lived experience. Thus if you ask him: 'How were you dressed on that day?', or 'At what point in the room were you at that moment?', this information has never been learned, but has probably been memorised. If the informer agrees to reply, he will spontaneously carry out the interior gesture of coming back into contact with the corresponding lived experience, where the possible answer is situated. He will carry out involuntarily and effectively the interior gesture of evoking and placing himself back in the situation in which he can discover elements of answers by apprehending them in secondary remembrance. But this technique assumes that one has already been focused on a singular situation in the course of the interview. If this is not the case, and if the person has difficulty in putting himself back in the situation, it is then possible to mobilise the awakening properties of retentions by 'empty focusing'.

The third technique is based on the possibility of awakening retentions which are relevant to the introspection targeted. It is based on a phenomenological idea: the possibility of 'empty focusing'. I can ask an informer to 'let come back the last time when he did x'. When I give this prompt, I propose to the subject to focus on something which is not yet appearing, but which we are sure exists because he must have experienced 'the last time he did x'. The attention is thus provisionally guided towards a target, which is supposed to exist, but which is not appearing, which leads to the idea of a provisional 'vacuum'. If we now concentrate on the idea of 'focusing', we enter the associative model of passive memory, and of the dynamic of the transition from the predonation field (phenomenological unconscious) to intentional seizing (transition to consciousness, at least pre-reflective) (Husserl, 1975). The hypothesis is that all this retention-related material can be mobilised by resonances and similarities, in short that these retentions and their interrelations have a form of sensitivity to everything which corresponds to them. Thus in the example of Proust, the taste of the present 'madeleine' awakens the same taste in the past, and brings with it the lived experiences which were attached to it, or in other words produces secondary remembrance. This example shows the classical case studied by the psychologists of the time (Gusdorf, 1951), in which the trigger occurs by chance. On the other hand it is possible to try to trigger such an awakening, by launching an intention. We have here a type of act to which early 20th century psychologists were attentive, 'the intellectual sentiment' (Vermersch, 1998) of which good descriptions may be found in Burloud (Burloud, 1927a). This act is characterised by the fact that I can launch it, intend it, and it unfolds without me having any grip or control on its execution, while

DESCRIBING THE PRACTICE OF INTROSPECTION   45

obtaining a result which is relevant to the intention. Here, what one is trying to mobilise in the informer, is an intention whose purpose is to awaken retentions linked to a particular past lived experience. This may be used to focus on a situation or a specific moment in a situation, but also absent information. For example, I may ask myself 'What happened just before?' when what was just before was not being given.

The contributions of Husserl's phenomenology of memory are manifold; the idea of retention considerably widens the potential field of what can be recalled from my lived experience. But as retention is always retention of lived experience, this also strongly emphasises the very specific nature of lived experience as an object of recall, as a subjective anchoring. Finally, the contribution of Husserl suggests and founds practical ways of working on retrospective introspection, of making it possible, of overcoming subjective difficulties relating to inadequate prompts or efforts. There are indeed as many things to do to help the subject stop from preventing himself from producing introspective data as there are things to do to elicit from him an amplification of the data.

One final point we must consider is not directly related to phenomenology, although the work done over a ten year period with Natalie Depraz and a group of researchers about the descriptive practice of Husserl has shown us technically admirable examples. If introspection is indeed a perception in the evocation of a past lived experience, then like any perception its fecundity and effectiveness will be commensurate with the categories which guide this perceptive activity.

3. Methodological conditions for to the description of all lived experiences

Schematically, it will be agreed that one can only describe what one knows how to recognise, what one has descriptive categories for. But if we were satisfied by this assertion, this would limit us for ever to what is 'already known'. We also need to be able to conceive of the appearance of something 'new'. In fact every description as well as every speech act may be inventive and creative in so far as the emergence of new sense is not a process which is under control. In the practice of the explicitation interview, the one who masters categories for the description of lived experience (and thus in structure[9]) is the researcher, for his informer usually only has naïve categories, which have in most cases not been subjected to in-depth conceptualisation, or expert categories which are strictly linked to the content of his activity. However, the interviewee remains the informer, and it is from him that the researcher will learn and discover things which he did not know, which he could not imagine. However the fact of guiding him in structure will also make the informer discover descriptive spaces which he would not spontaneously have ventured into.

I propose to draw a distinction between two sets of descriptive categories: categories which are specific to a subject of research, and generic categories which are appropriate for all descriptions of lived experience.

Categories which are specific to a subject of study

These categories constitute the specific theoretical expertise of the researcher, and the purpose of his research. For each new subject of research, they must be invented and discerned; the first descriptions, the first questionings, are a matter of trial and error. It may be the aim of an initial research, beginning a new programme, to discover what are the stages, properties, and variants of the realisation of a material or intellectual task, of the consciousness of an internal state, of an egoic property.

Practice shows that — after a first gathering of data based on the presuppositions which initiated the research — the first stage of analysis of verbalisations reveals descriptive traits of the lived experience which had not been imagined at the outset. This results in the need to start again the interview and the description, and also to invent new concepts, and modify theoretical needs. It is the aftermath of the first gatherings which is the time for the descriptive and theoretical invention. These are the moments which best demonstrate the role of the expertise of a professional researcher, through his experience in analysing the data, in allowing himself to be overwhelmed by the unexpected, as well as through the potential field of theoretical knowledge that he masters, and which enables him to subsume verbalisations into abstract categories. It is here also — if the object of study is not related

---

[9] Guiding 'in structure' signifies privately, not inducing content in the formulation of the question; positively, designating a possible place for new information, naming a possible container. For example, by asking questions without content, such as 'and there, what were you paying attention to?', or 'and just before that, what were you doing?'. This is inductive of a moment or a theme, but does not contain any suggestion about what it contains. 'What were you paying attention to?' opens up to the whole realm of possibilities in terms of sensorial channels and contents.

to an excessively specialised experience, as may be the case of leisure or professional 'micro-worlds' (for example learning scores by heart in the case of professional pianists, or practising movement play in rugby) — that self-explicitation is invaluable in that it can combine in the same subject an expert informer and an expert analyst, while in the second-person it would be necessary to find again the informer and question him again.

As far as these 'specific categories' are concerned, being an expert in introspection and introspective guidance is not enough if they are not mastered. I mean that expertise in the practice of introspection is a necessary but not sufficient condition for producing research. For example, Francisco Varela was a trained biologist and was expert in the experience of Buddhist meditation (which requires a specific form of introspection). When he began to describe how he would get his bearings in analysing a geometrical figure (a pretext task) or in describing an experience of listening to a sound, he was relatively ill-equipped[10]. I am not saying this as a criticism of Francisco, but for the value of this example, as because of his meditative experience, I could suspect that even without being trained in the explicitation interview, he had a good degree of introspective expertise. And clearly he did. But this expertise, developed in connection with a particular type of experience, Buddhist meditation, was not preparatory to its immediate application to another type of experience. If he had been a trained psychologist, he would probably have been familiar with the description of problem-solving behaviour. On the other hand, for Francisco, it was clear that his introspective skills enabled him to adapt very rapidly, depending on the thematic indications suggested. This is not an isolated example, I relate it both as a friendly sign and as something exemplary because it is so unexpected. I have had the same experience of being ill-equipped, and others have been like me, in the context of the Grex, each time we have approached experiences which we had never yet studied (evocation, attention, modes of addressing, prompts effects, empty focusing, etc.). Although we were a group of co-researchers who were expert in interviews and in introspection, to acquire this expertise on a new specific subject, it was necessary first to discover, create, and invent the descriptive thematisation specific to this new subject of study.

Introspective expertise, or the expertise of an interviewer, does not give someone universal thematic expertise. To be effective with 'new'

---

[10] I am referring to 'Ateliers de pratique phénoménologique' ('Practical phenomenology workshops') which were organised by three of us — Natalie Depraz, Francisco Varela and myself — over a period of 5 years in Paris.

subjects of research, it is essential to construct the interaction between the generic competence specific to mastering the explicitation instrument and the specialised competence given by the study of a new subject. On the other hand, upstream of expert knowledge of a field, there is a generic introspective expertise which enables one to easily get one's bearings; it is based on universal descriptive categories of the description of a 'lived experience'. This may seem a little contradictory, but I will explain further under the next heading.

Universal descriptive categories for the description of all lived experiences

Unlike perception which is related to objects whose appearance varies indefinitely, introspection is always fundamentally related to the same object: lived experience. Whatever the type of lived experience, its originality, its particularity, its character (rare or common), in all cases it is a 'lived experience'. In fact all lived experience has *the same basic structure*, a knowledge of which can provide guidance, and into which are inserted the more specific categories which we have just indicated.

What are these universal categories? I would suggest that there are mainly two which are specific to the object 'lived experience', and a third which is specific to the expert intent by which all descriptions are organised.

- The first is based on the fact that all lived experience is inscribed in temporality, all lived experience is a process, and describing a process can (or must) always consist of the description of all the stages of the process. This makes it possible in real time, and at a later stage in the analysis, to recognize what is not said, what is lacking (in the structure).

- The second takes into account the general components of the description of all lived experience, on the basis of the fact that all subjectivity will have cognitive, sensorial, thymic, corporeal and egoic aspects, in whatever way you wish to make this division as a matter of principle in order to remain coherent with your theoretical research framework.

- Finally, the third takes into account that (1) there exists an indefinite number of descriptive viewpoints relating to the same lived experience, and (2) all descriptions can be carried out according to various degrees of 'granularity', each one indicating properties which are invisible at other levels of fragmentation. Every description must be carried out at a degree of detail which is useful, relevant and elucidatory.

Let us reconsider these three points:

The descriptive basis of the structure of all lived experience: temporality.

All lived experience can/must be described in accordance with its temporal structure, as its basis. All lived experience is a process whose primary universal property is that it unfolds over time and whose seizing must be related to temporality. Several cases are possible: serial structures, i.e. one moment after the previous moment, one act after the previous act; but also synchronous structures, i.e. acts or states which unfold over the same time in a more or less complex way like overlapping tiles (one act started before another and continues at the same time as another, or ends after another which was taking place at the same time), and in some cases also durations, envelopes (like curves of sound, variations of intensity, expressive nuances), and tempos.

This does not mean that we will be shut inside a linear representation of time as a model for the intelligibility for all lived experience; this would be far too rigid and restrictive, and indeed false. Temporal, serial linearity is the basis of descriptive structure, and there is no other such basis, but it is not the basis of the structure of the analysis and interpretation of what is described. Cycles, repetitions, transpositions, and hidden non-linear correspondences will appear commensurate with the competence of the researcher. To better understand the meaning of this 'non-linearity', let us consider an analogy in the field of writing music, which is also intended to represent in a temporarily linear way the unfolding of a piece of music.

> A musical score describes in a strictly linear way what must be played, note after note, and part by part for synchronous scores[11]. But musical analysis will know how to distinguish all sorts of non-linear events, transposed themes, quotations, canons, tonal correspondences, rhythmic shifts, etc. The linearity of the temporal dimension is a guide to knowing whether the score (for us the description of a lived experience) is complete, coherent, consistent, with a start, an end and an intelligible process which links them at the level of events. In the same way as a score could not be written in a non-linear way, to be used as a guide to its reproduction by a musician who discovers it for the first time.

---

[11] This example based on a musical score is developed in Vermersch (2007b), pp 28–29.

Reciprocally, in the course of the interview or self-explicitation, everything which is described must be able to be marked in the succession of stages of the process, so as the researcher perceives its relative situation, but also the degree of completeness of the description, as well as its lacunae, contradictions and impossibilities. Listening to the other person in an interview with the use of these markers enables the identification of many items of implicit information in real time and in structure (i.e. without knowing the answer to the question which one considers necessary to reveal what is implicit).

> For example, one person describes what comes after a change of state for which he tries to understand how it was set up, insisting on the affective and reactional dimension of the new state. Through listening, it emerges immediately that what is to be questioned and described is situated both before the change, in order to hope to access what caused it, and at the very moment of the change, to better apprehend what the interior transformation consists of.

This does not mean either than in the course of an interview or self-explicitation the description must be accomplished while strictly following the time scale, for example from the start to the finish, but that the verbatim must make it possible to *reconstitute* the 'time line', as the police say in referring to a crime. And the guiding of the questioning must be carried out with the consciousness of the completeness or non-completeness of the stages of the process, of the lived experience.

The possible descriptive layers of all lived experience.

Any description can always be carried out from different perspectives, there is never a single description, and this means that the same moment of lived experience can form the subject of a multiplicity of complementary and successive descriptions (cf. the concept of 'layers of lived experiences' (Vermersch, 2006c). This is similar in a way to a map, which relates to the same region or country, but which may be a road map, an economic map, a geological map, a hydrological map, a botanical map, and so on. In the same way, a description of lived experience may choose different viewpoints: following acts which may be either cognitive or material; taking into account the body in its postures, tensions and gestures; taking an interest in thymic values, and valences; looking for the egoic dimensions related to beliefs, values and identity. And even if one only chooses one of these layers which are always present in all lived experience, for example the cognition layer, there is a multiplicity of possible co-occurring activities; as I perceive visually, at the same time I hear, I feel corporally, I smell or I taste something else. These large categories which designate layers of lived experience are intended only to make the interviewer or describer become aware of which layer of lived experience he is giving precedence to, and to question the legitimacy of not taking into account the other layers with regard to the purpose in mind. Technically, each viewpoint requires a further description of the same moment of lived experience. It turns out to be very difficult, or impossible, to carry out a description simultaneously on several layers at once.

Granularity of the description and fragmentation/expansion

Not only must the change of viewpoint be taken into account depending on the layers focused on, but also the change in the granularity of the description. Any description can be repeated by fragmenting the temporal stages into finer elements. Then at a moment when temporality is stopped, the description of each element may be expanded through a description of its qualities. Anything described — whether it is acts, perceptions, affects, corporality - inside a stage can always be fragmented, i.e. in terms of descriptive verbalisation can always be subjected to a descriptive expansion, as when the scale is changed with a geographical map. Each parcel of land, each property of that parcel, may or may not be represented, depending on whether the map is large scale or small scale. There is not *one* description of an object, but as many possible descriptions as there are points of view and scales or granularities that one decides to adopt.

But furthermore, it is the place to show that what we are concerned with is not only recollecting the past, but also questioning it according to the information which is sought. Mastery of descriptive categories is as important in successful introspection as having a memory in a good condition. Mastering generic categories for the description of lived experience makes it possible, from the same mnemonic base, to go much further in the description, for the single reason that the information is sought; if not, it would not be 'forgotten', unknown, but simply not processed. It is not a matter of describing an extraordinarily precise and complete memory, but of taking into account an ability to *retrieve* pre-reflective information.

Part Three: Conclusions

1. Questions of validation and limits of subjective seizing.

In seminars and colloquia doubts and critical questions about introspective verbalisation data, whether or not they are taken from explicitation interviews, are always concerned with the same issues: Can one trust what the subject says? Is what he says true? Can it be proven? How can we be sure that what he says is true? That he is accurately describing what really happened? Is he not making it up? Can we validate what he says? The questions are essentially sceptical.[12] In this conclusion I would like to show that most of these general questions are based on erroneous presuppositions.

But beforehand, it is first necessary to reconnoitre the terrain from which we are starting out when we study subjectivity, i.e. the viewpoint of the subject, what he can describe according to him. Subjectivity is radically and constitutively 'imperfect' in relation to a determination for objectification, a project to grasp a scientifically based truth. There is no point in dreaming that subjectivity could one day become 'perfect' and prove directly useful for research. I am not stating this in order to draw sceptical conclusions which would lead to an a priori denial of the possibility of research taking subjectivity into account, but to consider in a realistic way the difficulties which must be borne in mind. We have to begin from this native imperfection and learn to work with it, because it is, specifically, what makes it 'subjectivity'. Subjectivity is what is specific to the subject, and relativises everything he may say, because it is 'according to him' that he is describing. So, subjectivity is often not very sensitive, in the sense of not very discriminating, because the quality of attention is fluctuating, and may be very mechanical; conversely, it may be far too sensitive and thus be so invaded that it overestimates or ignores many aspects. It is not very faithful, it mixes the lived moments, presents them in a confused way, and bundles them together. We know that memory may be defective in many ways (Schacter, 1997): it may have gaps, it may be infiltrated by presuppositions, indeed we know that the subject may project his naïve theories and filter what he has lived,

---

[12] I term a 'sceptical' viewpoint, a viewpoint which is based on a negative a priori prejudice, based on a belief (I don't believe it). Husserl had clearly pointed out that such a view destroys itself, i.e. easily leads to a performative contradiction. In other words, can one trust memory? If I suppose that a priori it cannot be trusted, I cannot even understand how I remember the question I have just formulated or heard! Or all the forms of the statement 'The subject is not reliable'. Yes, what about the value of what you say? Is it reliable? In which case, the subject is reliable. Or is it not reliable? In which case the question you raise has no value.

reconstructing according to what he understands, and producing a retrodiction (Piaget & Inhelder, 1968); the subject's recollection is limited because he cannot describe (recognise) what he does not know or does not understand, etc. There are no mechanical processes to resolve this problem from the outset: the subject will never be a tape recorder or a video recorder which records everything accessible to them. The picture is bleak, and may lead to the temptation to do without what the subject says, *but in no science has one ever abandoned studying a field on the grounds that it was difficult to grasp!* For more than a century, the reaction of rejecting introspection in favour of behavioural data has merely avoided the question of understanding the experience of the subject as he lives it, and the work of methodological improvement enabling the taking into account of these native imperfections.

But the analysis of these imperfections, and the importance attached to them, are based first of all on the presupposition that it is the informer who provides us with the truth, immediately, simply because it is he who is speaking. But truth, in the sense of adequation to reality[13], can only be established indirectly, after the time of the event, by an expert third party (researcher, judge, historian). There is a confusion between an everyday, conversational meaning of the criterion of truth, and the use of the term in connection with scientific research. In the latter context, it is not the informer who establishes the truth, but the expert third party, and he is subject to the same requirements in finding evidence which supports his conclusions as any other researcher. These are the requirements of reason, based on the critical analysis of the data gathered. I thus place the establishment of truth in a second stage.

I therefore propose to draw a distinction between two approaches to the truth:

The first is to wait for it, or to ask for it; this is what I would call the ethical dimension of truth. It is an injunction on the enunciator (witness, informer) to express himself while attempting to tell the truth, whether in relation to external factual data or states and thoughts. This is explicitly what justice does when it asks the witness to tell 'the truth, the whole truth, and nothing but the truth'.

The second dimension of the truth is epistemic. It is not a request made to the person who is bearing witness, but a request made to an

---

[13] This idea of 'adequation to what is real' to characterise the criterion of epistemic truth does not presuppose in my mind the postulation of a 'reality' of which one must discover the properties, but rather that all knowledge founded in reason gives a hold on the world through its pragmatic adequation.

expert third party to establish the truth, on the basis of what the witness or the informer has said. 'Telling the truth' in this epistemic sense means producing an utterance of which one can ensure in a more or less gradual way that it is adequate to what it is referring to. But this epistemic value is never in the order of immediacy, it is in justice, as it is in history or in scientific research, the indirect product of applying a method of providing evidence whose requirements with regard to reason are the same for everyone.

I am fully aware that by drawing a distinction between the ethical dimension of the requirement of truth and the epistemic dimension of the necessarily indirect establishment of truth, I am shaking up our representations. It is like emerging from a comfortable cocoon of certainties about what or what is not the truth, and the naïve legitimacy of expecting it immediately. The conflicts between enunciation and the establishment of the truth only appear clearly when one explores the criteria of acceptability of a testimony; in everyday life, expecting someone to be truthful, having confidence that what he says is the truth, seems to be a minimum requirement, and can fortunately often be ensured. But in research, in justice, in history, this cannot be the case.

However, in the gathering stage, the researcher may take a critical view of the quality of verbalisations (see also the article by M. Hendricks in this issue). He may both judge them because he has criteria which enable him to do so, and act to improve the quality of verbalisation produced. In this appraisal, what will dominate will relate to the authenticity of the verbalisations, i.e. 1/ the degree of clarity of the intuitive filling-in of the recollection, 2/ the accuracy of the verbal expression, and 3/ the fidelity of verbalisation to what appears in recollection. The more introspective verbalisations appear to be authentic, the more we will be able to establish the existence of what the subject is describing according to him. Existence is not truth, it is only 'his truth' i.e. 'subjective truth', but for research it is an important basis as it informs us about what appears to the subject, according to him. In these different research frameworks which take into account the first person viewpoint, authenticity is the criterion which enables the attribution of information value to the descriptions produced. Authenticity is not ersatz truth, but it is the criterion which establishes the descriptive value of the verbalisations produced. It should not be confused with sincerity. The criterion of authenticity forms the basis of the value of the data. If it is not recognised and mastered, the subsequent analysis will have little meaning in so far as it is founded on information which is not faithful to what appears to the subject. The analysis must be able to base itself on this certainty of a translation which is as accurate and faithful as possible to what the subject effectively experienced according to him. It must be stressed that the criterion of authenticity is not a criterion related to the exactitude of what is described being adequate to what was experienced, but that it is related to the aperceptive act when it is related to a past lived experience; it relates to the accuracy with which what appears is put into words.

Obtaining this result only produces raw data, and from a research viewpoint a large proportion of the work remains to be done: constructing the temporal unfolding, understanding each of the events forming the lived experience, inventing new categories to precisely indicate the meaning of what is expressed, etc., i.e. conducting the whole analysis of the results right up to the conclusions and to their discussion.

2. In conclusion: introspection considered primarily as a perceptive act

For a long time, I considered retrospective introspection primarily as a question of recollection, related to the field of memory precisely because it is always a matter of relating to the past. But by working on the implications of the authenticity criterion and the importance of mastering descriptive categories, I have come to realise that introspection is a perceptive act, and that authenticity is primarily the appreciation of the quality of the perceptive act. Even if it is a perceptive act in the past lived experience. Once the condition has been met that access to this past lived experience is indeed lived experience, and thus a singular moment, and that the intuitive donation is sufficient in the evocation (first part of the authenticity criterion), the other theoretical elements can be considered as means to be taken into account to enlarge possible perceptions, and to deploy the perceptive possible. Accordingly:

The whole of the unreflected field[14] is a kind of invitation to grasp that which is not yet in the reflected consciousness mode. This leads to the perception of an immense deposit of data, available in the subject

---

[14] I propose to use the term 'pre-reflective' only for consciousness in action, and to use the term 'unreflected' only to designate everything which is not reflected, i.e. not only that which has already been subjected to an intentional seizing and has become pre-reflective, but also that which falls under the heading of phenomenological unconscious, which Husserl calls the predonation field, and which has not yet been subjected to an intentional seizing although it is already active in 'passivity'.

unbeknownst to him, and whose access is merely subordinated to a mutation of consciousness, a hold towards reflective consciousness.

The theory of passive memory, retention, and its possible awakening, opens up another field of possibility, that of extending the types of data potentially available when we bring the process of becoming aware into play. So many pieces of information have been deposited in us at each moment in our lives!

Finally, the taking into account — which is just as operative and fundamental — of the generic descriptive categories of all lived experience gives rise to many elements to be described, provided that one is informed of the fact that they exist as sources of information, and that one directs one's view in the right direction. The expansion of the description of something which is already described is largely based on this possible abundance of categories, if it is mastered.

These points open up an immense range of possibilities which can be questioned, and described, and which of course will be revealed in an act of memory, but above all will be the product of a shift in view inside the secondary remembrance, based on the evocation.

References

Ancillotti, J.-P. & Morel, M. (1994), *A la recherche de la solution perdue* (Paris GREX: Collection Protocole n° 4).
Binet, A. (1922), *L'intelligence* (Paris: Costes).
Burloud, A. (1927a), *La pensée conceptuelle: essai de psychologie générale.* (Paris: Alcan).
Burloud, A. (1927b), *La pensée d'après les recherches expérimentales de H-J. Watt, de Messer et de Bühler* (Paris: Alcan).
De la Garanderie, A. (1989), *Défense et illustration de l'introspection* (Paris: Centurion).
Depraz, N., Varela, F. & Vermersch, P. (Ed. 2003), *On Becoming Aware: A Pragmatic of Experiencing* (Amsterdam: Benjamins).
Fraisse, P. & Piaget, J. (1963), *Traité de psychologie expérimentale* (Paris: PUF).
Gusdorf, G. (1951), *Mémoire et personne(2)* (Paris: PUF).
Humphrey, G. (1951), *Thinking: An Introduction to its Experimental Psychology* (London: Methuen).
Husserl, E. (1925/ 2001), *Analyses Concerning Passive and Active Synthesis: Lectures on transcendantal logic* (Boston, MA: Kluwer Academic Publisher).
Husserl, E. (1975), *Experience and Judgment* (Evanston, IL: Northwestern University Press).
Husserl, E. (1989), *Ideas Pertaining to a Pure Phenomenology and to a Phenomenological Philosophy. First book: General introduction to pure phenomenology* (Boston, MA: Kluwer Academic Publishers).
James, W. (1901, 1890), *The Principles of Psychology* (London: Macmillan).
Lyons, W. (1986), *The Disappearance of Introspection* (London: MIT/Bradford).
Mandler, J. & Mandler, G. (1964), *Thinking: From association to gestalt* (New York: John Wiley & Sons).

Maurel, M. (2008), 'Repères chronologiques pour une histoire du GREX', *Expliciter*, 75, pp. 1–30.
Nisbett, R.E. & Bellows, N. (1977), 'Verbal reports about casual influences on social judgements : Private access versus public theories', *Journal of Personality and Social Psychology*, 35, pp. 613–24.
Nisbett, R.E. & Wilson, T.D. (1977), 'Telling more than we can know: Verbal reports on mental processes', *Psychological Review*, 84 (3), pp. 231–59.
Piaget, J. & Coll (1977), *Recherches sur l'abstraction réflechissante 1/L'abstraction des relations logico-mathématiques tome XXXIV des EEG* (Paris: PUF).
Piaget, J. (1974), *La prise de conscience* (Paris: PUF).
Piaget, J. & Inhelder, B. (1968). *Mémoire et intelligence* (Paris: PUF).
Reber, A.S. (1993), *Implicit Learning and Tacit Knowledge an Essay on the Cognitive Unconscious* (Oxford: Oxford University Press).
Reder, L.M. (Ed. 1996), *Implicit Memory and Metacognition* (Mahwah, NJ: Lawrence Erlbaum Associates).
Schacter, D.L. (Ed. 1997), *Memory Distortion: How minds, brains, and societies reconstruct the past* (Cambridge, MA: Harvard University Press).
Smith, E. & Miller, F. (1978), 'Limits on perception of cognitive processes: A reply to Nisbett and Wilson', *Psychological Review*, 85 (4), pp. 355–62.
Titchener, E.B. (1912), 'Prolegomena to a study of introspection', *American Journal of Psychology*, 23, pp. 427–48.
Titchener, E.B. (1913), 'The method of examination', *American Journal of Psychology*, 24, pp. 429–40.
Underwood, G. (Ed. 1996), *Implicit Cognition* (Oxford: Oxford University Press).
Vermersch, P. (1994, 2008), *L'entretien d'explicitation*, Nouvelle édition augmentée d'un glossaire ed. (Paris: ESF).
Vermersch, P. (1998), 'Le sentiment intellectuel', *Expliciter*, 27, pp. 1–4.
Vermersch, P. (1999), 'Introspection as practice', *Journal of Consciousness Studies*, 6 (2–3), pp. 17–42.
Vermersch, P. (2000), 'Définition, nécessité, intérêt, limite du point de vue en première personne comme méthode de recherche', *Expliciter*, 35 (mai), pp. 19–35.
Vermersch, P. (2004), 'Modèle de la mémoire chez Husserl. 1/ Pourquoi Husserl s'intéresse-t-il tant au ressouvenir', *Expliciter*, 53, pp. 1–14.
Vermersch, P. (2004), 'Modèle de la mémoire chez Husserl. 2/ La rétention', *Expliciter*, 54, pp. 22–28.
Vermersch, P. (2006a), 'Les fonctions des questions', *Expliciter*, 65, pp. 1–6.
Vermersch, P. (2006b), 'Rétention, passivité, visée à vide, intention éveillante. Phénoménologie et pratique de l'explicitation', *Expliciter*, 65, pp. 14–28.
Vermersch, P. (2006c), 'Vécus et couches des vécus', *Expliciter*, 66, pp. 32–47.
Vermersch, P. (2007a), 'Approche des effets perlocutoires: 1/ Différentes causalités perlocutoires: demander, convaincre, induire', *Expliciter*, 71, pp. 1–23.
Vermersch, P. (2007b), 'Bases de l'auto-explicitation 1', *Expliciter*, 69, pp. 1–31.
Vermersch, P. (2008a), 'Analyse des effets perlocutoires: 2/ Englobements, intrications, complémentarités', *Expliciter*, 76, pp. 1–9.
Vermersch, P. (2008b), 'Introspection et auto explicitation. Bases de l'auto explicitation 2', *Expliciter*, 73, pp. 42–55.
Vermersch, P., Faingold, N., Martinez, C., Marty, C.& Maurel, M. (2003), 'Etude de l'effet des relances en situation d'entretien', *Expliciter*, 49, pp. 1–30.
White, P. (1980), 'Limitations on verbal reports of internal events: A refutation of Nisbett and Wilson and Bem', *Psychological Review*, 87 (1), pp. 105–12.

Maryse Maurel

The Explicitation Interview
Examples and Applications

Abstract: This article summarily presents the explicitation interview with some examples of interviews. In the first part, referring to three excerpts from protocols, we consider some of the techniques used to guide a subject into an introspective posture. We show how these techniques create conditions conducive to access to pre-reflective knowledge, knowledge stemming from a moment of action experienced by the subject, of which the subject has no knowledge in the mode of reflective consciousness. Some of this knowledge is in fact surprising both for the interviewer and for the interviewee. The experience or the expertise of the subject interviewed is invariably increased as a result. In the second part, we provide a brief insight into the fields of application of the explicitation interview, with reference to three case studies, which are presented in a vivid and detailed way (in the fields of sport, health and training, and artistic creation). We conclude with a very brief panorama of the various known fields of application of the explicitation interview.

Key words

Explicitation interview, pre-reflective, explicitation techniques, reflection, verbalization.

This paper sets out to answer two questions:
- How does the explicitation interview make it possible to guide a subject towards an introspective posture enabling access to pre-reflective knowledge?

- What use can researchers and practitioners make of explicitation data?

Before answering these questions, let us consider briefly what an explicitation interview is. The explicitation interview is a form of guided retrospective introspection, writes Pierre Vermersch, also in this issue. As a result of the passive synthesis described by Husserl (Husserl, 1998), the subject constitutes for himself (or herself) continuously and involuntarily a passive memory, an autobiographical memory of which a large part is, for the subject concerned, pre-reflective, i.e. the subject is not aware that he (or she) has this information available, it is not reflectively conscious for the subject.[1] The explicitation interview makes it possible to support the subject, without induction, as he makes the transition from pre-reflective consciousness to reflective consciousness, about a specified lived experience in the past, and more specifically a lived experience of an action. To this end, the framework created by the interview provides the conditions for the possibility of the provoked awakening of recall. After concluding a communication contract with the subject and after expressing an intention of awakening recall,[2] the interviewer guides the subject towards the evocation of this specified lived experience and towards access to an intuitive donation[3] of recall, so that he carries out the intuitive filling-in process[4] and acquires reflective consciousness of this experience. We say that the subject carries out a reflection[5] of the past lived experience.[6] The final stage is that of putting into words or verbalization. The verbalizations gathered supply data to the researcher or practitioner about the action and the subjective experience of the subject interviewed. They also enable the subject to gather

---

[1] The existence of this pre-reflective knowledge is well known to ergonomists, who observe the gap between 'enacted knowledge' (i.e. what the subject has really done and can be observed by a third party) and 'professed knowledge' or 'declarative knowledge' (i.e. what the subject says he has done, which in most cases corresponds to institutional professional knowledge). The first example (When the gesture speaks...) is a perfect illustration of the existence of this gap.

[2] 'I suggest that you take the time to allow what comes back to you, as it comes back to you, about the moment when ...?' or 'What comes back to you first when you take the time to think about the moment when ...?'.

[3] This intuitive donation is triggered by sensorial elements or by elements of the context, elements of concrete memory. In this case, 'intuitive' means without words, unspoken.

[4] The interviewer guides the subject through his exploration of the field of attention in recall, to help him rediscover, in an unspoken mode, all the information whose recovery is desired.

[5] In this text, we say 'reflection' to mean the product of the reflecting act.

[6] All the subject's actions in this phase are referred to as a reflecting act.

information for himself about what he really did and experienced at the moment in question. It is important to note that for the interviewee to gain access to his pre-reflective knowledge, he is required to establish a special relationship with his past, and to place himself in a special discourse position, here termed the evocation position,[7] drawing on concrete memory (Gusdorf, 1951). It is important to stress that for the interviewee it is a matter of being present in relation to his lived experience as a lived experience, and not of thinking about his lived experience, which is something quite different.[8]

The three examples in the first part have been chosen to show the very technical nature of the guidance during the interview, and to show that the interviewer's expertise is of essential importance.

The three examples in the second part provide a glimpse of the fields and ways in which the explicitation interview is used, and are based on interviews concerning: sport, health and training, and artistic creation.

1. How Does the Explicitation Interview Make It Possible to Guide a Subject into an Introspective Posture to Gain Access to Pre-Reflective Knowledge?

Based on three examples, we will provide some indications of how the explicitation interview functions, of the expertise contained in the prompts and in the guidance used, and of ways of gaining access to pre-reflective knowledge. We will present, in each case, the context, the exchange, and the results we can draw from them.

1.1. When the gesture speaks...

The context

During a training course aimed at improving professionals' control of industrial facilities in malfunction situations on a simulator, the following event takes place: during the exercise, the head of the auxiliary circuits of the facility receives an order to cool the facility down. In the facility's operating guide, it is indicated that cooling is obtained by opening up a steam discharge circuit. As temperature is linked to pressure, the pressure merely has to be reduced to reduce the temperature. Unfortunately the operator carries out an inappropriate action which

---

[7] Vermersch tends to use the expression 'position de parole incarnée' ('embodied discourse position') to accentuate the link with concrete memory.

[8] For theoretical questions linked to the affirmations in this paragraph, see the paper by Vermersch in the present issue.

causes the circuit pressure to increase until a circuit protection valve opens. This is what happened in the debriefing of the situation, so that the operator was brought to a consciousness of his error (Blanc, Desjardin, 1997).

The exchange

Instructor:
>When you applied the operating guide, what did you start with?

Operator: *(after thinking for a moment)*
>We were at section x and I was asked to cool it down.

Instructor:
>And when you cool it down, what do you do?

Operator:
>I use the vent to atmosphere circuit and I request a lower pressure. *(As he replies, he mimes the gesture which he carried out on his control panel. His gesture corresponds to a gesture requesting a higher pressure, i.e. it is the opposite of what he is saying, but he does not realize this.)*

Intervention of station head:
>Look at the gesture you are making. It is contradictory with the objective of lowering pressure!

Results

This short interview, in which the instructor gives only two prompts, underlines the highly technical aspect of the explicitation interview: the two prompts are open, they do not offer an alternative choice, they request information about the operator's action. They do not induce anything, they simply place the operator back in front of his action in the situation that he has just experienced. They are precise. The first part of the first prompt 'When you applied the operating guide', refers the operator back to the specified moment when the error was committed. The second part, 'what did you start with?', focuses the subject on this moment which is identifiable by him, guiding him away from making any judgment or commentary and towards the description of his action. The second prompt, 'And when you cool it down, what do you do?', takes on board what the operator has just said and requests specification by an action of the verb 'to cool down' in this context. The operator gives a verbal response and pronounces a piece of professional knowledge. At the same time he replies corporeally and repeats the gesture which he did in fact make on the simulator, a gesture which denotes knowledge in action; the gap between the two is obvious. The intervention of the station head refers the operator back to the comparison of the two items of information, verbal and non-verbal, which he has just given. The instructor's prompts have supported him in the evocation of the action carried out on the simulator to 'cool it down'. The reflection occurs when he sees his gesture, i.e. when the pre-reflective knowledge of his action on the simulator is brought to his reflective consciousness and contradicts what he has just said. As we say in everyday language, he becomes immediately conscious of what he did.

1.2. Claire and her keys

The context

The interview excerpt presented in this example is taken from a series of research interviews about the mathematical activity of students entering university.[9] Claire has volunteered for these interviews. She wants to become a teacher. She is very interested in the way thinking functions in mathematics and in what she can discover about the way she herself functions. On the day in question, however, she resists the support from the researcher who tries, at Claire's request, to make her focus on a moment when she says she has understood in a flash the significance of a mathematical symbol.[10] As she comes out of the evocation, she says she is unable to recall what she was thinking and doing at the moment in question. To overcome this belief, the researcher proposes to her a second interview about a subject from everyday life. Claire agrees. The researcher then concludes a new communication contract, the aim being to find out what Claire was thinking at a moment of her own choice, in order to show her that her belief is not valid (Maurel, 2009).

---

[9] In the context of the CESAME research group of the IREM (Institut de Recherche sur l'Enseignement des Mathématiques and the IUFM (Institut Universitaire de Formation des Maîtres) of Nice. The working documents concerned have not been published. CESAME is an abbreviation for 'Construction Expérientielle des Savoirs avec Autrui dans les Mathématiques Enseignées'.

[10] It was in fact the definition of the existential quantifier.

The exchange

Claire chooses to recall what she was thinking when she went home at midday. She left the university on foot, and she bought a loaf and a cake (a 'galette des rois').[11] She arrived in front of her door, she had 'My bag on one side, the loaf and the cake balanced *(she makes the gesture with the left hand)*, I put my bag down because I had the keys in the left hand pocket, I took the keys *(she makes the gesture with her right hand, moving it in front of her body, and going to the left hand pocket of her coat)* and I opened'. She describes her bunch of keys and her entry into the apartment. She is in evocation, which is shown by the fact that, for example, she counts the keys in her bunch, 'One two three four', by going to find this pre-reflective, and thus unavailable, information in the past lived experience which she has made present for herself in the evocation position. The researcher points out to her that she has described in fine detail her arrival at and entry into the apartment, and that what she expects is a similar description of a moment when she is doing mathematics.

100. C   Wait wait, you want me to describe my way of thinking, in the same way that I have just described what I did just now at midday

[…]

105. M   I did not ask you what you were thinking when you had your keys and your cake, I did not ask you to do it but

106. C   Well, but I would be quite unable to say, even though it was at midday

[Claire's belief is present and very strong in this reply. However, in around forty short and precise replies and in a few minutes of interview, Claire will recall what she thought would be impossible to recall].

[In the replies which follow the one in which Claire reasserts her belief (reply 106), the support from the researcher involves several specific techniques used in the explicitation interview (Vermersch, 1994)

- the interviewee's consent for recontacting a past lived experience,
- the choice of a specified situation,

---

[11] The interview took place in the afternoon of 6 January (Epiphany holiday).

- a verification that Claire is indeed in the evocation position by non-verbal indicators (her rhythm of speech is slow, she is searching information which is not already available, her eyes are not focused),
- the resumption of the gestures,
- the holding in place on the moment when Claire puts the keys into the lock,
- access through the sensorial (by feeling the weight of the cake balanced on her left hand, a kinaesthetic feeling which triggers the vision of the trace of lipstick on the key), until the moment of the reflection of what she was thinking when she put the key in the lock].

[References to these techniques, or commentaries, are indicated between square brackets. The 'stage directions'[12] inserted during transcription are shown between curved brackets and in italics].

107. M   You are going to go back to the moment when you arrive in front of your door, the loaf and the cake *(I repeat her gesture)*

[The initiation of the awakening intention is a little sudden here, but it is situated in the confidence and consent horizon of the interview which authorises it; it is accompanied by the resumption of Claire's gestures.]

108. C   Mm

109. M   You take the keys *(I repeat her gesture)*

[The researcher helps Claire to rediscover the elements she has already given to create the conditions necessary for the reflecting act, hoping that one of them — or other new ones which will come later — will open up the path towards what Claire was thinking at the moment in question. She is creating the conditions needed for the reflecting act, and supports Claire in the intuitive filling-in.]

110. C   Yeah yeah

111. M   You take the key

112. C   For the top of the door

---

[12] By analogy with the stage directions of a play (acting indications given by the author), we use this term to denote information about the non-verbal behavior of the interviewee or interviewer in our transcripts.

[Claire's eyes are unfocussed, she is in evocation, and is searching for the information before replying.]

113. M   For the bolt at the top of the door

114. C   Ah I took it with my mouth in fact

[Claire is astonished as she recalls pre-reflective knowledge.]

115. M   Yes

116. C   I know because that put lipstick on it

[Claire justifies, spontaneously, how she knows that she took the key with her mouth, she is so associated to her past experience that the non-verbal attunement with the researcher is sufficient to support her: the researcher adopts the same body position, talks with the same rhythm, resumes the gestures, and in short acts like a mirror image of Claire.]

117. M   And before they were in the mouth, the keys were where

118. C   I took my keys, I took them out *(gesture of the hand)* and to sort them out, to find the right key out of four, I did this *(she mimes with her hands and her mouth)* finally I got the right one out, and after I took it with my hand

119. M   And at the exact moment when you put the key in the lock

120. C   Well

121. M   You were thinking of what, put yourself back in front of your door, you have the cake, you feel it, you feel the weight.

[The researcher reminds Claire of the purpose of the interview, and asks her to return to a moment slightly before when the key was put into the lock, she supports her and suggests that she should direct her attention towards the bodily feeling at the level of the left hand which is carrying the cake and the loaf laid on top, to recall this feeling and complete the recall.]

122. C   Mm

123. M   You can feel *(I repeat her gesture)*

124. C   Yeah yeah

[Prompt 123 encourages Claire to take the time to relive this feeling, and supports her by repeating the gesture.]

125. M   The key you took in your mouth

126. C   Yes

127. M   You take it back in your hand

128. C   Yes

129. M   You are going to put it into the lock

130. C   Yes

[The researcher describes the gesture Claire carried out at 118, she induces nothing else except what Claire has already mimed or verbalized.]

131. M   At that moment

132. C   Well just at that moment I saw the lipstick and that's when I saw it

133. M   Yes you have seen the lipstick, you feel the cake there, it feels heavy

[The researcher helps Claire to complete the sensorial information and to put it together.]

134. C   No it is balanced rather

[The researcher helps Claire to complete the kinesthetic feeling.]

135. M   It is balanced, you put the key in

136. C   Yeah

137. M   And you see the lipstick, where is it the lipstick

[The researcher helps Claire to complete the visual dimension in the intuitive filling-in.]

138. C   Just on the teeth of the key *(she seeks the information before answering)*

139. M   Yes

140. C   And I say to myself *(laughter),* yes but it's really stupid

[This precise moment is the moment of reflection of what Claire was saying to herself as she opened the door, on that day, on 6 January, shortly after midday. Intuitive filling-in is sufficient to obtain the information sought. Claire has just recalled what she was thinking about. Claire blushed, as this thought was perhaps difficult to say in a recorded research interview. The researcher puts Claire at her ease, the content is not important, the aim has been achieved, it has been proved to Claire that she can recall what she thought in a past lived experience that she thought had been forgotten. What has been done once can be repeated. Claire now knows, in the pre-reflective consciousness mode, experientially, because she has just done it, that she can recall information of which she does not have reflective consciousness. The researcher will use this lived experience as the basis for resuming explicitation interviews about Claire's mathematical activity, which she sets out in a performative way at the end of the interview by renewing the contract in 151 to return to the objectives of the research.]

143. M   And there you are, you have recalled what you were thinking when you put the key in the lock. That's all, you keep it for yourself, what interests me is that you have recalled it for yourself

144. C   Yeah

145. M   If I ask you brutally 'hey, you know, when you put the key in the lock at midday what were you thinking about', you'll tell me: 'I don't remember', that's only to be expected, everyone gives the same answer

146. C   Yes

147. M   If we put ourselves back there, rediscovering the body's feelings, which we saw, you saw the lipstick, you said to yourself something which made you laugh and which you keep to yourself, but you have recalled what you were thinking

148. C   Yes yes

149. M   At that precise moment

150. C   Yes yes, yes but there, there was that little detail, that there was lipstick

151. M   Yes and well I look for the lipstick in the analysis exercise[13] and I couldn't find it.

Results

We have pointed out in this example some of the techniques of the explicitation interview. Claire's final reply (reply 150) confirms that the reflection was triggered by the vision of the lipstick on the key. This vision followed the physical sensation of the weight of the cake on her left hand.

In most of the interviews, after the awakening intention of the interviewer, the subject addresses her lived experience, and initially nothing comes.[14] Remember that this belief is not valid, the recall is not immediate and its possibility is counter-intuitive. Furthermore, the recall cannot be the result of a deliberate act on the subject's part; it is necessary to create the conditions for emergence by expert support. And perhaps the recall will take place? This is what happens here. The recall takes place despite Claire's belief, expressed in 106: 'I would be quite unable to say'.

Note that this interview was not intended to gain access to the content of Claire's thoughts, but to work with her on a limiting belief which prevented her from accessing her past mathematical activity. The real purpose of the interview, in agreement with Claire, was to get over this limiting belief and enable the continuation of the explicitation interviews about her mathematical activity. For Claire, who was interested by its functioning in this field which she adored, and which she had chosen against the wishes of her family. For the researcher, who had a research program in progress.

1.3. Sybille's table

The context

The psychologist Guillaume, in his manual of psychology published in 1932 (Guillaume, 1948; 1932), suggests a simple task, the learning by heart of the following matrix of numbers:

---

[13] Analysis is a field of mathematics.

[14] It is therefore essential that the interviewer helps her to explore possible ways of access: 'Perhaps you hear something, perhaps, perhaps not...'. The same thing applies to seeing and feeling. The interviewer may draw on observation of sensorial predicates in the language of the subject, or on the subject's eye movements (techniques borrowed from NLP).

12	8	9
4	21	6
7	15	11

We have used this task a great deal in the research group led by Pierre Vermersch, to obtain protocols for explicitation interviews about the lived experience of actions. The interviewer asks the interviewee to learn by heart the table of numbers, and during the process, observes or films the interviewee. Immediately after the memorization of the table, the interviewer carries out an explicitation interview so that the interviewee can make explicit the details of how he learns the table, and particularly the end criterion (how did he know that he knew?) It is this part of the interview, the final part, which we will look at here. The interview is conducted by Catherine Le Hir and the interviewee is Sybille. Sybille has just described in detail how she memorized the numbers, some of which were easier to memorize than others (Le Hir, 1999).

The exchange

[Sybille said, at 517]

517 S: in fact I have the impression that the numbers are in front of my head and that as I repeat them, they enter. Those which have really entered go to the back, and those which have not really entered, they are on the sides or the edges

[At the end of the interview, Catherine's aim is to obtain the end criterion. She accompanies Sybille in this effort. She reformulates with Sybille's words what Sybille has told her earlier.]

548 C: those that enter immediately, they go immediately to the back

549 S: those I know well, whose place I know, they go immediately to the back

550 C: all right

551 S: those I know less well, they are on the side

552 C: all right, OK

553 S: that's right

554 C: so there are those that go to the back, and those that are on the sides, and that's when you know that those ones are less well installed

555 S: yes

556 C: mmm, that's when you start reciting more slowly

[Catherine here again uses a piece of information Sybille gave her earlier in the interview.]

557 S: yes, until those on the edges enter

558 C: yes

559 S: and afterwards, well, it goes a bit quicker

560 C: all right

561 S: afterwards I say to myself 'I know it', so it's OK, usually I say to myself 'I know it', I recite it one more time and afterwards

[By a succession of prompts using the words 'how do you know that...', repeating the very words of Sybille, Catherine now keeps Sybille on the precise moment where she knows that she knows, she does not let her go, she continues until the criterion has been elucidated, without inducing, without interpreting, merely by repeating the very words of Sybille.]

562 C: and *how do you know* then that it's OK when you recite them?

563 S: after I have said 'I know'

564 C: yes

565 S: because it comes of its own accord

566 C: because it comes of its own accord

567 S: yes

568 C: *how do you know that* it comes of its own accord

569 S: because it runs through like that

THE EXPLICITATION INTERVIEW 71

570 C: because its runs through like that, of its own accord like that?

571 S: yes

572 C: *how do you know that* it runs through of its own accord and that it's OK

573 S: because I don't think

[Sybille says she does not think; we know that denegation masks what exists; when Sybille does not think, she is necessarily doing something else. Catherine takes on board what Sybille is saying, and searches for what Sybille is doing, by getting around her denial.]

574 C: because you do not think, and *when you do not think, what do you do*?

575 S: in fact, I know it's OK because I'm able to recite them on my own, I'm able to hear them in my head, and then if there are other noises, I'm able to hear other noises at the same time

576 C: all right, you can be both in your head and outside at once

577 S: that's it, at the same time

578 C: well, thank you for all these details, you know it's really interesting.

Results

In this protocol, we have no indications about the non-verbal dimension but we can imagine from the quality of the information gathered that there was postural agreement between Catherine and Sybille, and that Catherine repeated the gestures of Sybille, and copied the tone of her voice and her speech rhythm to provide her with support. We have noted in the course of the exchanges the repetition of Sybille's words by Catherine, the non-inductive character of the prompts, and the holding in place on the moment when Sybille knows that she knows to elucidate the end criterion: Sybille knows she has completed her memorization of the table of numbers when she knows it sufficiently well to be available for another activity, such as listening to other sounds, as she hears the numbers in her head.

2. What Use Can Researchers and Practitioners Make of the Explicitation Data?

To answer this second question, we will provide examples taken from practitioners or researchers, specifying the context, the information gathered in the exchange, and the results we can draw from it. The first two examples concern action situations, while the third draws on an explicitation interview to document an artistic creation. It is important to stress that the explicitation interview does not exclude all the other kinds of expertise of the people who use it. It is just one more tool to explore a new field of data, that of the world as it appears to the interviewee.

2.1. The hurdle race of a top athlete

The context

The example is that of a top woman athlete, who produced some of the best French performances in 2000. She thus has a very high level of expertise. She is running a 100 meter hurdle race shortly before the Sydney Olympic Games. The hurdle race is an extremely standardized exercise during which the athlete jumps ten hurdles of identical height with fixed intervals between them.[15] The race in question is the first important competition of the season. The competition takes place in two races. The athlete chooses to be interviewed about the one race of the two which 'left a bigger impact on her than the other'.

The athlete agreed with great interest to an explicitation interview with Jean-Louis Gouju (Gouju, 2001), as what she felt about the race was extremely negative. And yet, she had just produced her best-ever performance, and her coach was positive about it. Watching the video film, there was no indication of any justification for the athlete's negative judgement about her race. Nor had the coach seen anything visible or observable about the race to justify taking this view. Uncovering pre-reflective knowledge by the mediation of the explicitation interview would inform us about what could not be observed by a third party. The athlete contacts her past lived experience[16] with a specific relationship to the past, that is the evocation position. She carries out the reflecting act on her lived experience of the race at the moment she jumps the fifth hurdle and just afterwards.

---

[15] The course is 100 meters long, with 10 hurdles 0.838 meters high, separated by a fixed interval of 8.50 meters. The distance between the start and the first hurdle is 13 meters, and the distance between the last hurdle and the finishing line is 10.50 meters.

[16] The race only lasted 13.35 seconds.

Information gathered

The beginning of the interview explores the moment before the start, getting into the starting-blocks, the start of the course and the jumping of the first four hurdles. The athlete talks about jumping the fifth hurdle, and a 'black hole' after this hurdle. She provides a piece of information: 'it's the girl next to me'. The interviewer asks her if she agrees to reconsider this moment. He gathers the following items of information:[17] 'Well, when I jumped the fifth one *(silence, leaning forward)*, it was as though I was frozen, you know, I didn't react in fact. After that, I let the hurdle take over because I saw her, that is I did not see her, but felt her, the girl there, the girl *(gesture with the left hand)* because we're about at the same time, she maybe has a very small lead, but nothing at all, you know... and then, she shoots off *(rapid gesture with the edge of her hand, and her eyes wide open)*. I feel like I'm standing still. And her, whoosh. Because I'm in my thing you know, even so. Then I see her, I see her front leg, I see her leg, her right leg, I see the leg and I see that she is off. And then I lose my temper, well, I don't lose my temper but *(laughter)* I don't feel good *(laughter)*, I don't feel good at all, because then I get angry with myself in fact, I get angry with myself. Because I concentrated on her and not on what I was doing myself, as a result I was surprised and *(silence)* I didn't give up but I said 'oh shit, I'll keep going, but well, heck *(gesture of annoyance and giving up of the hand, which moves away upwards and backwards)*, I'll finish the race, you know'. And I feel that I am not fighting. The rhythm, I can't even hear the rhythm any more, and I continue, you know, I finish my race'.

The athlete then says that she doesn't feel the sixth hurdle, 'she passes', 'No, I can't see anything, I can't hear anything, not even the spectators, I think they're shouting however, usually they always shout, I can't hear anything at all.'

When the interviewer asks her to describe her bodily sensations at the end of the race, she says: 'At the end of my race, *(silence)* I don't feel like I'm fighting, I don't feel like I'm fighting as I should do. I have the impression of being heavy in fact, as though I was letting things happen rather than anything else. At the end of my race, it's coming back, I feel it's coming back *(rotating hand gesture)*, but at a certain moment, I have a black hole, in the middle, between the fifth and, I don't know, about the ninth, I don't know exactly, I don't really know but I feel I have a black hole'. The interviewer keeps her

---

[17] Only the informative passages of the interview have been kept, and placed one after the other, with all the rest of the discourse and the prompts being deleted.

focused on the bodily sensations of the moment in question, which makes it possible to gather the following information: 'it's as though I had lost concentration, and *(mouth noise of annoyance)* and afterwards I... *(rotating hand gesture)* I don't know. I have the impression that I did not attack *(hand gesture)* that is the impulse, I can't manage to *(gesture)* as I should and everything, and throw everything into it, you know *(gesture)*, <u>I have lost concentration,</u> *(silence)* I'm hot, I'm hot, I'm hot, yeah, and I have the impression that my arms are doing *(gesture of the arms)*, I'm hot. I have the impression that my arms are going off in all directions. When I attack the hurdle, I have the impression that *(gesture of opening the arms)* I can't control it. <u>I can't control what I am doing</u>. I let it go *(gesture of the hand)*, there's a moment when, like that, I don't know why, I get back into it. I don't know why it came, and then I make a sprint *(rapid gesture in parallel of the two hands held forwards)* but I don't know, I rush *(laughter)* and *(silence)* as though I have the impression that I have wasted time and I have to make up for it in fact, even if it can't be made up, you know, but on the flat, I tell myself, it's my strength,[18] I must make up for it, you know'.

Results

The key event of this race, from the athlete's viewpoint, is the existence of the 'black hole' after the fifth hurdle. This 'black hole' — and the loss of concentration which results — is triggered first by a feeling, and then by a vision of the right leg of the girl in the next lane, by the sensation of the girl who heads off, who is going faster than the athlete interviewed. The 'black hole' begins with a feeling of the opponent and her speed. 'It's the girl next to me'. This triggers a feeling of total loss of speed. 'It was as though I was frozen'. 'She shoots off', 'I feel like I'm standing still', 'And her, whoosh', 'I see that she is off'. In this 'black hole', the athlete cannot rediscover the expected feelings, which are coached in the work of training.

It is an accompanied return to this moment which enables the obtaining of interesting verbalizations. Everything happens as though the 'black hole' characterized something which the interviewee does not know. From then on, the feelings of heaviness, of being hot, of arms not being held, are not considered as forming part of the race. The interviewee then says she had lost concentration. She is no longer present in the race. Everything suggests that this incident led to her losing contact with the world of action as she had constructed it. But there is an important item of information which is not in the interview,

---

[18] The athlete is also a very good sprinter over 100 meters.

and which could have been sought in a second interview if it could have taken place. We do not know what happened just before the 'I let it go' which marks the emergence from the 'black hole'. What does the athlete do just before? what does she say to herself? what does she feel? what is her inner condition? what does she perceive? what does she pay attention to? to sum up, what triggered the emergence from the 'black hole' and the transition to the 'I let it go' for the final sprint.

It is worth noting the pointing up of a difference in tone between the positive external judgment of the coach and the chronometer concerning the race described — it leads to a personal record and a performance of a very high national level — and the negative subjective lived experience of the athlete — a 'black hole' lasting for more than four hurdles, an impression of heaviness, a lack of fighting spirit, a lack of control, a sensation of being hot — which she stresses at the end of the interview: 'And *(silence)* afterwards, I was really not happy, I go off, I get changed, I take my time because I am angry well, my coach comes and says to me 'why are you in a bad mood?' I tell him I really didn't feel good and everything, 'but no, you did 13.35 seconds', I say 'really', and it's the first time in fact that I break a personal record and I don't express great joy, you know'.

The athlete had not been overtaken in a race by an opponent for two years! So she had not anticipated what happened and what she experienced in the race. She did not know how to (or was not able to) incorporate it into her lived experience during the race.

We consider this interview to be extremely characteristic of the type of data gathered by explicitation interviews, data which cannot be observed or accessed by other means. There is no perception of this data by the coach, the video shows nothing. The researcher can enter into a dialogue with the coach and offer him these data so that he can decide how to use them. We have here two complementary kinds of expertise: that of the researcher who gathers the data and that of the coach who will be able to incorporate them in his coaching.

2.2. *Jeannine's expertise*

The context

Jeannine is a trained nurse. For twenty years, she has been an instructor, and head of training for paramedics at the University Hospital Centre (CHU) of La Rochelle. Jeannine wanted to better understand how she went about making intravenous injections, which she always succeeded in doing, even in difficult situations. This knowledge would help her in her teaching, and in the instruction she provides.

Maurice Lamy carried out an interview with her. The purpose of the interview is clearly defined. Jeannine is not certain that she is teaching the gesture used to put an intravenous injection in place well. She wants, through the mediation of the explicitation interview, to find out what she knows how to do (knowledge in action) but does not know how to transmit it (declarative knowledge).

Information gathered

The interview protocol is very long, effective and richly informative. We will present the situations explored and some pre-reflective expert knowledge which is made explicit, without showing how it has been obtained (Lamy, 1998). We will limit ourselves to what Jeannine has discovered during the interview about preparation, quality of interpersonal relations, and the putting in place of the tourniquet.

The first specified situation described is that in which Jeannine takes a blood sample from her son. The boy is very tense, he fears the injection. Jeannine describes how she uses both her hands to manipulate the equipment with her right hand and maintain the arm, by gently massaging to establish a relationship and provide relaxation and instill a sense of calm.

The second situation, which emerges during the interview, is that of the moment in which an anesthetist taught her what she knows how to do very well, and, above all, how he taught it to her. She was a student at La Pitié Salpêtrière hospital, she was 19 at the time.

In the third situation, she is at the hospital, she shows a 'nurse in difficulty' (who is unsuccessful in all her attempts to set up intravenous injections) how to go about it.

Jeannine describes in great detail all her gestures in the first situation, she confirms them in the third situation, and she compares the pre-reflective knowledge they have just uncovered with what she says when instructing her students. She also compares what she does in training and how she does it, with what was passed on to her by the anesthetist and how he passed it on to her.

First situation: overcoming the patient's reticence and stress

This is the preparation of the injection with someone who is reticent, which was the case of her son on the day in question: 'I sat down next to him,[19] I put both my hands closer, I take his hand. He was extremely tense, I spoke to him, but as I touch him, I feel that I have someone

---

[19] Only the informative passages of the interview have been kept, and placed one after the other, with all the rest of the discourse and the prompts being deleted.

who is under stress under my hands *(she takes an imaginary hand between her two hands)*, I have something which is holding back, which is contracted, there is a little muscle which is hard and which is contracted. And this is what I massage. I was talking to him. Little by little, I felt that his arm was relaxing. In fact, to take a blood sample, the arm must be extended. When I put tourniquets on, in general, I always massage the arm, moving upwards, that is while feeling the veins, and I put the tourniquet on. In fact, it is rather caressing. I have two hands and I use them.'

Jeannine comes out of the evocation to make a comment: 'I hadn't realized that I use both my hands, but that is extremely important! Because one of them provides reassurance and the other carries out the action. Finally, that's the word I should have used with the students. In fact, when you move your hand upwards, the person does not only feel the tourniquet, the person who is tense also feels something else'.

Jeannine returns to the evocation position: 'I take it fully in my hand... I don't work with the tips of my fingers, but with the hand, moving upwards. I take the rear of the arm. I have my tourniquet in that hand *(she looks at her left hand)*. I always keep my right hand under the arm of the person. I take the end of the tourniquet. I draw out only one end. I move it upwards. In fact, I have one hand which acts, and the other which hardly moves at all, and which holds, which only holds. And I pass, still with the same hand, I pass the tourniquet under the loop... *(she carries out the gesture)*. And I tighten with my left hand. Like that *(she again repeats the whole of the gesture)*. In fact, I take my tourniquet like that, I hold like that, I take this one, and hop, I pass it through like that. I still have my hands on the arm. And I don't tighten hard! I take care that there should be no wrinkles in the arm. I pay attention to the suppleness of the skin. Because I see again the anesthetist[20] telling me: 'Be careful with that, if you tighten it too hard, you damage the veins. If you're taking one blood sample, it doesn't matter, but if you do several, you damage them'. Afterwards I do not let go, when I remove my hands, I don't remove them like that *(she raises the two arms high in front of her)*, that is I do not raise them into the air, I remove them by lowering them, *(she taps her hand on the table)*, with my left hand, I tap a little bit on the arm *(laughter)*, on the inside of the forearm.

---

[20] Jeaninne talks about the anesthetist for the first time in the interview.

Second situation: the anesthetist at La Pitié Salpêtrière hospital

'In fact, looking at my hands, I can recall the hands of the anesthetist who showed me that. It was at La Pitié Salpêtrière hospital, I was 19 years old. Those were my first intravenous injections. And I remember I put the tourniquet on in front of him. I remember I pulled the tourniquet, at right angles to the arm, it was crazy! From such a height! Perhaps I'm exaggerating, I couldn't say, but I have the impression as I see the tourniquet again as if I had pulled on some chewing gum! *(laughter)* It's just crazy! It had frightened him to see me do that. He said to me: 'You're wrecking all the patient's veins. Wait a minute!' And as he realized I was embarrassed, he said to me: 'Look...' He took me by the arm, he stood me next to him *(as though to himself)*: he stood me next to him. He says to me: 'Stand there! And watch!'. So he showed me, and he said to me *(barely audible)*: 'A tourniquet, you put it on like a ribbon'. And I was amazed, subjugated to see his hands, gentle. When he had finished showing me, he had this gesture on my arm. *(She mimes the gesture on his arm)*. He did it on my arm in the same way'.

Return to the first situation

Then 'I took the tourniquet off very very gently... Super gently, it's an extremely slow gesture, because if you take it off too quickly it can make the needle move. I put my hand back under his arm... I took the cotton wool which had remained in my hand. I applied gentle pressure, I asked him to press on it and not to bend his arm. This is extremely important. I asked him to apply pressure and not to bend his arm. Never bend the arm, because the vein has just been weakened, and if you weaken the vein, if you bend the arm, that makes it burst, and a bruise can form. Never. Never!'

And Jeannine comments on this pre-reflective knowledge which she has just brought into her reflective consciousness: 'And that should be taught, that should... That, I've just realized that it is very important to teach. Because everyone can understand it. When you take the needle out, just apply pressure, the bruise will form with the blood cells and the fibro. If you bend, the hole will be made larger. When you unbend, the clot which is in the process of forming will be destroyed, and a bruise will form. The blood will go under the skin.

In fact, it's crazy all the gestures I can make... When in fact it all goes incredibly quickly! And something extremely important I have just realized also, the bevel of the needle has to be facing upwards. Even if you are injecting on the side, it has to look at you, this bevel!

You need to have a space between the body and the syringe, or if it is a vacutainer, an assembled system, you need to have the space practically for a finger below. And I should have told them that...'.

Comparison of what Jeannine says and does when training

Jeannine has already recalled and identified knowhow which she puts into practice but which she does not teach. She goes further with this idea: 'It takes me back to the time I was teaching, I was telling them it wasn't difficult! *(laughter)*. I went too quickly with the gestures, and I should have done it in a way enabling the other person to appropriate the gestures. Because it's not easy putting a tourniquet in place, I've just realized. I went too quickly. And then also, I think also that I thought that because I could do it, the others would be bound to be able to do it.'

Third situation: the nurse in difficulty

She recalls another moment: she is at the hospital, she is showing what to do to a 'nurse in difficulty' who fails in all her attempts to set up an intravenous injection. Jeannine confirms everything she has just said by describing the setting up of an intravenous injection on a lady whose vein had been badly damaged by the unsuccessful attempts of her colleague: 'So I caressed with the hand. I spoke to the lady. I took my time, I let the arm rest a little bit, I massaged the arm in a horizontal position, not at all with the hand low down, with the hand flat against the bed. When I say I took my time, I took a good ten minutes. I sat down next to her. I did nothing. I massaged her arm. And I spoke to her. I used a very small piece of cotton wool dipped in alcohol moving upwards, and never moving downward, that is from the bottom towards the top. I held it with my hand, I did not rub, never, never. I held her vein with my hand, I put my hand round her arm, I remember I was unable to put my hand completely around, as she had a fat arm. So I held her vein just as it should be done. I took a little bit of an angle, with the vein, I know that pushed it, and hop, I straightened it up, and I slipped into the little vein, the blood came out into the epicranian immediately, but immediately, I took off the tourniquet. I didn't hurry up, I continued to touch the lady's arm in the right way. Hop, I connected the drip feed.'

Results

At the end of the interview, Jeannine sums up the key points: 'Never move from the top to the bottom. Do not tighten the tourniquet... too much! Or tighten it, but not too much. Do not make the patient tighten his hand like crazy. Do not make the patient put his hand too low. Do things quickly. And make use of this little gesture which means that you hold on properly to your vein, you take it a little bit from the side. So as not to take it against the grain of the fibers. We call that a "moving vein". If it's a moving vein, it will move and you go through it. So instead of having one hole, you have two. And after when you pierce it again, that makes a third hole. And when you put the drip feed in place, it's porous.'

She comes back to the transmission given to her by the anesthetist at La Salpêtrière hospital.

'That's someone who succeeded in passing on the right gestures to me, he did something to me which I should have done to others, that is, he said to me: "Look at what you are doing". And the fact that I had realized from the outset that I was tightening the tourniquet too much, that I was going too fast, that I was not paying enough attention to the other person, well, that made me go over all the gestures again. On the other hand, what I can't understand, is that I taught it in fact for 15 years, or even 19 years, this gesture, and I am not certain that I transmitted it completely.'

She draws conclusions of what the interview has done for her: 'I think that the quality of the preparation, the putting in place of the tourniquet, that, I was not aware that I was carrying out so many gestures. And also the end of the blood sample, or the intravenous injection, is extremely important. You have to think of the other intravenous injection which will come afterwards.'

Jeannine concludes: 'On the other hand, I would repeat what I said: it's extremely simple and extremely difficult…'

2.3. Explicitation in the performing arts

The context

During the academic year 2007–2008, Frédéric Borde took part in the artistic project of the Sylvain Groud Company, a choreographic company based in Normandy (Borde, 2008). This was the result of a partnership between the company and the Rouen university hospital centre (CHU), under the auspices of a ministerial convention on 'Culture in the hospital'. The partnership took the form of a one-year residence, during which the company provided performances, workshops and improvisations in departments which wished to receive it. This period of immersion led to the writing of a choreographic and theatrical show on this subject. During the period of residence, Frédéric

Borde was a permanent liaison officer between the company and the CHU. His function was to propose explicitation interviews to the nursing staff in order to document the play on the aid relationship. His active participation in the various workshops enabled him to make contact with the departments, and to meet enough volunteers for the interviews. In a few cases, it was possible to carry out several interviews with the same person, but in most cases, there was a single interview lasting about one hour. Frédéric proposed to his subjects that they describe 'professional lived experiences in which the body holds an important place'. However, it was less a matter of documenting the lived experiences of the 'physical' body than that of the 'flesh', that is the subjective body, according to the phenomenological expression.

In this example, the format of the interviewer's prompts guides the subject towards exploring and describing other layers of lived experience, rather than the lived experience of the action. We are entering a new field here: that of meaning. I chose this example because it seemed to me to perfectly illustrate the use of explicitation techniques and of the interview posture needed to provide information about the phenomenological lived experience of the body of the interviewee, and to take the troupe's artistic creation project forward.

Information gathered

The following excerpt comes from the second interview with Franck, a voluntary visitor to people who are HIV-positive, who works with the association AIDES.[21] Franck is talking about his first vision of Cyril, from a distance, at the moment when Cyril comes out of his room in a wheelchair, and he perceives him as 'young and old', with 'debris of youth, blond hair, a quite lively look in his eyes and an old emaciated body', 'damaged, wounded, humiliated... a physique which is moving towards death... definitely...'.

[Frédéric keeps Franck on this moment when they first exchange looks, and supports him in the description of the bodily elements of his emotional lived experience. The dotted line indicates pauses in Franck's words. We write A in place of Franck and B in place of Frédéric in the following exchanges].

60. A – I feel... I see in his face a great deal of violence... an enormous amount of violence... a revolt, an aggressiveness...

61. B – Mmm... and when you see this face of revolt and aggressiveness, what effect does that have on you?

---

[21] AIDES is the french name for the association helping HIV-positive people.

62. A –   I am fascinated... that is I am... completely drawn... I feel I am drawn, there...

63. B –   When you feel you are drawn, what does that mean for you?

64. A –   Well, when I feel I am drawn, it is... the body extended towards... that is... how could I say it... as though it is an essential encounter... an encounter you cannot miss... something... as though I had come for *that*... not for him, but for *that*...

65. B –   Mmm...

66. A –   But not at all in... with the feeling, in fact... with the motivation of being a voyeur... That is... to make... it's very powerful, anyway I'll say it... to move towards a merging with *that*... *that* being everything he lets me see at that moment...

[Franck is in evocation, he is very closely associated to his past lived experience, he is in a quasi-reliving experience, what he is recalling is something inexpressible, unutterable. He is in the setting of the interview and of the communication contract that Frédéric has agreed with him; we should not forget either that he had asked for this interview. He is therefore consenting to verbalize, but this verbalization is difficult for him, he is looking for words to describe what he is contacting under the effect of reflecting act. We see clearly here, and in the rest of the interview, that words to describe may be difficult to find, that appropriate words, at least the words which are most appropriate at the moment in question, only arrive after several rejected attempts at verbalization].

67. B –   All right... and when you are attracted by a merging, what is that for you... what do you do when you are attracted by a merging like that...

68. A –   Well, my body... in my body, anyway... I feel it in my body, a great receptiveness...

69. B –   Yes...

70. A –   An ability to... to be in contact with the other person... with the skin of the other person, with... after, all that is more or less restrained, censored, but... at any rate, it is...

THE EXPLICITATION INTERVIEW

71. B – I suggest that you take care to stay with that moment... what is it for you at that moment, stretching out to him for a merging...

72. A – *(silence)* It's a little bit like lacking oxygen...

73. B – Lacking oxygen...

74. A – Yes... being out of your depth...

75. B – Mmm... when you are out of your depth, what happens for you?

76. A – Well... you're no longer in control...

77. B – At that moment, at the moment you go out of your depth, what is it for you at that moment...

78. A – What I feel?

79. B – Yes... how do you know you go out of your depth?

80. A – Because, because at that moment I am no longer reasoning... I am no longer in thought at all... and it's the body, the flesh, the skin, which... which vibrates...

81. B – Mmm... when the flesh vibrates, what happens?

82. A – It's something that tears, in fact... like a tearing, in fact, it's... something tearing, which opens up, which... which offers itself, which... like a great freedom of the body...

[Franck knows that, after this first exchange of looks, he has entered into a relationship with Cyril, he knows this because he has given him a pullover, 'a pullover which I liked a lot' and he recalls a moment when he saw Cyril wear the pullover. This commitment was judged to be dangerous by people 'who were voluntary as I was, and who said I was doing it all wrong, and that I was going to get my wings burnt'. Franck then describes a moment with two volunteers who are also friends, who remind him of the volunteers' basic training].

220. A – She tells me something is wrong, that I can't do that, that... that I'm going to hurt myself, that I'm going beyond the... the framework of my intervention, that I... am a volunteer, that...' Remember your training, support, empathy...', that you're like a helicopter, you don't guide, you take him by the hand but you are above and you... you want to stop him falling into the ravine and that's the role of the volunteer...

you are in empathy but you can't be in support, and that me, I hold out my hand, there... I take the hand instead of being above, of listening to him... of listening to the other person and... of being there more to hear than to guide, to advise, etcetera... and that I am getting it all wrong and that I can't do that... she also tells me that I may hurt the other person, by instituting a relationship like that... a close relationship...

[Franck hears but does not listen to the two volunteers who want to protect him].

230. A – I can't hear anything... I... I close up, without aggressiveness, but... I smile... convinced that my approach is right... nothing can stop me...

[It is then that Franck remembers that Cyril had become a symbol of his own revolt against AIDS. He realizes, in the aftermath of this recalled moment, that this moment corresponds to the period during which he believed he was HIV-positive, without daring to take the tests. When, after ten years, he decided to take the test which turned out to be negative, Franck continued his voluntary work, but this time following the recommended conditions, in a way he considers to be appropriate, and of which he is very proud].

Results

The interpretation of the data presented below is mainly the result of the work of Frédéric Borde. Here, as in the other examples, it is important to note that the interview of Franck provides us with information about his lived experience. The researcher receives what Franck has experienced, as he experienced it, from his viewpoint. Once gathered, these data, like the third-person data, form the object of the researcher's analysis and interpretation, no more and no less.

This interview is a perfect example of the inadequacy of the resources made available and the declared purposes of a person. Franck's motivation, which centers on his personal relationship to the pathology, leads him to subvert the deontological framework of his practice, and finally to put himself in danger and endanger the person visited. He acts with this person as he would with a person close to him, he forgets his status as a volunteer and the training he has received to fulfill this role. This example clearly shows the point at which the balance tips from 'therapeutic distance' to the horizon of 'burn out',[22] this illness which affects those who work professionally in interpersonal relationships, which is frequently encountered amongst carers. Resources of a personal nature gain the upper hand over professional resources to the point of sweeping them away. This opens the door for all kinds of dangers for the two protagonists, as no rule now governs what they invest in the relationship.

This issue is a deep one because the carer has to call on his personal resources, and this everyday aspect of his work is not taken into account, supervised, supported. This is probably why this difficulty of being divided between the personal and professional fields is the topic which has emerged in the great majority of interviews. This is why Sylvain Groud and Frédéric Borde have chosen this issue as the main topic of their play, entitled 'If you would like to follow me…' ('Si vous voulez bien me suivre…').

Conclusion

We hope we have demonstrated in the first part how technique comes into play in an explicitation interview, and how it operates to enable access to the pre-reflective dimension of the subject's experience. Without this access possibility, a great deal of our experience escapes us. These examples demonstrate this. We should also point out the amazement and the pleasure of the interviewees who discover, in contact with their past experience, biographical elements which they have experienced, but only in the mode of pre-reflective consciousness.

In the second part we set out to show how researchers and practitioners/researchers with different backgrounds use the data obtained form explicitation in their work, and how they extend explicitation in order to achieve professional goals.

The article format is not conducive to covering the whole field of explicitation interview applications. Many researchers and practitioners have in fact taken advantage of this interview technique in a wide range of fields: education, training, analysis of practices and debriefing (Vermersch & Maurel, 1997), educational sciences and psychopedagogy, cognitive sciences, the control of industrial facilities, major companies, sports (athletics, rugby, football, refereeing, swimming), justice, health, bodily awareness and arts including performing arts.

---

[22] 'Burn-out' is the final and catastrophic stage of specific work-related stress. It mainly affects those whose professional activities call for a strong level of relational commitment in an aid relationship, such as social workers, the medical professions and teachers. It affects individuals who are committed and devoted to a cause.

A few examples are listed below:

- The thesis by Alain Mouchet (Mouchet, 2003) takes as its starting point the apparent contradiction between the discourse and the approaches of a number of top rugby coaches: they focus on the planning of the team's decisions and actions in several game phases; but at the same time they aim to create a maximum of uncertainty in their opponents, and deplore a lack of creativity and adaptation in their own players. Based on this observed situation, Alain Mouchet explores, for top rugby players, the connection to be found between the necessary degree of collective organisation and individual initiative in some game phases. This work is currently being reinvested in the teaching, training and coaching of an experimental team.

- The thesis by Armelle Balas (Balas, 1998) on metacognition, and more specifically on becoming aware of one's own way of learning, provides, through the analysis of explicitation interviews with adults, some indications which can help in answering the question: what does it mean to become aware of one's way of learning, and what role does this awareness play in learning?

- The thesis by Sylvie Coppé (Coppé, 1993) studies mathematical verification processes among pupils in a supervised assignment setting, with reference to the papers and roughs of the pupils, and explicitation interviews carried out with them.

- The thesis by Yves Champlain (Champlain, 2008) is a research/training work of a music teacher in primary education, which radically calls into question the legitimacy of his practices. This questioning forms part of a project to find what makes practical sense; it leads the author to delimit an epistemology which is specific to the analysis of practices, to explore the embodied and pre-reflective nature of action, and to question the very specific phenomenon of the articulation which can exist between a pedagogical gesture and an 'education feeling'. It opens the way towards a practical and continuous education system.

- A thesis is in progress in cognitive sciences, to apply explicitation techniques to issues of knowledge management. This is the work of Anne Remillieux, which is aimed at eliciting, and modeling knowledge for the management of change at

SNCF,[23] which is largely pre-reflective, in order to facilitate its sharing inside the company.

- Other major French companies have initiated research and training work carried out using the explicitation interview, but the results of this work belongs to the companies, and cannot therefore be made public.

- A research project has been carried out in response to a call for tender from the training department of the Judicial Protection for Young People unit (*Protection Judiciaire de la Jeunesse*) (Faingold, 2008 a, b). An initial phase of data gathering, carried out through explicitation interviews of experienced educators, has enabled a detailed analysis of their activity in educational aid in an open setting. [24] A second phase of work, involving a reflective analysis group working on practices which drew on data gathered through explicitation, has encouraged the uncovering of invariants and the formulation by professionals themselves of statements reflecting shared professional knowledge. The results of this research will be used to draw up a new training program for the educators of the Judicial Protection for Young People unit.

Articles on all this research can be found in the journal Expliciter, in published theses and memoirs, and in books. On the site www.expliciter.fr you will find an exhaustive list of the research, of which we are aware, in which the explicitation interview is used to gather data.

The journal Expliciter and the site of the same name are published by the Groupe de Recherche sur l'EXplicitation (GREX), under the scientific responsibility of Pierre Vermersch, a researcher at the CNRS.[25] The GREX is made up of practitioners, instructors and researchers involved in a very varied range of fields. The group leads training courses in explicitation aid techniques, it guarantees the certification of the leadership of the training courses, and it is the benchmark group for the analysis of explicitation practices. It is also the

---

[23] SNCF is the French national railway company (Société Nationale des Chemins de fer Français).

[24] Educational Aid in an Open Setting ('Aide Educative en Milieu Ouvert') is a judicial measure ordered by the children's court judge in the case of children who are in danger. The aim is for the social worker (specialist educator or social assistant) to eliminate danger by means of an educational action directly inside the family, or in a protected situation outside the family.

[25] French National Centre for Scientific Research (Centre National de la Recherche Scientifique).

place for the development and dissemination of research on the practice of introspection (explicitation of explicitation). Pierre Vermersch leads five seminars a year in Paris, and a 3-day experiential summer school seminar once a year at Saint Eble, in Auvergne.[26]

Finally, we should mention the research training and support work of Maurice Legault in Quebec, Canada (Legault, 2004, 2006). Mention should also be made of the dissemination and training work in Switzerland of the Swiss branch of GREX, Antenne Suisse, under the presidency of Mireille Snoeckx, with the participation of Vittoria Cesari. The translation into Italian by the latter of the book by Vermersch (2005) has opened the door in Italy for our work on explicitation and the practice of the explicitation interview.

References

Balas, Armelle (1998), 'La prise de conscience de sa propre manière d'apprendre, de la métacognition implicite à la métacognition explicite'. Thèse de doctorat en Sciences de l'éducation, Université Grenoble II.

Blanc, Philippe & Desjardin, Daniel (1997), 'Quand le geste parle', *Expliciter*, **18**, p. 16.

Borde, Frédéric (2008), 'Un explicitation interview dans le contexte d'une création', *Expliciter*, **73**, pp. 16–31.

Champlain, Yves (2008), 'Le sentiment d'éduquer. Une approche acousmatique de conscientisation du geste pédagogique d'un enseignant en musique au primaire'. Thèse de doctorat en psychopédagogie, Faculté des sciences de l'éducation, Université Laval Québec.

Coppé, Sylvie (1993), 'Processus de vérification en mathématiques chez les élèves de première scientifique en situation de devoir surveillé', Thèse de doctorat en didactique des mathématiques, Université Claude Bernard Lyon 2.

Faingold, Nadine (2008 a), 'Les pratiques éducatives à la Protection Judiciaire de la Jeunesse dans les services de milieu ouvert', *Expliciter*, **73**, pp. 1–10.

Faingold, Nadine (2008 b), 'Etudes sur l'analyse de l'activité des éducateurs de la Protection Judiciaire de la Jeunesse dans les services de milieu ouvert (suite). Méthodologie de présentation des exemples', *Expliciter*, **74**, pp. 1–14.

Gouju, Jean-Louis (2001), 'Objectivation de l'organisation de l'action, contribution à l'intervention didactique en athlétisme'. Thèse de doctorat en STAPS, Université Paris XI.

Guillaume, Paul (1948, 1932), *Manuel de psychologie* (Paris: PUF).

Gusdorf, Georges (1951), *Mémoire et personne*, (Paris: PUF, 2ème édition 1995).

Husserl, Edmund (1998), *De La Synthèse Passive* (Grenoble; Millon).

Lamy, Maurice (1998), 'Transcription intégrale d'un entretien sur la pratique experte d'une infirmière', *Expliciter*, **26**, pp. 4–16.

Legault, Maurice (2004), 'La symbolique en analyse de pratique. Modélisation des étapes du retour vers un vécu singulier dans la suite du pré-réfléchi au réfléchi', *Expliciter*, **57**, pp. 47–52.

Legault, Maurice (2006), 'Analyse évolutive d'une pratique scientifique en recherche qualitative et phénoménologique', *Expliciter*, **67**, pp. 1–11.

---

[26] Auvergne is a region of France.

Le Hir, Catherine (1999), 'Explicitation de la mémorisation de la grille de chiffres', *Expliciter*, **28**, pp.51-58.
Maurel, Maryse (2009), 'Claire et ses clés', *Expliciter*, **78**, pp. 22–25.
Mouchet, Alain (2003), 'Caractérisation de la subjectivité dans les décisions tactiques des joueurs d'élite 1 en rugby'. Thèse de doctorat en STAPS, Université Victor Segalen Bordeaux 2.
Vermersch, Pierre (1994/2003), *L'entretien d'explicitation* (Paris: ESF).
Vermersch, Pierre & Maurel, Maryse (1997), *Pratiques de l'entretien d'explicitation,* (Paris: ESF).
Vermersch Pierre (1997), 'Questions de méthode. La référence à l'expérience subjective', *Alter: Revue de Phénoménologie,* **5**, pp. 121–36.
Vermersch, Pierre (2005) *Descrivere il lavoro. Nuovi strumenti per la formazione e la ricerca: l'intervista di esplicitazione (*Roma: Carocci Faber).

Natalie Depraz

The 'Failing' of Meaning
A few steps into a 'first-person' phenomenological practice[1]

Abstract: *The experience I am going to go into refers to a process of emergence of meaning in consciousness. More particularly, what was given to me in terms of 'meaning' was the very lack of meaning of what was happening to me in the very moment. There is a crucial hypothesis here: this is the discovery of one's own experience and the production of a personal description of it within the framework of a disciplined practice. It is the only way to check the effectiveness of my first-person access to my unique and irreducible experience. After having written a lot 'about' the necessity of such a putting into practice, after having 'claimed' it as an absolute requirement, after having checked it recently in the light of a step-by-step reading of a book of Husserl and having contended that as* <u>the</u> *genuine approach of Husserlian phenomenology, here I am one who ends up revealing a bit of herself while risking such a putting into practice. It is one thing indeed to 'account' for the first-person experience by relying upon the utterances of the phenomenologists who write about it, as is often done today in the context of crossings between phenomenology and the cognitive sciences; it is quite another thing, which is epistemologically quite*

---

[1] I want to thank Pierre Vermersch and Eve Berger for their precious comments, for giving me quite useful advice and for their on going exchanges. Without their help, such a contribution would not have been possible. I also wish to thank Claire Petitmengin for inviting me to contribute to the present issue, particularly requiring from me to write on the basis of my first-person account and not on the conceptual level, as it is still so usual today and so unrootable in my native philosophical academic context. Finally I want to thank Lester Embree for revising and correcting my English

different, to practise such a first-person experience while accounting via a self-elicitation for a <u>unique</u> example, which is <u>hic et nunc</u> situated, i. e., while using a descriptive tool which is faithful to it and thus closely attests to the practice in question by working with it.

Key-words

First-person experience, first-person method, phenomenology, practice, self-elicitation, description, creation of meaning, meditation, example

Introduction

The experience I am going to go into refers to a process of emergence of meaning in consciousness. More particularly, what was given to me in terms of 'meaning' was the very *lack of meaning* of what was happening to me in the very moment. In short, it corresponds to my experienced loss of meaning, which went hand in hand with a 'failure' of my ability to 'be there' at what was happening, again, with a deficiency or a collapse of my ability to remain in contact with the continuity of the on going experience. The challenge here of such an experiential self-elicitation of inner work is to try to reconquer the meaning of such a meaning-deficiency: it in no way amounts to observing an absence of meaning and just staying there. In other words perhaps more familiar to phenomenologists, what was given to me in such an experience was the very fact of the non-givenness of meaning.

Various methodological resources were taken into account for describing the differents stages of such an experiential moment. Either (1) they were given to me before the beginning of the work or (2) they emerged as useful in the course of it.

(1) Before the experience: (a) Since it is a *past* experience, I used a method of evocation and of re-evocation of this unique *hic et nunc* situated moment, thus endeavouring to come closer to it while putting aside any other moment which might at first sight look like it, and consequently trying to live again the proper quality of such a moment by suspending my spontaneous tendency to add reconstructed features to it that were not then available; (b) while starting with such way of access, I began to collect features of this moment while focusing on its situation in time: I thus gradually saw how this moment was temporally differenciated, it includes just-happening and going-to-happen stages, it reveals an immanent stratified dynamics that may be deepened further while carrying on the self-elicitation of this lived experience; (c) in the framework of such step-by-step writing down

elicitation, I used various strategies: sometimes I recreated a lived contact with my experience — such as being able to evoke it again — by first going through my previous notes; at some other moments, I just tried to evoke the very example spontaneously ('*à vide*'), that is, without previous re-reading; or I found a new impulse toward the living context with my experience by studying a text dealing with such a lived experience; (d) I finally used a method of finer and finer temporal phase-cutting of anterior, posterior and intermediate segments.

(2) In the course of the description, on the other hand: (a) I first found an experiential spur when a comparative experience emerged, which appears to be a mirror-experience, not of failing but of a becoming of meaning, and acts as a foil to it; (b) I felt I had to do justice to the global (synoptic and synchronic) quality of such a moment, as a further addition to the temporal cutting, which led me to see new contrasted components.

Such is the methodic framework of the immediate presentation of the 'material' of my experience as it was given to me as I gradually elicitated it. I am providing the reader with such a 'material', which corresponds to the native material, or to what may be called a '*verbatim*' as a fourth and final step.[2] As a first step (section 1) I will analyse the broader context of the research (at once genealogical, thematic, and also epistemological). In section (2) I will indicate the difficulties, obstacles, impossibilities, and emotional shocks I went through while I endeavoured to contact this very unique experience again and to elicit it descriptively, which refers to a non-immanent mode of account: to a more reflexive one. Besides, only such a critical distance will have allowed to bring out the reformed presentation of the example as it is offered in the following step, which extracts it from its comparative context and opens the way for a genuine deeper self-elicitation matrix, the latter remaining a here still undeveloped

---

[2] First I thought I would *begin* with such a 'raw material', then show how I had worked it out while decoupling both examples and leaving aside the one which had emerged afterwards in order to be able to dig further into the first one and finally build into it the temporal re-organization which furnishes the reader with the 'real' temporality of my experience. I finally thought it was more relevant to introduce this first example in its uniqueness while dissociating it from the second and reorganizing it in order to get the real temporality of the experience. However, since the emergence of the first example is also relying on the second, my contention is that the latter is intrinsically part of the very emergence of the first example. I therefore decided the following: I presented the *verbatim* at the very end, stressed eight different temporal sequences of the unique example I chose thanks to a drawn framework in **bold sans serif font** leaving outside the frame the other exampleand underlined the various phases of the real temporality of the experience. By putting together these three formal typed levels, I wish to provide the reader with the possibility to see better the whole emergent context of the example.

dimension that will correspond to a future step of the present research. At section (3), I will then be able to present the example in its singularity, extracted from its initial comparative strait jacket and reorganized along the lines of its real temporality. The the final step (section 4) will be dedicated to the mentioned three layered formal typing (normal, drawn framing, **bold sans serif font**), which show the different steps of building the example from the initial *verbatim*[3] onwards.

1. The Context of the Research and its Epistemological Status

My example was born in the framework of the research group initiated by Pierre Vermersch during the fall 2006: we aimed at carrying on the work that was opened up with *On Becoming Aware* (Depraz et al., 2003) and that consisted in the on hand descriptive account of the process of becoming aware and at doing justice to two main limitations of the book: on the one hand, it is meant to focus on the experiential language at work, in order to get away from the naive alternative dilemma between the contention about the apriority of language and the contention about the primacy of experience; on the other hand, we wanted to explore further the role of the examples in a process of validation: by using situated and individuated first-person examples rather than generic structural ones (as we mostly presented them in the 2003 work), we aimed at 'laying the path while walking'.

The following example as well as its experiential and descriptive laying out emerged directly from the work that was carried out within our small group, the members of which were then D. Austry, E. Berger, N. Depraz, F. Lesourd, B. Pachoud and P. Vermersch. While referring to M. Richir's philosophical research in his *Phenomenological Meditations*, we first focused upon the following linguistic expression: '*sens se faisant*', which P. Vermersch had taken up from Richir's work; it gave rise to many discussions based on the concern to refer to a philosophical thought that was considered by some of us as obscure and speculative, although it was not entirely lacking fruitful insights; E. Berger then suggested we label our research 'the creation of meaning', which had the advantage of stressing the inventive process at work, of dissociating ourselves from a reference to an author who was not bringing agreement among us, but situated us in the orbit of Merleau-Ponty's philosophy; the expression 'experiential meaning', which was for example recently broached by L. Tengelyi (2006), was

---

[3] From the latin *verbum*, speech; an adverb, which means 'word for word', 'literally'.

also mentioned.[4] These various references are approximations of the problem which is at the core of the present research, but they do it in a way that remains situated 'above' the first-person experience proper.[5] In effect there is a crucial hypothesis here: this is the discovery of one's own experience and the production of a personal description of it within the framework of a disciplined practice and it is the only way to check the effectiveness of my first-person access to my unique and irreducible experience. After writing a lot 'about' the necessity of such a putting into practice, after having 'claimed' it as an absolute requirement (Depraz, 2006), after checking it recently in the light of a step-by-step reading of a book of Husserl (see Depraz, 2008) and having contended that it is *the* genuine approach of Husserlian phenomenology (Depraz, 2009) here I finally am, the one who ends up revealing a bit of herself while risking such a putting into practice.

The experience of meaning understood as an emergent individuated process arising in my first-person consciousness is the only leading question. Why, however, choose the word 'meaning'? What does it add to the words 'consciousness' and 'experience'? As I have already mentioned, the word 'meaning' itself includes a reference to language, including in the broadest sense of non-verbal expressions, such as signs and symbols. Of course, I do not mean to reduce 'meaning' to a logical ideality nor to a linguistic signification. Beyond the 'semiotic' component *lato sensu*, which provides the experience with a kind of native intelligibility ('it makes sense'), the word 'meaning' is laden with a 'value' component, that furnishes such an experience with a specific 'relief' ('it matters to me') and with an 'affective' component ('it moves me'). The word 'meaning' thus includes these three components of 'sign', of 'value' and of 'affect', which allows one to clearly dissociate oneself from the sheer notion of consciousness, though relying upon the process of becoming aware as the very

---

[4] Tengelyi's leading question is: 'comment un processus de formation de sens spontanée, dont l'initiative se soustrait à la conscience, s'impose pourtant à celle-ci ?' ('How a process of spontaneous building of meaning, for which consciousness has no impulsive dynamics, nevertheless requires the latter? My translation.)

[5] It is one thing indeed to 'account' for the first-person experience by relying upon the utterances of the phenomenologists who write about it, as it is much done today within the context of crossings between phenomenology and the cognitive sciences (for example in Zahavi, 2006, includingly in order to attribute to Husserl — a bit too quickly to my mind — the contention of a 'first-person phenomenology', whereas Husserl's referring to his own first-person lived experience is quite often 'generic', that is, non-individuated), it is another thing, which is epistemologically quite different, to practice such a first-person experience while accounting *via* a self-elicitation for a *unique* example, which is *hic et nunc* situated, i. e. g., while using a descriptive tool which is faithful to it and thus closely attests to the practice in question by working with it.

method for approaching the experience of a first-person emergent meaning.[6]

I was greatly advantaged by the regular meetings of our research group, which played the crucial part of 'framing' my individual work, allowing each of us to go into his or her experience without having to care for such a framing. Some of us had already produced detailed descriptions[7] and the goal of such monthly meetings was to enable each of us to enter his or her own experience in his or her own way. I then felt again the exploratory flavour of the seminar of 'phenomenological practice' of the Nollet street which took place during 1997–1998, but I could see how careful and disciplined the experiential and descriptive first person method had become insofar as what was at stake was a deliberate production of a first person description. During the meetings, each of which provided the renewed opportunity to immerse myself again in my experience, and to bring out its new phases each time, I gradually gave birth to the first segments of what was to appear as a preliminary work of 'self-elicitation'.

A few theoretical references also gave a more systematic frame to the still fragile first person methodology: D. Austry introduced us to Y.-M. Visetti's and to V. Rosenthal's work, and I presented W. James' epistemological perspective, as possibly enlightening our collective research.

2. The Difficulty of First-Personal Experiential Going Into Action: Meeting Obstacles, Living Emotional Shocks and Creating a First Critical Distance

Having established the context of the present research and indicated the epistemology I prefer (and which I will identify by the term 'practical phenomenology'), I would like to express the crucial difficulty of such a change of attitude with regard to my own personal experience, which is considered by many philosophers and scientists as belonging to the field of privacy.[8] The mere fact of stressing the difficulty of such a change of posture relative to myself already amounts to entering into the intimacy of my own experience, i.e., to *vividly contact* what's happening in myself when I accept the discipline of no longer using words

---

[6] Such a terminological clarification was drawn from a discussion I had with E. Berger, B. Pachoud et P. Vermersch during a work-session (February 8, 2009).

[7] P. Vermersch and E. Berger, respectively *Expliciter* no. 61 and no. 68.

[8] Expressions like 'private world' or 'private thought' are often used by the 'attackers' of the relevance of a first person experience: to begin with, in a radical way, by Wittgenstein and some of his eminent interpreters (see Bouveresse, 1976).

and concepts as an inner protection that acts as a psychic screen between myself and my experience. In that respect, I suggest making a distinction between 'privacy', which refers to the particular content of my personal anecdotal experience and therefore does not need to be communicated and 'intimacy', which involves an ability to connect myself to an inner part of my self. With this distinction I do not mean to produce another artificial construction that would support the *a priori* inaccessibility of the private lived experience, but rather to show factual limitations: obviously the latter may be moved, but still, they remain as operative limits. It might be useful and even necessary to put my private experience to work in order to account for the intimate mode of being, that is, for such a lived connectedness with myself, but, again, I will not focus on the particular private content (which would be inappropriate or self-intrusive), but rather on my lived and living ability to connect myself to it: in other terms, by 'first person experience' I understand 'intimacy' and not mere 'privacy'.[9]

Now, given the initial presentation of the research context, if the reader looks at the *verbatim* postponed until the end, it might appear that, except for the inner work linked to the initial 'choice' of the example, which I accounted for at the beginning of the *verbatim* and which attests to a genuine structural difficulty of 'letting emerge' a relevant example, the whole of the elicitation movement seems to spontaneously unfold from meeting to meeting. In that respect, the apparent smoothness of the directly growing description I am presenting at the end may appear misleading, i.e., as if the experience was sheer and transparent, as if the very bareness of my experience as it is offered to the reader unconsciously erases my own resistances and incapacities. Such a risk is paradoxically generated by an unfolding which faithfully takes again the immanent self-elicitating movement, with the first motivation not to build any speculative construction. Now, again, such a faithfulness, which includes respect for emergent

---

[9] The words 'intimate' (*intime*) and 'intimacy' are not new : Husserl's French translator of the phenomenology of inner time-consciousnes early (1966) chose the adjective '*intime*' for the German '*innig*' ; still earlier it is to be found in Augustine's *Confessions* in the famous expression : '*interior intimo meo*'; it is used by Paul Ricœur in *Soi-même comme un autre* in the framework of what he calls a '*altérité intime*'; besides it emerged for me in the context of a discussion group around the 'living connection', which seeks to understand what is precisely such an ability to be livingly connected with ouselves, to be present to ourselves. In this regard, I want to thank the participants, who have been meeting for a year and a half now in Souvole, at the Ligugé Monastery and, more recently, at the Convent in Martigné : Christine Delliaux, Jacques Lefèvre, Père Jean-Pierre Longeat, the Père Abbé from Ligugé, and Frédéric Mauriac. The operative distinction between privacy and intimacy however emerged recently in the course of a recent discussion with E. Berger in the context of a research meeting of the above mentioned work (February 8, 2009).

contents, was at the same time unfaithful to the inner events that revealed constitutive difficulties or emotional shocks and thus attested to a rupture of the apparent continuity of the current emergence. I would like to do justice to such ruptures while paying attention to the moments where self-elicitation was impossible or difficult on the one hand, to my emotional reactions on the other hand. In this way I hope to account for a genuine first person experiential practice.

The first difficulty I encountered was my sheer repeated inability to put myself to work outside the meetings. I became gradually aware that I programmed each time that I would have gone forward in the process of the self-elicitation of my example for the following meeting and found myself reading again my notes just before the meeting without any real progression in-between; my observation (that is, my 'explanation') was that I needed the frame of the meetings to guide my self-attention and to provide myself with practical tools of evocation; I was also claiming (in the less relevant way) that I could not find time enough to immerse myself in the past moment in order to re-evoke it: was this a rationalized pretext or a genuine lack of time? Whatever the true reason, I was not able to put myself to work and progress by myself. The *verbatim* results from a series of self-elicitation moments which only took place during group meetings.

The second difficulty I could see — with P. Vermersch's and E. Berger's help — lies in the meaning of the comparison which early emerged within the *verbatim*: indeed a second example (Jouvernex's dream) comes out as a contrast with the first one (Dechen Chöling's meditation): I first used the former as an opening that enabled me to better identify the singularity of the latter and chose to let them unfold as mirroring parallels. My hypothesis in the following, while dissociating them, is that the second example, instead of enriching my access to my first person experience, prevents me from moving forward in the self-elicitation of my first example. Of course, comparing amounts to opening, but it also contributes to confusion and explosion of meaning. Maybe the enriching hypothesis is an illusion and rather amounts to a '*fuite en avant*', the second example allowing me not to confront the bareness of the first one.

Such inner resistances went hand in hand with small emotional shocks linked to the unveiling of words or expressions that came back to me as I went into the evocation of the process: first, the expression 'same village' came to my mind and immersed myself back into the happiness of such a meditative moment; still stronger, the word '*sheshin*', as it came to my mind, resulted in jubilation: I then became aware of the intensity of such a moment. The expression 'subtle elation' astonished me as it suddenly occurred in myself: I then lived again the mixed feeling of uneasiness and attraction I had when it was referred to by the Sakyong. The lived associations themselves, the second example first of all, the images of the cocoon and of giving birth then let me feel how fragments of myself still scattered in myself were gathered and given as a dynamic unity.

3. The 'Shaping' of my Example Thanks to a Double Extraction from the Strait Jacket of the *Verbatim*: The Genuine Time of the Experience (May 2000)

The goal of this third step consists in presenting the *verbatim* again while (a) dissociating the first example from its comparative emergent context and (b) reconstructing the genuine experiential time so as to make it stand out as an ordered singular time. Such a method of presentation amounts to 'dismantling the continuity' of the self-elicitation process, which may at first sight seem more real, insofar as each detail of the experience is kept, in order to stress the singularity of the situated example, that is, to show its most outstanding meaningful features. My contention is consequently is that I will better see the shadowy parts of my experience, the still obscure phases of my consciousness; besides, the result of the temporal reorganisation is different: I am able to distingush the chronology of my evocation and elicitation processes and the effective temporality of my experience, thus offering the reader from the start a 'real time' experience.

1. **Dechen Chöling, May 2000. First meditation retreat with the Sakyong: intense meditation time (10 hours a day).**

2. **A talk each afternoon. The Sakyong is teaching, he lets us see the nine stages in shamatha. He lets us feel and see the inner path within the space of mind, I am going into it with him, living it with him.**

3. **His way of talking comes back again to me, a modality of speech which is at once smooth, light, and slow. Yes, he speaks slowly but without ever repeating himself. He leaves some time between his utterances, but not much, for you never feel any gap, you never feel you are waiting for the following utterance. You always feel related to him and at the same time, what he says inhabits you: he takes his time in order for you to have what he says resonate in yourself.**

THE 'FAILING' OF MEANING 99

4. I am following his track while he brings me from the first stage to the second one, then to the third one, each time, I am saying to myself: yes, that's it, I know that, that's what I am living.

5. I am attuned with him, he talks about something that I know because I lived it, I went through it again and again, in the same way as a friend of mine tells me about an experience she had and you can really see what she talks about because you already had such an experience. My attunement to him is such that I could nearly talk instead of him: words are coming to my mouth at the very moment when he pronounces them, almost before him. I have a feeling of a dense presence, of inner warmth, like when you are with dear and close friends.

6. Such a contact with myself pops up as a feeling of being related, of living something like a deep unity between myself and what I am living; such a unity appears through an inner warmth and density.

7. In the moment just before there is a very strong tension, a deep awaiting, an inner relaxation linked to the very long previous time of meditation; there is the Sakyong's smile, his slowness; an expression comes back to my mind: the 'same village' with Trungpa, a quality of presence which I feel as paroxystic.

8. The words of the Sakyong while I am related to his talking: the 'same village'. He talks about his relationship with Trungpa; I am looking at him, I am making notes, I am intensively focusing towards his speaking presence, an invisible thread is linking me to him. He only speaks for me; he speaks of it: stage 1: he places my body; stage 2: he places my breath, he helps me link myself to my breath. I am going through the stages exactly while he 'speaks them'. I am doing what he says to do and I do it at the very moment when he says it: it provides me with an inner experiential texture of 'dense presence'. I don't do it afterwards, I even do it a little bit just before, I know what he is talking about. He recreates within myself something I know quite well, he furnishes it with a specific thickness; stage 3: he places my thoughts upon my breath; he places the dis-synchronicity, the unsteadiness, the to and fro moves, the fluctuations: presence, non-presence.

9. I prepared myself to experience what he now speaks about: observing the arising thoughts, seeing them fade away, not being aware when I am not there any longer, becoming aware of it too late, observing thoughts again, feeling that I am elsewhere, feeling frustrated because I failed again to grasp the arising thought, because I was not able to welcome it without grasping it. I have been going through all these thoughts again and again for hours. His speech therefore comes to me as just ripe fruit that only waits for being plucked.

10. He talks about me. Great feeling of familiarity.

11. Then he talks of the 'observer' (*sheshin*), who is both inside/outside, and then, I have the feeling that I enter an unknown space, something new, which attracts but does not fit into my lived experiences.

12. Somehow, I know it quite well such an enigmatic *sheshin*. At the very moment when he mentions it, I try to identify it within my lived experience. I am endeavouring to approximate it — such a magical word and experience — within my well-known familiar experiences and words; he also calls it an 'observer'; I know very well it is not exactly the right word. Of course I can also name it thus, which means that it grasps a fragment of my lived experience. I try to catch it that way, which I feel that it is definitely not the right word. The word '*sheshin*' is beating in my head in a compulsive manner, in an almost panicking way, like an empty space that the word does not fill out, and it even seems as if the wording still increases the gap, still makes it more open (wide-open, gaping: '*béant*'). A kind of opening of something abyssal, which is related to a radical lack of experiencing. My own experience of *sheshin* appears to me blurred, fragmented, scattered, confusion-ladden, I sometimes half-see it as the very temporal quality of my being always too late to what arises in myself as thoughts-events: again, I am structurally late to what I am present, the move of my becoming conscious is always too late. I just become aware (too late) that I have been there when the thought arose. Of course, if *sheshin* embodies such a structural dynamics of belatedness, I can only crash down when hearing it being named by the Sakyong, since I am precisely lacking such an experience. Like the very presence of absence — the mode of being of what is not there — death.

13. Then, when he moves on to the stage 4, then, a hole, void, — I feel a hole in my stomach.

14. He talks of 'subtle elation': I get lost, I can't catch any meaning, I feel that I enter a more delicate space, something lighter that I don't know.

15. I don't see anything more, what happens, that, I don't know, I never lived that.

16. I am not linked to the lived words, I can only listen to 'words', I make notes without embodying his words.

17. I look around me to check if the others live through the same thing as I do, but I only see heads bent over their sheets making notes or looking towards Sakyong and listening to him.

18. I feel I am lost among strangers, I am not there any longer, I am lost in the memories of meditation and try to find again something that would be like what the Sakyong is talking about, but, in a sense I feel it also, it is too late.

19. Nevertheless, I read what the nine stages are, I thought I knew what they were, I really try to catch them again, I look all around in my lived experiences, but I don't find anything, or it is very obscure and full of confusion, where does he bring me, I thought I knew this place, I feel frustrated, even desperate, I thought I knew this path, but I actually did not go through it; such a inner space, such a path within my mind is literally failing.

20. Then I let it go, I am listening differently, I am listening to somebody who is giving a talk, who is talking to me, but in another manner. His way of speaking has changed for me, his words are not relying on my lived experiences, are not embodied any longer.

21. Very well, I observe, I am there in my exploration of meditation. I will need to explore deeper the space of my mind in order to see if I can find again his description of the following stages. After crashing down because of losing the experiential thread, because of my not following any more, I realize that I could at least identify where I am. I am certainly disappointed to be so far short, so little advanced. However, I feel a genuine satisfaction to know at which stage I am.

4. The '*Verbatim*' of the Example and Its Double Shaping

I will now show how the *verbatim* may be doubly shaped and framed in order to let appear the genuine temporality of the example and its singularity. As I said, the *verbatim* is the initial material of the elicitation of my experience. I used it as a basis in order to extract my example from its mixed comparative emergence together with a second example and to frame it thanks to eight sequences in which I presented the genuine experiential phases of the experience (in **bold sans serif font**): I distinguished them from the aftermath commentaries on the one hand; I reorganised them according to the real experiential time on the other hand. Now, such a temporal reorganisation, which explicitely unfolds above (step 3), re-appears here thanks to the numbers (1) to (21), which are also mentioned in **bold sans serif font**. The font-difference along with the redistribution of the numbers reveals the existence of two non-coïnciding temporalities, the one of the experience and the one of the evocation/elicitation. I am only indicating here the distortions of the temporal phases thanks to the numbers, the order of the time of evocation/elicitation being altered by the other order of the time of the genuine experience: I will take such an 'inordinance of time' into account at a later stage of my research, and will be able to examine the meaning of such changes of temporal phases for the understanding of the present experience.

A. Going into the experience[10]

1. The time of gestation

During spring through summer 2006, all kinds of experiences pass through my mind, which may refer to what Pierre Vermersch has in mind with the expression 'emerging meaning' ('*sens se faisant*'); as a matter of fact, I notice in myself that most thought processes are driven by a meaning that is not known yet as such, that is not named or identified, that is in the course of becoming conscious, a 'working' meaning that I did not yet identify.

Such an experience appears to me so obvious because so familiar that examples of it overwhelm me and, then, none of them end up more relevant than any other. None of them stands out, each of them could be relevant, none of them catches my attention in an exclusive way.

After some time of confusion and perplexity, I just feel I had better go along with such a confusion, which fundamentally refers (but I

---

[10] Beginning of the taping of my notations: Tuesday, July 1, 2008.

only realize it now while writing) to an inner state where the meaning is still unborn; in this way, the discriminative work may operate on its own and give rise to a meaning of such an 'emergent meaning'.[11]

2. The putting to work just before

During a meeting at the Grex,[12] Eve Berger presents the moment of the emergence of meaning as a process of creation, endowed with a potentiality of opening.[13] I realize that the word 'frightening' (*l'effroi*), that Pierre used in order to name the initial feeling of void in the process of emergence of the meaning produced a hindering effect in me, in virtue of the negative meaning of the word, which made it impossible in part for me to find an exemplary (meaning, pregnant) situation for me. The way Eve named such a process of emergence of meaning as an 'inner move' by which 'we enter a space of the mind where we usually don't go', from which 'we do not know what is going to come' and 'if it will come',[14] here is what moves me (moved me then) and builds in me the conditions of motivation of the emergence of an experience for which the meaning was under way in a part of consciousness which is still governed by unsaying. Eve's first-person experiential narration was what brought me into my own experience, in a kind of isomorphic way, from experience to experience, in a verbal though pre-conscious and mimetic way. Thanks to her way of naming her lived experience, she helps me feel a part of myself that refers to a taste, to an intensity of meaning that has something of the vital, crucial, and archaic.

3. The instant of emergence

'That's it! I got it! *Eurêkâ!* Eve opened a door…'

4. The immediate context of the situation[15]

Extract 1 (October 2, 2006)

(1) Dechen Chöling, May 2000. First meditation retreat with the Sakyong: intense meditation time (10 hours a day). (2) A talk

---

[11] Friday, July 4, 2008.
[12] Beginning of my making notes: Monday, October 2, 2006.
[13] July 4, 2008.
[14] July 4, 2008: lived again comment.
[15] Notes from October 2, 2006: 11.50–12.00.

each afternoon. The Sakyong is teaching, he lets us see the nine stages in shamatha. He lets us feel and see the inner path within the space of mind, I am going into it with him, living it with him — (4) I am following his track while he brings me from the first stage to the second, then to the third one, each time, I am saying to myself: yes, that's it, I know that, that's what I am living, (13) then, when he moves on to the stage 4, then, a hole, void, — I feel a hole in my stomach, (15) I don't see anything more, what happens, that, I don't know, I never lived that, (19) nevertheless, I read what the nine stages are, I thought I knew what they were, I really try to catch them again, I look all around in my lived experiences but I don't find anything, or it is very obscure and full of confusion, where does he bring me, I thought I knew this place, I feel frustrated, even desperate, I thought I knew this path, but I actually did not go through it; such a inner space, such a path within my mind is literally failing. (20) Then I let it go, I am listening differently, I am listening to somebody who is giving a talk, who is talking to me, but in another manner. His way of speaking has changed for me, his words are not relying on my lived experiences, are not embodied any longer. (21) Very well, I observe, I am there in my exploration of meditation. I will need to explore deeper the space of my mind in order to see if I can find again his description of the following stages. After crashing down because of losing the experiential thread, because of my not following any more, I realize that I could at least identify where I am. I am certainly disappointed to be so little far, so little advanced. However I feel a genuine satisfaction to know at which stage I am.

Immediate comment [October 2, 2006: 12.30.]

Writing on the go, I am not being careful about how I write, I leave behind all my ideas about how to write! About what I have to write! I am not cautious at all, I only forget completely my ideas about how I write! About what I am writing! The experience alone leads me. I know that, but in some contexts of poetic writing, or of pregnant phenomenological themes. I have the deep feeling that the content only is able to serve as a leading thread.

B. Entering into the experience as a concret space

1. Notes from October 2: 17.20–17.35[16]

While reading again the extract from *On Becoming Aware* which deals with the phase 3 of the *épochè*, i.e., letting-go, I suddenly realize the very quality of the experience of a direction and of an orientation without any fulfillment or satisfaction: it refers to a kind of awaiting that is emotionally coloured, to a sort of quiet impatience. I hear within myself a great deal of moments emerging back, which possess the same 'colour': in the first place, in my village (Jouvernex) as I was having breakfast in the gallery, I had the sensation of a very important dream for which I still have no words but which I know is about to come back, the deep joy together with a light disappointment in the background: it was it! In the second place, very close to it, behind it, I had a great number of dreams coming back again, which had popped up some time ago during quite an intense period of my life which a more stable relationship with my oniric life got structured and where I had the feeling of contacting an unknown though familiar part of myself: a feeling of opening, as if a fragment of myself was sticking out from myself, then I had the content of this ever-coming dream which had been living with me for months without me being conscious of it: I am taking off. I am running, running, running and, at a certain moment, I feel it, I open my arms while I am leaving the soil, I go up, I am flying over at a certain altitude, I have the feeling of keeping, keeping flying, I know how to keep flying at the same altitude, I held my breath and go up a little more, and its lasts very long; the moment just after that, I catch the awaiting relaxed feeling linked to the awaiting in pregnancy (mixture of weight and of being carried) in the dreamy half-dream of the afternoon-nap; but just behind, I get a quality of quiet impatience I feel when welcoming the sure/unsure coming of pleasure during sexual intercourse, its to and fro moves, its uncertain rhythms of intensity.

2. Notes from October 14: 17.50

While reading again the previous moment (October 2), I observe that there is a related network of moments, of qualities which slowly begin sticking out from myself, like particles of a pill which get suspended in water and become visible, tangible, whereas they were until then building a unity and did not appear as separate particles. I also get the

---

[16] I am carrying on making notes.

feeling that both native fragments do not have the same 'colour': are they different, various, divergent!

C. A first return to my initial notations

> **Extract 2 (October 23, 2006)**
>
> I read again my first description of Dechen Chöling. I say to myself: what do I mean when saying 'the Sakyong *let us see*' (repeated twice)? **(3) His way of talking comes back again to me, a modality of speech which is at once smooth, light, and slow. Yes, he speaks slowly without ever repeating himself however. He leaves some time between his utterances, but still not much, for you never feel any gap, you never feel you are waiting for the following utterance. You always feel related to him and, at the same time, what he says inhabits you: he takes his time in order for you to have what he says resonate in you.** I read: 'I am following his track'. What do I mean? **(5) I am attuned with him, he talks about something that I know because I lived it, I went through it again and again, in the same way as a friend of mine tells me about an experience she had and you can really see what she talks about because you had already such an experience. My attunement to him is such that I could nearly talk instead of him: words are coming to my mouth at the very moment he pronounces them, almost before him. I have a feeling of a dense presence, of inner warmth, like when you are with dear and close friends.** Then I read: 'I feel a hole in my stomach.' What do I mean? I believe I remember, **(17) I look around me to check if the others live the same thing as I do, I only see heads bent over their sheets making notes or looking towards the Sakyong and listening to him. (18) I feel I am lost among strangers, I am not there any longer, I am lost in the meditation memories and try to find something that would be like what the Sakyong is talking about, but, in a sense I feel it also, it is too late.** I get now two more associations with two other experiences: 1. a feeling of my stomach dropping on a circus wheel in London, 2. a feeling of void (but also of rage) as I was late and could not catch my train at the East Station in Paris.

D. The aftermath of the experience: a beginning discrimination work

> **Extract 3 (November 20, 2006)**
>
> *Strategy* — I read my notes again — I find again the different aspects (bodily, emotional, rhythmic) of the context which preceded this event.
>
> **(6) Such a contact with myself pops up as a feeling of being related, of living something like a deep unity between myself and what I am living; such a unity appears through an inner warmth and density. (7) In the moment just before there is a very strong tension, a deep awaiting, an inner relaxation linked to the very long previous time of meditation; there is the Sakyong's smile, his slowness; an expression comes back to my mind: the 'same village' with Trungpa, a quality of presence which I feel as paroxystic. (9) I prepared myself to experience what he is now talking about: observing the arising thoughts, seeing them fade away, not being aware when I am not there anylonger, becoming aware of it too late, observing thoughts again, feeling that I am elsewhere, feeling frustrated because I failed again to grasp the arising thought, because I was not able to welcome it without grasping it. I have been going through all these thoughts again and again for hours. His speech therefore comes to me as just ripe fruit that only waits for being plucked. (10) He talks about me. Great feeling of familiarity. (14) He talks of 'subtle elation': I get lost, I can't catch any meaning, I feel that I enter a more delicate space, something lighter that I don't know.**
>
> T1: to be related
> What happened between these two moments? I don't know.
> T2: to lose the thread

Notes from November 20, 2006

'Surprise': here is the word that gathers both experiences (Jouvernex's dream and Dechen Chöling's meditation). Such a word suddenly comes to my mind when writing part of an article on the experience of 'self-previousness' (*auto-antécédance*), which provides the lived body with an extraordinary lucidity.

> **Extract 4 (January 29, 2007)**
> **(10.30–11.45 at P. Vermersch's home)**
>
> *Strategy*: I am reading my notes again; my goal is finding the intermediary moments between T1 and T1/T2.
>
> T1: **(8) The words of the Sakyong while I am related to his talking: 'same village'. He talks about his relationship with Trungpa; I am looking at him, I am making notes, I am intensively focussing towards his speaking presence, an invisible thread is linking me to him. He only speaks for me; he speaks of me: stage 1: he places my body; stage 2: he places my breath, he helps me link myself to my breath. I am going through the stages precisely while he 'talks them'. I am doing what he says to do and do at the very moment when he says it: it provides me with an inner experiential texture of 'dense presence'. I don't do it afterwards, I even do it a little bit just before, I know what he is talking about. He recreates within myself something I know quite well, he furnishes it with a specific thickness; stage 3: he places my thoughts upon my breath; he places the dis-synchronicity, the unsteadiness, the to and fro moves, the fluctuations: presence, non-presence.**
>
> T1 and T2: **(11) Then he talks of the 'observer' (*sheshin*), who is both inside/outside, and then, I have the feeling that I enter an unknown space, something new, which attracts but does not fit into my lived experiences.** My desperate breakdown will be due to the fact that I feel I am unable to be part of what he is *saying* while living it as my *lived experience*, for I do not possess it in myself as an available lived experience. I can only listen to it and try to understand without having a corresponding lived experience at my disposal.
>
> T2: **(16) I am not linked to the lived words, I can only listen to 'words', I make notes without embodying his words.**
>
> From T1 to T2: there is a link with the lived experience, but it is not a full and continuous presence: 1) intuition of a lived experience; 2) attraction towards such a lived experience.

1. The common point between both situations: there is the creation of a contact with a place in myself which I did not enter yet, although it refers to two different modes of givenness of the contact.

The dream of Jouvernex: the contact is being created through the sticking out process of fragments of hidden lived experiences, which come out and give way to a similar sensation of density and of inner warmth when becoming conscious.

2. The immediate context just before:

The dream:

T1 refers to the sensing of an important dream, the content of which is not available yet, but appears as just about to be given.

T2 is the popping up of the image of the dream.

What happened between T1 and T2? I get it, I lose it, I go away, I come nearer.[17] It lasts a long time: I am feeling I am in an heterogeneous space, which is pluridimensional, very thick, very dense, very heavy.

The dream of Jouvernex enlightens the meditative situation of Dechen Chöling: the quality of the link, of the connexion, creates a space which is quite heterogeneous in itself; it is made of to and fro moves, of alternating presence and absence moments, from a tension which is full of fluctuations.

Dechen Chöling and Jouvernex offer two versions of a unique dynamic structure, the name of which would be 'surprise'. In Dechen Chöling, 'being there' (T1) is the time of a being related, whereas T2 embodies a loss, an experience of not catching any more; in Jouvernex, T1 refers to a 'patient awaiting', while T2 corresponds to a 'sudden arising'. Their structural common point lies in temporal double move : the continuity and duration of T1, as opposed to the falling ove rand isolated instant embodied by T2. The difference, however, consists in the *modality* of the passage from T1 to T2: in Dechen Chöling, we have to do with a all of a sudden unique 'jumping', while the passage consists in Jouvernex in to and fro moves enacting phases of losses and reunions; besides, the Dechen Chöling unique and sudden passage from T1 to T2 is a going from fullness to emptiness, whereas the Jouvernex circularity between T1 and T2 ends up in a move from emptiness to fullness.

Jouvernex

T1: I am sitting at the table in the gallery, on the chair in front of the kitchen door. The children are having breakfast. While acting (putting

---

[17] Like in the game in which you look for an object and the other person says : you 'are getting warmer', you 'are getting colder' (comment: July 7, 2008).

a teabag in my cup, preparing for myself a piece of bread with strawberry marmalade), I say to myself: I had an important dream. But I can't remember its content. I know that it was meaningful, however. I am having an *inner* research-time, while having breakfast. It lasts a long time. I know that my dream is close, just there, but I don't know what to do in order to have it come back. *I keep paying attention to this feeling that it is there*, not very far away, I have the feeling of possessing something very important — a treasure — which is there and not there, which remains at a distance from myself.

T2: *at one point,* I catch a bit of it (its orange colour), but it goes away as soon as it appeared, I feel both attracted and frustrated, I feel torn and innerly tensed, then other bits appear, like pieces of a puzzle (I have a feeling of lightness, I am in the cabin of a plane), but I only have fragments which don't build a picture, and then, here is the dream, suddenly coming, I feel inhaled: I am flying just above the ground; and thus I am gathering all kinds of sensations: inner bodily struggle to keep flying, my arms open in order to keep the right position with the wind flow, the landscape streaming through below me, the goings up and down, the inner tension which alone enables me to maintain the direction and the altitude, or at least to choose it.

The dynamics from T1 to T2 lies in multifarious moves from T1 to T2 which correspond to multiple gains and losses. Such inner moves are the following: (1) I feel attracted and frustrated at the same time; (2) I am confident about the coming back of the process; (3) I also feel a general tension.

Extract 5 (March 12, 2007)
(11.15–12.00 at P. Vermersch's home)

Dechen Chöling

Strategy: looking for what happened between the intermediary time between T1 and T2, that is, $T^{1/2}$ *and* T2. I name the intermediary of the intermediary time: $T^{3/4}$.

Beginning from the phrase 'something new, which attracts but does not fit into my 'lived experiences', something comes back, which emerges again from that moment: **(12) Somehow, I know it quite well such a enigmatic *sheshin*. At the very moment when he mentions it, I try to identify it within my lived experience. I am endeavouring to approximate it — such a magical word and** experience — within my well-known familiar experiences and words; he also calls it an 'observer', I know very well it is not exactly the right word. Of course I can also name it thus, which means that it grasps a fragment of my lived experience. I try to catch it that way, but I feel that it is definitely not the right word. The word '*sheshin*' is beating in my head in a compulsive manner, in an almost panicking way, like an empty space that the word does not fill out, and it even seems as if the wording still increases the gap, still makes it more open (wide-open, gaping: '*béant*'). A kind of opening of someting abyssal related to a radical lack of experiencing. My own experience of *sheshin* appears to me blurred, fragmented, it is mixed up, fragmented, scattered, confusion-ladden, I sometimes half-see it as the very temporal quality of my belatedness to what arises in myself as thought-events: again, I am structurally late in relation to what I am present, the move of my becoming conscious is always too late. I just become aware (too late) that I have been there when the thought arose. Of course, if *sheshin* embodies such a structural dynamics of belatedness, I can only crash down when hearing it being named by the Sakyong, since I am precisely lacking such an experience. Like the very presence of absence — the mode of being of what is not there — death.

My question is: what happens between this intermediary time ($T^{1/2}$) embodied by sheshin and T2 (the time of the loss)? I am looking for the intermediary time between the first intermediary time (*sheshin*: $T^{1/2}$) and T2 (not being able to catch any longer), what I call $T^{3/4}$, that is: a being present at my being late, or again, a mode of presence of my being absent.

Jouvernex

Strategy: endeavouring to describe more closely these different movements which occur between T1 and T2.

While reading my notes again, I begin immersing in my lived experience at the very moment when I read the following utterance: 'I keep paying attention to this feeling that it is there.'

What I find again immediately is the nearly bodily inner state which I just got closer before the emergence of the dream. I can describe such a state in the following way: my look fades away, goes very far away, becomes blurred and confused: I am looking without seeing;

besides, I feel in my head a kind of density, which provokes an effect of relaxing and interrupts any will of focalisation. I just stop moving internally, I just rest and I begin to feel vibrations — a kind of state of lethargy.

Comparison between the two fragments of lived experience which came back to me:

Immediate comment

> *Dechen Chöling*
> The search for the intermediate state and then for the intermediate state of the intermediate state reveals and provides the quality of the lived experience which occured just before my state of desperate breakdown with more detailed micro-phases.

Jouvernex
A similar research opens up the possibility for getting the general continuous state which let bits of the dream emerge. Such a state appears as a global bodily disposition of openness.

Conclusion: contrasted modes of temporal cuttings are thus revealed: is it linked to such an experience, to its particular quality each time?

E. Another strategy of spontaneous evocation: 'à vide' (unprepared)

> **Extract 6 (May 14, 2007)**
>
> *Strategy*
> — Spontaneous evocation '*à vide*' (unprepared), this time without any previous re-reading of my notes; nevertheless, this evocation is not completely spontaneous, unprepared ('*à vide*'): it is interwoven in the background with my re-reading of W. James' chapter of *The Principles of Psychology*, entitled 'The Stream of Consciousness'.
> — Putting aside the model of the temporal dynamics, which is the basic method I spontaneously made use of till now, for it naturally emerged. Why? I feel the risk of introducing a methodological artefact.[18] I feel the risk of exhausting the richness of the experience due to its excessive formalisation.

---

[18] Notes from July 18, 2008

— Goal: immersion in the global immediacy of the concrete experience.

Dechen Chöling

(1) Feeling of density, of being envelopped, of warmth

(2) Impression of being dragged out, of getting out of this warm bath

I am experiencing pregnancy, I then say to myself: (1) envelopment, it is the gradual development of meditation, the 'being one with the Sakyong's words'; then, (2) it is the going out of the envelopment, the delivery, the birth, and the feeling of dragging out, even though I still remain stuck: the umbilical cord? From (1) to (2), there is not a rupture, but a continual transition: the gateway toward the exit (i.e. the delivery), and the discovery, not of something void in contrast with something full, but of something else. I am leaving a shell, I am venturing outward, I become aware of the fact that my desperate breakdown is in fact a way out; maybe the previous moment, when I felt attuned, related, connected, being at one with the Sakyong was in fact an illusion. Maybe my feeling of breakdown is a genuine experience of getting free. The intimate link with the Sakyong's words maybe results enslaving, the shell results a prison, constraining frame. I discover something that does not stick here with what I evoked until now from my lived experience. Is the dragging out of the 'warm bath' of the Sakyong a breakdown or rather a liberation?

Extract 7 (June 19, 2007)

Strategy: the spontaneous evocation '*à vide*' (unprepared), without any former reading. Just a try. A somewhat painful effort to remain connected, to keep attuned. It is not so immediate nor spontaneous as that. I feel a great tension, I apply concentration, I feel the artificial aspect of the presence of the Sakyong, which is linked to the compelling framework.

I find it extremly difficult to keep attuned to the arising thought, like it is difficult to keep attuned to, in phase with the Sakyong's words. Both difficulties go hand in hand: I feel the intensification of the quality of presence, but I also feel overburdened by the very possibility of being there.

Comment: the meaning of this moment comes back to me in a fragmented way, but such fragments are linked together. For example, today's 'fragment' is 'linked' to the fragment that was evoked during the previous session — which I do not remember in the first place, before I contact the moment itself in Dechen Chöling, which I somehow use as a transition in the evocation, as a transitory phase where I am involved again in the experience, but in a mediate way — it was linked to the other in fact, because the image of the 'shell' and the feeling of being trapped related to it lets appear again the quality of effort and of difficulty, whereas this moment had a positive color till now. Valences here are inverted. The following moment, where I feel I get lost, am not attuned, am not there, appears to me now as a moment of 'relaxation', where I feel a 'void' linked to my being no longer concentrated, which is given to me as a liberating phase. What I named then a 'liberation' comes to me now as the experience of a paradoxical lightness: the lightness of the no longer obsessive compulsion of being present. Retrospectively, I feel how hypnotising the previous moment was: inertia, somnolence, lameness. From the first moment to the second, I feel an awakening and an openess, and not a loss or a discordance.

Extract 8 (June 24, 2007)

Strategy: I read the whole again, in order to put myself to work while I am evoking the situation.

I come back to a wordless awaiting time, where the lived experience is fully given. In a sense, the detailed and refined notations is a burden for me, it disturbs me and prevents me from unearthing again the freshness of the experience. I feel that the language is always inadequate with regard to the lived experience, either because it does not say enough (the saying is too poor), or because it says too much (the description is too fully complete, it leaves no space to think). I look for the right balance, but it is difficult.

To be sure, words arise, which are meaningful: 'surprise', also '*sheshin*', but they are still too dense, they need to be unfolded.

Overview about the temporal process at work in both examples:

+ in the example of the dream at Jouvernex, the becoming of meaning in me refers to a process of generation of yet-not-given to my consciousness, which is fulfilled when the meaning is finally given,

THE 'FAILING' OF MEANING   115

whatever the mode of givenness may be, partial at the beginning (as we saw), gradual in any case, sometimes even regressive, not necessarily full even at the end.

+ in the example of the Sakyong in Dechen Chöling, the meaning of what happens to me appears to me as an event which creates a rupture with the continuous presence to what occurs and requires me patiently to reconstruct the temporal phases of the previous appearing, until I discover how the two main phases may be inverted as far as their valence-ladenness is concerned : the continuity results a closure, the rupture a release.

The temporal contrast between the two examples is striking: the first one suggests an *emergence* of meaning which follows the time of the evocation of the remembrance, although such an emergence refers to something that is pre-conscious and appears as such to my consciousness, according to and fro moves that express the non-linear way of meaning for me; the second one offers a description of the break of meaning, which gives birth to an experience of 'failing' and then creates another meaning, which is unexpected and, as such, surprising.

5. Provisional Conclusion: Some Notations as a Starting Point for a Future Analysis

What strikes me after having proceeded to such a working out in real time of the example is the importance of verbal segments that do not refer to an immediate and singular lived experience: indeed I chose the **bold sans serif font** for emphasis. Multifarious utterances occurred while eliciting this experience that refer to something quite different from a direct written 'account' of my experience: they are inner 'comments' that amount to a private conversation I had with myself while I was eliciting my own experience. I had to give way to rationalized productions in the aftermath, which helped me explain to myself what I had then lived through (or, again, what I had precisely not lived through!) or justifying for myself such and such an astonishing or distorted lived experience.

These comments in the aftermath took on various forms: sometimes they are directly linked with my experience, although they may occur six or seven years later, but they may also be reflective comments I am producing while eliciting, which may have no clear link with what I then lived. Besides, these comments are to be distinguished from inner comments I produced at the very moment when I had the experience, which as such belong to the latter, are lived experiences as such although in discursive form: this only attests to the fact that my experiential inner life is permeated by inner discussions, which are as such in **bold sans serif font**. Such an observation accounts for the intricate existence of extremly powerful layers of inner discursivity at the core of the first person lived experience, be they immanently inherent in it, or be they arising in the aftermath, or again, be they operating as reflective overviews separated from the experience.

In other words, after having disected both examples, after having extracted the various comments in the aftermath, after having identified my multifarious discussions, my first-person lived experience finally yields extremly poor results. In any case, it is definitely often built up together with an inner discussion, at least as long as I did not explore the process of creation of meaning at work in such a failing meaning.

What has still to be done — I realize it right now as I notice the preliminary aspect of what I presented above — is to embody again while re-living them the different phases of elicitation *via* the evocation of this experience of a failing meaning, in order to try to emphasize the steps of its semantic creation; in short, the next step is to put myself again in living contact with my elicitating and describing phases (October 2006–June 2007), as I did for the Dechen Chöling experience proper (2000), in order to make vividly emerge the different inner procedures of creation of meaning through mental wording and handwriting during these eight phases. While contacting my writing experience in 2006–7, the challenge is to let emerge the different ways (emotional, bodily, temporal, intersubjective) along which the meaning of the Dechen Chöling experience were given to me. The idea then is to be able to account for the detailed texture of the meaning in its processual generation to my consciousness. Then I might be able to take again the various moments of the 'naked' experience in its genuine time of emergence, that is, the ones that are in **bold sans serif font**, in order to begin analysing them and endeavouring to produce their reflective meaning.

References

Bouveresse, J. (1976), *Le Mythe de l'intériorité. Expérience, signification et langage privé chez Wittgenstein* (Paris: Editions de Minuit).

Depraz, N. (2006), *Comprendre la phénoménologie: une pratique concrète* (Paris: A. Colin).

Depraz, N. (2008), *Lire Husserl en phénoménologue* (Paris: PUF/CNED).

Depraz, N. (2009), *Husserl: une phénoménologie expérientielle* (Paris: Eds Atlande).

Depraz, N., Varela, F.J. & Vermersch, P. (2003), *On Becoming Aware: A Pragmatics of Experiencing* (Amsterdam: John Benjamins).

Tengelyi L. (2006), *L'expérience retrouvée. Essais philosophiques I* (Paris: L'Harmattan).

Zahavi, D. (2006), *Subjectivity and Selfhood* (Cambridge, MA: MIT Press).

Charles Genoud

On the Cultivation of Presence in Buddhist Meditation

Abstract: *This article is an exploration of the nature of consciousness. The author draws in depth from works of philosophy, psychology, literature, and meditation practice to examine a subject so subtle that we may overlook it.*

Consciousness, in the Buddhist tradition, cannot be held as merely another object of knowledge, a thing to be known, because it is not located in time or in space. Some modern philosophers seem to arrive at the same conclusion. Consciousness cannot be discovered through common scientific strategies. Only presence—being conscious of being conscious of something—allows one to realize what consciousness is. And this can only be discovered by an exploration in the first person. Buddhist meditation offers a skillful means of investigation.

> Huike said to Bodhidharma, 'My mind is anxious. Please pacify it.'
> Bodhidharma replied, 'Bring me your mind, and I will pacify it.'
> Huike said, 'Although I've sought it, I cannot find it.'
> 'There,' Bodhidharma replied, 'I have pacified your mind.'

Essentially, the Buddhist path is an investigation of consciousness. Knowing the nature of consciousness and how it functions, according to this tradition, can free one from illusion and bondage. On the Buddhist path two general forms of meditation are practiced. Samatha, through the development of concentration, aims to bring stability to the mind so that it may be used in a more skillful way. It is not directly concerned with the investigation of mind. In Vipassana, the path of clear seeing, meditative presence is cultivated so that one may discover the nature of mind.

Practices that develop concentration are not difficult to understand as they are similar to the ways the mind is used in daily life. Stability of mind after all is needed so that our activities may be accomplished. The required technique is a simple one: the meditator chooses an object of interest, and keeps it in mind. One may focus on the breath, or on some positive emotion, like compassion. One may recite a mantra, or concentrate on a colored disk. Again and again, whenever the mind wanders, one reels it back. Over time, after long practice, the meditator can remain fixed for hours to the object, without wavering.

There is fundamental difference between concentration and meditative presence, or simply, presence. (There is no difference between meditative presence and presence.) The mind holds, through concentration, to an object; it holds to contents, to something that it knows. In meditative presence, the mind is concerned by itself. It rests upon itself. This does not mean something vague. The difference between concentration and meditative presence is not a matter of exchanging one kind of object for another — that would be a serious misunderstanding. Rather, it implies a difference in attitude.

Concentration requires aim; it requires effort. Concentration requires that attention be directed toward a specific object. In meditative presence, however, the mind is its own end, and does not require any specific orientation, any effort toward the accomplishment of anything.

— Imagine a tennis player. Perfectly aware of how she holds her racket, aware of the other player and of their intricate play together, the movement of the tennis ball — perfectly aware of everything during the course of the game — she may completely forget herself. This is an example of concentration, not presence. During the game she had no clear consciousness of herself.

It is a characteristic of concentration to become absorbed in the chosen object. When meditators develop this capacity of mind to an uncommon degree, this characteristic may be more evident. One meditator, for example, practiced concentration for several months on a yellow disk. This implies fixing the mind from 16 to 18 hours a day upon a yellow disk, avoiding any fluctuation, any move to another object, such as sounds or pain in the body, thoughts. His mind became so focused on the yellow, he reported, that when he later saw the yellow of an egg he felt as though he was being inhaled, or swallowed; he felt bound to disappear. — At this point, there is no sense of presence. As concentration implies grasping to an object, there is therefore a lack of presence, which can be partial or near-total.

> To study Buddhism is to study oneself.
>
> — Dogen

As the aim of meditation is not ultimately to know the world around one *or any specific object* but rather to know oneself, another orientation is required. One needs to look within. Looking within does not mean looking within the body, but within the mind. *Within* means that the looker, the mind, is looking at itself. In such way, one shifts beyond the practice of concentration to meditative presence, to awareness. But this represents only a step, a way to withdraw the mind from its fascination with external objects. It is a means of opening to discovery. When the mind is not pushed by fascination in any direction, neither to external objects, nor to internal objects, like thoughts and emotions (treated as external objects), there will be no object, no aim. Notions like 'within' and 'without' will lose their meaning.

The mind is so used to being directed toward some object that it is hard to understand how to proceed in the exploration of mind. Even thoughts are treated as if they are external objects.

Jean Piaget, the Swiss naturalist and philosopher well-known for his work with children, and for his work in cognitive development and genetic epistemology, asked children which was heavier: the name *feather* or the name *stone*. The children said, *Stone*. Names were confused with the objects they were referring to. As adults, we are not entirely free from this type of confusion.

Freud noted:

> By their interposition internal thought-processes are made into perceptions. It is like a demonstration of the theorem that all knowledge has its origin in external perception. When hypercathexis of the process of thinking takes place, thoughts are actually perceived — as if they came from without — and are consequently held to be true (Freud, 1990, p.16).

Mostly, we relate to thoughts and to mental images as if they are concrete objects, or real people. Based on such mistaken assumptions, we react with desire or aversion, anger or sadness.

In some meditation manuals, meditators are invited to uncover the source of their thoughts: Do thoughts come from outside the meditator? Does a thought come from fire, earth, water or air? Can a thought be traced to a mountain, a river, or a tree? Only once it has been ascertained that thoughts are not to be confused with tangible objects, is the meditator invited to check within.

Before we look for consciousness, let us see how the Buddhist tradition defines it. Dharmakirti, the seventh-century Indian philosopher whose work became normative in Tibet, has much to say on this point. Georges Dreyfus, in his book *Recognizing Reality: Dharmakirti's Philosophy and its Tibetan Interpretations*, offers rich examination of Dharmakirti's work, and this will help nourish our discussion. In *The Transcendence of the Ego* and *Being and Nothingness*, Sartre also brings incisive commentary to this matter. In some respects, Sartre seems to express a vision similar to that of the Buddhist tradition, although in a more contemporary language.

In Tibet, debates were held for centuries about the way to define consciousness. There was much at stake. How meditation would be practiced was dependent on the outcome. Some scholars described consciousness as 'that which knows an object.' In other words, that there is always an object of consciousness. We may find something similar in modern philosophy. In phenomenology, as Husserl tells us, 'all consciousness is consciousness of something.' This points to intentionality. Consciousness, in this view, always aims at something which is not itself. It aims at something transcendent.

But this definition does not account for an awareness of consciousness itself. For those Tibetan scholars and practitioners who held to this definition, it was not possible to cognize the mind directly. Only through concept, according to this position, only through cognizing a previous moment of consciousness, can consciousness be known. The Dalai Lama, describing the gelupga view of meditation on the nature of mind, explains: 'In the meditation of Mahamudra, we may use either a moment of consciousness to focus on the remembered experience of a preceding moment of mind, or we may use one part of consciousness to focus on another.' (Dalai Lama, 1997, p. 133) But a previous moment can only be known as a concept. It is not a direct awareness of consciousness; it is only the trace of consciousness. Tibetan masters who believed it possible to know the mind directly, without concept, did not find this an acceptable definition. 'Sapan (Sakya Pandita, of the 13th century, one of the most respected philosophers of Tibet) rejects the definition of mind as that which cognizes an object since it does not include self-cognition.' (Dreyfus, 1996, p. 403)

Another definition of consciousness — *that which is clear and knowing* — is less restrictive. It is also more widely accepted by Tibetan scholars of the Buddhist tradition. Even if we were not concerned with the knowing of consciousness itself, it seems that to describe a consciousness that could cognize an object without knowing that it is cognizing this object would amount to a useless cognition. There would be no difference between cognizing and not cognizing an object. If we were to state that a second instant of consciousness that knows the first instant is needed for consciousness to function, then we would need a third instant to know the second, and so on. Sartre was well aware of this problem. 'Consciousness of self is not dual,' he said. 'If we wish to avoid an infinite regress, there must be an immediate, non-cognitive relation of the self to itself' (Sartre, 1960, p. 12).

> Consciousness is aware of itself in so far as it is consciousness of a transcendent object. All is therefore clear and lucid in consciousness: the object with its characteristic opacity is before consciousness, but consciousness is purely and simply consciousness of being consciousness of that object. That is the law of existence. (Sartre, 1960, p. 40)

From the Buddhist point of view as expressed by Dharmakirti:

> Consciousness does not apprehend external objects directly but only through the mediation of aspects. An aspect is the reflection or mark of the object in consciousness. To be aware of an object means to have a mental state that has the form of this object and is cognizant of this form. (Dreyfus, 1996, p. 336).

Dreyfus goes on to explain this aspect as:

> ... the aspect of the object in the consciousness as well as the aspected consciousness itself. Awareness takes on the form of an object and reveals that form by assuming it. In the process of revealing external things, cognition reveals itself. (Dreyfus, 1996, p. 336)

But the mere arising of this aspect in consciousness is not enough to provide cognitive context. The aspect needs conceptualization to endow it with a meaning.

> For Dharmakirti perception does not identify its object but merely holds in its perceptual ken. Hence perception does not provide any cognitive content by itself but merely induces conceptual activities through which content is constructed. (Dreyfus, 1996, p. 219)

Conceptual activities may be similar to what phenomenology calls intentionality.

A concept induced by perception can be stored by memory. Of course such concept is no longer dependent on the presence of physical elements, like light, and so on. This may be why there is confusion between what is thought of and what is perceived. The concepts are the same, but the conditions for their arising are different.

Intentionality, as noted earlier, signifies that consciousness always aims at something which is not itself, something transcendent. Such conceptual activity is needed for cognitive content, and this creates duality. Duality, between consciousness and its object. But consciousness can furthermore be placed at the level of an object through the construction of the concept *I*. Now we have the duality of an object and I.

We commonly speak of *my* thoughts, *my* sadness, *my* pleasure, *my* vision. We take the I to be consciousness. Sartre also pointed to this misconception.

> Everything happens, therefore, as if consciousness constitutes the ego as a false representation of itself, as if consciousness hypnotized itself before this ego which it has constituted, absorbing itself in the ego as if to make the ego its guardian and its law (Sartre, 1960, p. 101).

> The ego is not the owner of consciousness; it is the object of consciousness (Sartre, 1960, p. 97).

*

Buddhist meditation is an exploration of the nature and function of consciousness. As consciousness is not an object, the exploration of consciousness needs an uncommon approach.

In opening to such exploration, one main difficulty is the tendency to fall back on the attitude commonly associated with the exploration of objects.

Consciousness cannot be the aim, the object of a quest. As soon as there is an objective in mind, one is dealing with an object. Therefore, any wish, any desire or hope to discover what consciousness is—veils it. Meister Eckhart, the 14th century Christian philosopher and mystic, expressed this in a paradoxical way: 'We should pray to God,' he said, 'to free us from God.'

It is not through the cultivation of a specific objective that the mind can be known. But the mind *is realized* when one drops all aim and objective. It is a *via negativa* well-known to mystics. But this is not to suggest any negative objective, that is, the wish to get rid of any contents of the mind regarded as an obstacle. There is nothing to get; there is nothing to get rid of; there is no hope; no fear. Tibetan meditation texts repeat this endlessly.

Sartre was aware of the need to have no intention, no motivation:

> A reflective apprehension of spontaneous consciousness as non-personal spontaneity would have to be accomplished *without any antecedent motivation*. This is always possible in principle, but remains very improbable or, at least, extremely rare in our human condition. (Sartre, 1960, p. 97)

But Dharmakirti, who was certainly used to the practice of meditation, points to this possibility:

> Due to the speed of the mental process, the untrained person usually cannot differentiate conceptual from non-conceptual cognition. Only on special occasions, such as in some form of meditation, can a clear differentiation be made. (Dreyfus, 1996, p. 351)

In vipassana, the main aspect of Buddhist meditation, it is possible for the meditator—through the very sharp cultivation of mindfulness—to be aware of the first instant of perception before the arising of a concept: to be mindful means, precisely, to be present at each instant. This allows the meditator the possibility to not buy into objectification of the perception. But this requires a state of mind that is totally balanced: a mind that is not engaged in the object, either positively, through desire or attachment, or negatively, through aversion. It requires a mind that is not dulled through indifference. It requires a mind, in fact, that is free of intention.

The Burmese meditation master Mahasi Sayadaw describes one facet of the process through which the meditator is aware of the arising of any experience in the mind:

> As the practice get more refined, at times the number of different objects to note may shrink to one or two or all may even disappear. However, at this time, the knowing quality is still present. In this very clear open space of the sky (-like consciousness) there remains only one blissful consciousness, which is very clear without comparison (Mahasi Sayadaw, unpublished material).

A Thai master, Achan Mahabowa, spoke of meditation on the breath. —Mindful of all the physical sensations that accompany the inflow and outflow of breath, the meditator simply rests. After a while, as the meditator's mind becomes more deeply attentive, and refined: perceptions become finer, more subtle still, until they disappear all together, and only the knowing quality of the mind remains. This is a pure knowing. Paul Valéry, a modern French poet, writes with extraordinary intuition: 'to feel the knowing itself and no object.' (Lafranchi, 1993, p. 23) In allowing for intimacy with the experience, objective content disappeared for this poet, and the mind suspended any involvement with the object. In another approach to meditation, meditators work on the attitude of the mind. Using modern terminology, we could say that it is the intentionality of consciousness which is suspended. That is, one does not take the duality of consciousness-object for granted. Meditators need to recognize how the mind constantly buys into intentionality, into conceptualisation.

Let us examine a few of the concepts that we impose upon our experiences: As suggested earlier, *within* does not clearly express what is at stake in meditation. 'The mind is neither within nor without, nor is it to be apprehended between the two.' (Thurman, 2001, p. 30) To look within, even when understood to signify within the mind, gives objective to the meditation: it gives intention. Looking for the mind, whether within or without, is to conceive of an object. Consciousness is not located in space as that is a characteristic of objects. There is nowhere to direct the mind. 'Don't try to place your mind inwardly. Don't try to observe an object outwardly. Rest in the observer, the thinker, mind itself, without fabricating anything.' (Patrul Rimpoche, p. 148)

Presence. — To be present means that we are conscious of being conscious of something. And this is entirely different from being absorbed in the object that is being perceived or thought of. Although the word presence, or present, may be used, one must be careful to not make it an instance of temporality. An instance between past and future. The word present is used merely to avoid being trapped in past and future; nor does it mean, instead, being trapped in another aspect of temporality, the so-called now. Temporality is a concept, a frame that is used to organize the recording of experiences: it is useful, and efficient, but it is nonetheless only a frame, framework, and nothing else.

Sometimes, the mind aims at past or future, and this keeps a concept in mind. Use of the word presence is an attempt to clear, dust off this misunderstanding. Lost in thoughts of the past or future is certainly a way to not be present. But temporality is perpetuated in less obvious ways, too. — Any attempt, for example, to transform or change an experience that is arising implies temporality. When we transform an experience, it means that we anticipate another experience that is not present, an experience that we project onto another time.

Saint Augustine, the 4th century philosopher and theologian, was puzzled by the notion of time. He said that if no one asked him, he knew what time was, but as soon as he was asked — he did not know. The past does not exist, he said, and neither does the future, nor is there a gap in-between for a present to exist.

Consciousness is not located in time; time is a content of the mind.

In meditation, the most common confusion is to believe that presence has a specific aspect, like vastness, peacefulness, or clarity. But this is to make an object of presence. Such notions arise when one does not recognize that no matter the experience, presence is the awareness of being conscious of this or that. But consciousness is not the content — it is the experiencer, the knower of the experience. This awareness implies that consciousness is not lost in its object.

The object is irrelevant for the knowing of consciousness.

It is possible to be present in any kind of experience — agitation, sleepiness, joy and sorrow — providing one's concern is not with the content of the experience but rather rests, simply, in the knowing of it. But the investigation of consciousness can only unfold in the first person.

*

In order to explore consciousness, one not only needs to disregard the object, but also pass beyond the tendency to personalize consciousness. When one identifies with this knowing capacity which is consciousness, thinking *I* know, *I* see, and so on, one projects a concept onto the experience, splitting it in two: Object and subject, with the individual in question as subject. It means that one is attached to the content of experience: the concept I. Lost in this content, awareness of the knowing capacity of consciousness is veiled. Consciousness appears in whatever aspect of the I. If the mind clings to this appearance, there is no awareness of the consciousness that appears as I.

Exploration of this knowing capacity of consciousness does not require a new technique, but rather the suspension of the habitual function of the mind by means of temporality, personality, and the duality of a subject facing an object. The notion of a technique is subjected utterly to purpose. It is subjected to an aim.

Can consciousness be sought out by seeing? Can it be known by hearing, touching, or thinking? If that were so, consciousness would be a shape and color, a sound, a tactile sensation, a thought. None of which is true. Treating consciousness as an ordinary object of knowledge splits consciousness in two. But consciousness is not breakable. — One does not have to get rid of any experience, only not be lost in it. Consciousness reveals itself at the moment of seeing, hearing, touching, thinking. In a sutra, the Buddha expresses this clearly. (Anguttara Nikaya IV.24)

First, the Buddha said that there is nothing in the universe that he does not perceive. This is to point out that he is free from any deficiency. 'If I were to say, "I don't know whatever in the cosmos ... is seen, heard, sensed, cognized ... pondered by the intellect," that would be a falsehood in me ...'

He goes on. 'Thus, monks, the Buddha, when seeing what is to be seen, doesn't construe a seen. He doesn't construe an unseen. He doesn't construe a seer.'

The Buddha continues, speaking of all perceptions, and thoughts. Clearly, the Buddha is describing an attitude that is free of duality. And yet his mind is not empty. He does not construct, when seeing, the duality of a seer and that which is seen. According to the Buddha, this is the attitude of freedom.

Sartre points in this way to the artificial nature, the split, the duality between world and I:

> It is enough that the *me* be contemporaneous with the World, and that the subject-object duality, which is purely logical, definitively disappear from philosophical preoccupation. The World has not created the *me*; the *me* has not created the World. These are two objects for absolute, impersonal consciousness and it is by virtue of this consciousness that they are connected (Sartre, 1960, p. 105).

— How is that possible when thinking?

The first step: understanding that a thought is not the object it is pointing at. For example, the thought of water isn't wet. But one needs to go further.

A thought is only an appearance taken by the mind. There is no duality between a thinker and a thought. The thought is the consciousness of a certain meaning, or rather, consciousness taking on the appearance of a certain meaning. There is no meaning that needs to be known. Meaning cannot be distinguished from consciousness of the meaning.

*

Let us explore consciousness of emotions. — Imagine an experience of sadness. If I wish to get rid of it, that would mean I believe it to have a concrete reality, an objective reality, something I really could get rid of. It would mean that sadness has an existence separate from that of the mind. But sadness is just a coloration that the mind has at this particular instant. At this instant, sadness is to the mind what temperature is to water. Consciousness is the *material* out of which sadness is made.

Imagine a houseplant not far from the living room window. Only a small part of it receives direct sunlight, and this part appears as bright green. But the rest of the plant seems rather dark, a darker green. It would not make sense to take a cloth to somehow rub away the brighter area. In order to get rid of this shade of bright green one would have to clip it away. Moving the plant slightly, turning it just so, would be easier. Instead of changing the plant, which remains exactly the same plant, we change the context.

We cannot act on sadness directly as with an object, but we can change the condition that causes sadness.

Our concern here, though, is not to imagine how we can get rid of sadness, but to know what consciousness is. If one thinks one needs to get rid of sadness in order to be aware of consciousness, this implies that one is dealing only with contents. When we do not make an object out of an emotion, we can experience it as the way consciousness appears at this instant. But this does not change what consciousness is. 'Pleasure cannot be distinguished — even logically — from the consciousness of pleasure. Consciousness (of) pleasure is constitutive of the pleasure as the very mode (of) its own existence, as the material of which it is made.' (Sartre, 1956, p. 14)

Another common mistake in meditation is to believe that in order to know consciousness, one must get rid of all contents—to have an empty mind. And so one tries to push away any experience that appears to the mind. Paul Valéry seems to fall into this trap:

> The soul enjoys its light without any object. Its silence concerns the totality of its speech... It feels equally at a distance from all names and forms. No image affects it or constrains it. The smallest judgement will spoil its perfection. (Lafranchi, 1993, p. 18)

We may wonder what Meister Eckhart means when he says to the mystic that she must give up temporality, multiplicity and personality. Does he mean to get rid of them, or to negate them somehow, or to simply let them be?

One must take nothing for granted to understand the nature and function of consciousness. It is not possible to meet with understanding when one frames one's search, narrows it, through the notions of temporality, multiplicity (duality) and personality. It is not that one needs to do something special. Rather, one simply needs to suspend any doing.

In their attempt to discover what consciousness is — whatever name they may have called it — scientists, mystics, philosophers and artists have all been confronted with similar difficulties. The solution that many have opened to is not drawn from a vast array of techniques, but comes rather from a shared willingness to go on with the quest in the most complete destitution — to let tools, skill and technique all fall away. As the modern French writer Maurice Blanchot tells us: 'Presence upon which we are without power.'

A recent description of the universe suggests that it is not expanding into something. It is unique, and comprehends everything. There is nothing outside it; it has no center, no periphery. As there is nothing other than itself, it is not located anywhere. This also seems an illuminating allegory for the mind.

References

Anguttara Nikaya IV.24 *Kalaka Sutta*: *At Kalaka's Park*, translated from the Pali by Thanissaro Bhikkhu (2002–2009)
http://www.accesstoinsight.org/tipitaka/an/an04/an04.024.than.html.
Dalai Lama (1997), *The Gelug: Kagyü Tradition of Mahamudra* (Ithaca: Snow Lion).
Dreyfus, G. (1996), *Recognizing Reality* (Albany, NY: State University of New York Press).
Freud, S. (1990), *The Ego and the Id* (New York: W.W Norton & Compagny).
Lafranchi G. (1993), *Paul Valéry et l'expérience du moi pur* (Paris: La bibliothèque des arts).
Patrul, Rimpoche (1986), *Self-liberated Mind* (Kathmandu: Rangjung Yeshe Publication).
Sartre, Jean-Paul (1956), *Being and Nothingness* (New York: Washington Square Press).
Sartre, Jean-Paul (1960), *The Transcendence of the Ego* (New York: Hill and Wang).
Thurman, R. (2001), *The Holy Teaching of Vimalakirti* (Pennsylvania: The Pennsylvania State University Press).

Marion Hendricks

Experiencing Level

An instance of developing a variable from a first person process so it can be reliably measured and taught

Abstract: The concept 'Experiencing (EXP) Level' points to the manner in which what a person says relates to felt experience. The manner is a first person process which is quantitatively measurable. Examples of low, middle and high Experiencing are given. In a high experiencing manner a person attends directly to a bodily sense of what is implicit and allows words (or images and or gestures) to emerge from that sense. The Experiencing Scale which measures the manner of process is a third person rating of a first person process, according to precise linguistic and somatic characteristics. A new rating method gives high reliability. I will briefly summarize several of the more than one hundred research studies which have used the EXP Scale or other measures of high EXP process. The high end of the EXP Scale describes what came to be called 'Focusing'.

Because EXP level is a variable of the <u>manner</u> of process, it can be applied to almost any <u>content</u> area. Examples from tape-recorded psychotherapy sessions, creative writing, and theory-building will be analyzed in terms of experiencing level. Having defined the variable in observable terms makes it possible to formulate exact steps for teaching high Experiencing. Two practices — Focusing and Thinking at the Edge — have been developed, which can be taught in precise steps. This kind of third person variable can be found only from first person process. Its value for studying living will be shown.

Keywords

Experiencing, Experiencing Scale, Experiencing Level, First Person Science, Third Person, Focusing, Body, Felt sense, Carrying forward

The Concept of 'Experiencing Level'

It is often thought that because a process is experiential it can only be measured by self-report, which is considered unreliable. Therefore (it is thought), 'subjective' experience cannot be studied in a scientific way. This is untrue. I will trace the development from first person experience to a reliable research measure, and to practices that can be taught.

The concept of 'Experiencing Level' points to the manner in which what a person says relates to felt experience. The manner of process can range from a pure narration of events with no reference to felt experiencing to a present exploration of meanings arising from felt experiencing. In a high Experiencing manner a person attends directly to a bodily felt sense of some situation and allows words (or images and or gestures) to emerge directly from that sense. Usually after some small steps of attending to the felt sense, it opens and *new meanings come into a thereby changed situation.* The body responds with a deep breath or tears or some expression of whole body relief.

Each manner of process has precise linguistic and somatic characteristics which can be observed. This specificity allows the 'subjective' first person process to be researched and taught precisely. Two practices — Focusing and Thinking at the Edge — have been developed. In each practice there are precise instructions for making touch with implicit felt experience which has no words as yet.

Development of the Experiencing Scale

The concept of Experiencing Level and the Experiencing Scale were developed at the University of Chicago by Gendlin and colleagues. Gendlin's philosophical model of how words function in relation to experiencing (Gendlin, 1962) was applied in the field of psychotherapy. At that time much innovative research had just been completed at the University of Chicago Counseling Center. For the first time in history therapy sessions were being tape-recorded and looked at to understand what helped people. There was an abundance of data — audio recordings and transcripts rather than descriptions by the therapist or client self reports. Gendlin came to this data with the beginnings of his 'explication model' already developed. This model developed out of his first person experience. It did not just exist 'out there' waiting to be found. Someone else would not have looked for or 'seen' what he saw in the data. But, once defined, anyone can see it, with training.

At that time, most research on the efficacy of psychotherapy examined the content of the client's verbalizations – *what* was discussed, e.g., one's mother, the relationship with the therapist, childhood memories. Because Gendlin's model makes the process of explication basic, it is possible to look at the *manner* in which *any* content is being discussed.

An Experiencing Scale (EXP)was developed which reliably measures the manner of process without the use of self reports. While clients' verbalizations in a therapy session might be considered self report, the variable we are observing is not what they are reporting. They are not saying, 'Now I am using language to point to a felt sense.' 'I am having a culturally prescribed emotion.' 'I'm relating events with no personal meanings.' It is important to distinguish the first person process and the process of measuring it. Clients are reporting on their lives. If we were measuring the content of their lives then we would be measuring by their self report. The process we are measuring itself is always first person, but it can be measured by trained raters who have no other contact with the situation.

Basic terms of the explication model
- '*Bodily Felt sense of*' refers to a person's immediately sensed, but implicit, experiencing of a situation, an issue, a creative task. One feels 'something' but does not yet know what. It is important to distinguish between the felt sense and an emotion. Emotions are a narrowing of the body sentience of a whole situation. They prevent us from being aware of the whole situation. A felt sense is a 'turning' one's attention on that which is implicitly present, and making it a datum, 'that whole thing about X'. See Gendlin (1997) for the philosophical derivation of this distinction between emotion and felt sense.
- '*Felt shift*' refers to the bodily felt release that occurs when words come to say exactly what was implied. This usually occurs after a number of small steps.
- '*Carrying forward*' is the effect of the explication in each step. What will 'carry forward' is found empirically. It is not arbitrary (not just any words will do), nor is it determined (only *these* words will do). Many words might carry forward what is implicit, but even one set can be hard to find.

Linguistic and somatic markers of experiencing level

I will illustrate these terms with transcript material, taken from psychotherapy sessions.[1] The observable linguistic and somatic markers of high experiencing (Focusing) lead to training procedures for therapists. The detailed markers help therapists recognize when a client has immediately sensed, but implicit, experience right now in the session. *This is the juncture at which something new can come.* I will also show one kind of therapist response that points toward the implicit, the felt sense, and will show the difference such a response or the lack of it makes to the client's subsequent responses. While drawn from psychotherapy sessions, the examples and the analysis of them in observable terms can help any person, including the reader, locate or learn this first person process in their own experience.

LOW EXP LEVEL Example

One day he [the doctor] called me and said, 'I'm afraid she won't last long. It's spreading like wildfire.' They couldn't get all of it. It was too late. And so that's about the extent of it, you know. She went into a coma, she lasted for about three or four months. Altogether from the time she became ill, the entire time was about two years. After he performed the operation he said, 'I'm surprised she lasted that long.' We didn't know it had gone all the way back. There was no sign of it, nothing. But it was there all the time. Can you imagine that.

MIDDLE EXP LEVEL Example

A____ and I ... .spent about two hours talking over the luncheon about his problem. And I've never known him, until that time to be so low and despondent about his future in science. He said, 'You won't believe this Dad, until I tell you, that it has been over six months since I had a test-tube in my hand' ... and after listening *I was very much disturbed* by what he said because this was a very serious conversation, and it dealt with what I felt had to do with a decision he had to make regarding his work and his marriage, and they were both at stake ... I said, 'But A____, don't you think if J____ were made to realize how desperate the situation is that she would elect to allow you to do more of your science?' ... And there was silence for a moment or two and he shook his head, and said, 'She will never change.' Now when he said that I felt he had already made a decision ... to divorce rather than to continue ... *I felt absolutely consternated* by that because I knew they really loved each other, I knew they could have a harmonious relationship for many years to come if only she could understand.

---

[1] I have excerpted this description from an earlier article (Hendricks, 1986) with some changes.

HIGH EXP LEVEL Example

It's almost like ... it kind of feels like ... sitting here looking through a photo album. And, like each picture of me in there is one of my achievements. And, I think [inaud] because I wasn't achieving for me. I was always achieving for ... someone else so they'd think I was good enough. It's like *it feels right to me to say ... that ... I don't know quite how to say it ... It's like the feeling is there, but I can't quite put words on it. It feels right somehow to say it's like* I've chosen this man as my challenge ... knowing that I'd be defeated. That this person wouldn't respond to me in the same way. So that I could kind of buy right back into the photo album being flipped through. I didn't have what it took (T: Uhhum) to get what I wanted.

Reading these excerpts side by side one can see the differences in the manner of relating to felt experiencing. I will point out the linguistic and somatic markers of the EXP process for each level.

Low experiencing level

This man is telling a series of events: the course of his wife's illness, her death, what the doctor said. A characteristic of low EXP process is that it is *externalized*. We learn some details about the events but not about any inner process. There are few, if any, self-referential statements. In spite of the highly painful content, the client does not name his feelings about the events or the inner meanings of the events for him. One can guess that he feels angry at the doctors and bereaved, sad, and lonely about the loss of his wife. But he does not tell any of this. The closest he comes is his statement, 'Imagine that.' One can hear a suppressed shock, outrage, anguish in this comment. Again one can guess what he would be feeling if he could 'open up' this statement. 'How could something so awful happen with no warning, no signs?'; 'It's terrible to feel so helpless to save someone you love'; 'I'm furious that they didn't diagnose her properly.' But he is not exploring any of this kind of inner detail.

We cannot know what his wife's death actually means to him. One gets a sense of his discomfort with his feelings when he tells about the doctor informing him of the terminal nature of the illness. In the midst of telling this surely grief-laden material, he says, 'So that's about the extent of it, you know.' It's as though at the point where feeling might break through, he flattens or distances from the feelings, as though he were saying, 'There is nothing *more* here; I've told you the whole thing and that's it.' He's closing down, moving away from any larger, implicit, textured sense of that whole situation. Events are described as flat and self-evident. One has a sense that this man's experience will remain blocked, silent, and pained for many years until time blurs its sharpness.

To summarize, Low EXP Level has the following characteristics:

(1) Most comments are in the past tense.

(2) One reports mostly external events.

(3) Events are described as flat and self-evident.

Middle experiencing level

Again, an event is being reported — this man's conversation with his son. He describes the setting, their behavior, and their exchange: 'He said ... and then I said ...' However, there is a difference from segment one. This man refers to his feeling about the conversation and his son's situation: 'I was very much disturbed by what he said ...' 'I felt absolutely consternated by that ...' At this middle EXP level the narration of events is interspersed, parenthetically, with the client's impressions, feelings and emotions. We get some account of how he is affected by the events he describes.

However, references to personal meanings remain parenthetical to the event-story. Each of these self-referent statements has the structure, 'I felt X because ...' and what follows is more about the son than the father. 'I felt disturbed because they (son's marriage and career) were both at stake.' 'I felt consternated because they loved each other, they could have a harmonious relationship.' We don't hear what it is that is disturbed in him in response to his son's situation. What is it about the potential divorce that so disturbs him? The therapist does not and cannot know unless she can get him to differentiate inwardly his whole sense of that situation, the sense that he is calling 'disturbed.' What is it exactly that feels so disturbing? Again we can guess: It hurts him to see his child in pain. He's scared his son's career will be jeopardized because he needs his son to succeed so he can feel like he is someone through his son. If his son claims what he needs, and divorces, perhaps it raises issues about the father's own marriage and how he stayed at too great a price to his selfhood. These are, of course, pure speculations. We cannot know what's actually in the 'disturbedness' this father felt as he listened to his son's struggle. Quite possibly, the client himself couldn't tell us what his 'disturbed' feeling was even if we asked him, or at least not at first. He would probably give us some obvious answer: 'Any parent would feel upset about his child's marriage breaking up. We want the best for our children.' Or some such 'commonsense,' 'self-evident' conventional answer. (And, of course, that would be true in a way.) A person at this middle EXP Level is not used to turning and attending to the body sense of a situation and letting it articulate itself.

As in the first segment, the past tense is used. Even when feeling is referred to, it is a present report about what was felt then. There is not now an ongoing sensing of the problematic situation.

Middle level EXP has the following characteristics:

(1) One gives mainly a descriptive narrative of events.

(2) Emotions are referred to, but briefly, without internal elaboration.

High experiencing level

Segment three illustrates a high EXP level process. There is almost no narration of events. It isn't even clear what the client is talking about in terms of time, place, event. There is only a brief, vague reference to 'a man' who 'won't respond' to her. This is the reverse of segment two. The events are parenthetical to the inner exploration, which is the main focus. If one had to summarize what each segment is about one could say: Segment one, 'wife's death'; Segment two, 'upset about son's divorce.' But what shall we say of the third? The first two are about someone else. The third is about the client herself, her own sensing of inner meanings. The entire process is self-referential.

In the other two segments one could make guesses about what the implied meanings might be, but here one can't even guess. She is working at a level where the process is unique, specific to the individual. What comes next can only arise out of her wholistic sensing of whatever situation/issue she is working on.

Much of the segment is in the momentary present tense, for example, '*if I could ...*' '*it sort of feels like ...*' '*The feeling is there.*' When the past tense is used it is to articulate a felt sense she experiences currently.

She isn't afraid to let something come — an image, a phrase for a whole sense of something. '*What comes ... what comes to me ...*' She is able to let new content emerge freshly from her immediate sensing. We see this again when she says, '*I don't know quite how to say it ... it's like the feeling is there but I can't quite put words on it ... it feels right somehow to say ...*' She has an immediately present tangible sense, but she does not yet 'know' cognitively what it is. She lets words (or images) come from it directly. When they come, she learns something about herself that she hasn't articulated previously. Her process is also characterized by pauses as she attends to her bodily felt sense and waits for words to come from it (instead of trying to fill in or deduce what it must be). She has to grope for words that will 'fit' the sense just right. This bodily sensing is individually specific. Clichés and ordinary uses of language have little power. She creates metaphors or similes to get at the exact specific quality of the experience. Metaphors and similes are a use of language marked by 'it's like ...' ('Your eyes are like stars'). She is using language this way when she says, 'it kind of feels like ... [pause as she gropes for words and lets them come] sitting here looking through a picture album.'

To summarize, a high EXP process has specific, observable linguistic and bodily characteristics:

(1) An inner exploration of personally felt meanings is the main focus. Events are referred to only as a base from which to sense inwardly into one's whole body sense of a situation.

(2) Present tense is used.

(3) There are pauses as one waits to let words or images come from the felt sense.

(4) One uses language metaphorically: 'The feeling is like ...'

(5) One uses language to point to the implicit: 'it,' 'that,' 'something,'— what is sensed but not yet known.

Therapist responses can increase or decrease client's experiencing level

While I am discussing this in terms of psychotherapy the same points apply to any interaction. Open pronouns and content free words are the most important words in Focusing-oriented psychotherapy e.g 'it', 'that' 'this" 'something' 'in some way'. They allow the therapist and client to stay in direct connection to that which is sensed but which does not yet have words. They help us not to prematurely name and thereby close what is emerging. Unfortunately it is often the case that a therapist does not know the high EXP process. Below is an example in which the client is at a high EXP level and the therapist is not familiar with pointing to or with speaking from the implicit.

Client: Yuh ... it's really gone... And yet, like I feel ... there's ... there's something underneath it all but I don't know what ... and if I kind of knew what it was ... I might feel differently, I don't know. But it's vague right now.

> Therapist: Okay, .if things could be a little more definite. If you were really able to identify the cause you really think that you'd be able to cope with it then. But right now you can't seem to put your finger on what the real problem is.
>
> Client: Yuh ... and ... that ... like when you say that ... that makes me mad because I feel ... you know like I'm ... intelligent. I can, figure things out. And yet ... right now I don't know what the hell's going on with me.

In the first statement, the client is in a high EXP level process. She literally describes having a felt sense, 'Something (there) . . . . but I don't know what.' She is concretely sensing the presence of some whole thing, but it is implicit. She does not yet know what is in this sense. Such an implicit sense is often felt as 'vague' initially. It doesn't yet have a sharp, definite, explicit form. The possibility of something new, some change, arises when working in direct contact with what is not yet known. The client can sense that if this felt 'something' would become explicit, it might shift her whole context or bring some release. Actually, she is telling the therapist exactly what needs to happen next — that she and he would stay next to the 'something' underneath so it could explicate. Notice the high EXP characteristics: pauses, not being able to find words immediately, the use of 'something' to point to what is there without prematurely labeling or imposing definition on it.

The therapist's response is not inaccurate. We can see what he responds to, with each of his phrases. His 'identify the cause' refers to client's 'if I kind of knew what it was'. His 'be able to cope' refers to 'then I might feel differently' and 'more definite' refers to 'vague'. However, every major word or phrase the therapist has chosen ('definite', 'identify causes', 'cope', 'the real problem') is closed, explicit, 'definite'. His message seems to be, 'Stop being so tentative and vague ... let's uncover and label the cause and solve the problem.' The therapist does not recognize the felt sense, He moves away from the implicit in his response and the client's EXP level is decreased.

The therapist is often defined by the client as having power and expertise. When there is trouble in the interaction, as there is here, clients may define it as something wrong with them. Most clients would feel vaguely put down without knowing why, give up the attempt to articulate the felt sense of the issue, and shift to a more cognitive, problem-solving, speculative manner of process, or feel badly about their ineptitude. This client is somewhat able to hold onto her experiential response, after her initial verbal agreement with the therapist. But he doesn't recognize the problem as a therapist error. She defends herself against the implied message that she is cognitively inadequate. 'I'm intelligent', 'I can figure things out'. Notice she has shifted to the therapist's cognitive framework, 'figure out', and away from her original felt sense, 'I feel ... I might feel differently.'

How would the therapist respond in this excerpt if he had recognized the client's high EXP process? He might have said, 'You can feel something right there ...' Or, 'You can feel it right there underneath ...' Therapists can use open pronouns that function as pointers *toward the implicit* without labeling or defining it. The therapist would acknowledge and reflect that the client has a direct referent, a 'something' concretely felt. He might say that neither the client nor he as yet knows what it is. In this way they both turn their attention toward it, to let words come from it.

Here is an exchange in which both therapist and client are in a high Experiencing process. The client has been discussing two issues.

> ML: (pause). I don't know how they're intertwined right now, but it... they're ... they feel ... what I mean is I don't know if they're dependent on one another, but, the way my hands are going right now, *somehow* they're, they're connected. And I, ... *tears come up and I feel a softening in my throat.*
>
> J: Yeah. There's a quality change, and tears come, and it softens somehow.
>
> ML: Yeah, (in a quavering voice) ... and (there is a) *wanting* that it could be this connection I keep. It could be this connection, and, and it feels broken, or withdrawn from, *or something*.

Notice the characteristic markers of High Experiencing in the first client statement. She is pausing, groping for words, letting her hand gestures explicate the felt sense of her situation. In her use of 'somehow' she is pointing to a sensed relation between two feelings, but she is holding it open what exactly that relation is. She is not prematurely naming her felt sense, thereby closing it. And so 'it' opens further and brings the whole body marker of tears, which often come when the felt sense begins to open into explicit symbolization. She makes a distinction between the thought that her two feelings may be dependent on each other ('I don't know if they are') and her gesturing which resonates in her body and brings the tears. Her body responds to the freshly emergent gesturing and not to the thought — the words 'dependent on each other' don't carry forward her felt sense right now. The therapist's response is gentle and exact. By repeating her words, he welcomes not only the content that comes, but also her manner of process. This non-intrusive response lets her continue in a High EXP manner and she finds that she cares more about this connection than she knew. She wants it to be the one she can keep. Her use of 'or something' is again this odd use of language which indicates that 'broken' and 'withdrawn from' don't quite fit her felt sense, or at least that there is more there than is explicated by these words.

The Experiencing Scale measures this first person process

Having shown experiencing level using verbatim tape recorded segments, I will discuss the Experiencing Scale (EXP) which was developed to measure the manners of process illustrated above. It has seven stages. The scale was tested until a successful method for attaining reliability was found. Samples of each experiencing level were excerpted from session tape recordings. They were rated by experts and then used for rater training. A rater is trained individually in a room alone until the ratings are reliable with the expert ratings of the standard segments. Given that training is to a standard, there is no necessity for raters to meet each other. This precludes a situation in which raters talk together and their ratings then correlate with each other, but not to the standard. This rater training procedure results in high inter-rater reliability, typically in the 80s. The rater training package[2] consists of tape recorded practice segments and transcripts, the EXP Scale, the history of the concept and a rater instruction manual which includes expert ratings with justifications for each practice rating. The rating procedure can be taught in eight training sessions. The scale can also be used to rate written material. .

The Experiencing Level variable has been widely used in research

The EXP Scale and several related measures have been used in over 100 studies. Researchers Lambert & Hill (1994, p. 94) state, 'Perhaps the most widely used and best-researched observer-rated measure(s) of client involvement in the therapy process (is) the Experiencing Scale …' The EXP Scale is available in Dutch, German, Japanese, and Spanish. A new study from Japan (Miyaki 2008) validated a five-step EXP Scale against the original seven-step scale.

Many studies (Hendricks, 2002) have found a positive significant correlation between measures of EXP level or Focusing and various psychotherapy outcome measures. For example, Goldman (2005) found that EXP levels, at Stage 4 and even more so at Stage 6 in the

---

[2] The training package is available from Dr. Marjorie H. Klein, Department of Psychiatry, Wisconsin Psychiatric Institute and Clinics, 6001 Research Park Boulevard, Madison, Wisconsin 53719-1179.

last half of therapy, were strong predictors for reduction in depressive symptoms, and Stage 6 predicted an increase in self-esteem.

In addition to psychotherapy outcome studies, EXP level has been shown to have a positive, significant correlation with measures of creativity, ego strength and psychological differentiation. Correlations with physiological, attentional, and cognitive variables have been found. I will give a brief overview summary of some of this work.

Focusing is based in the body. '*Bodily felt sense*' is one of the main terms in this model. The correlations between Focusing and physiological measures is not surprising. Focusers or high EXP subjects are better able to discriminate physiological states (Kolilis, 1988). The process of focusing is accompanied by body relaxation indicators (Gendlin & Berlin, 1961; Bernick *et al.*, 1969). The felt shift correlates with an increase in EEG alpha frequencies (Don, 1977). Lutgendorf *et al.* (1994) studied whether or not verbal disclosure of a traumatic experience would influence immune responsiveness. The extent of experiential involvement in the disclosure of the traumatic event was measured using the Experiencing Scale and focusing. Questions were used to increase experiential involvement in the disclosures. Her findings showed that disclosure alone did not affect the EBV-VCA antibody titres in a statistically significant way. However, greater experiential involvement, as measured by the Experiencing Scale, summed up across three disclosure sessions, was associated with increased immune function over the course of the experiment. This suggests that it is the *manner* in which one engages in the expression of the trauma that makes the difference in immune functioning rather than just talking or writing. Physical illness or injury is a trauma. Utilizing focusing to increase experiential involvement may be a key variable in the area of psychoneuroimmunology.

A series of five studies (Zimring, 1974; 1990) show that performance on complex mental tasks requiring attention to internally generated stimuli is increased by doing the first step of Focusing, Clearing A Space before the task. In line with the idea that focusing enhances cognitive process, focusers were found to do better on measures of creativity, intuition, flexible use of attention, and conceptual complexity . Focusers can maintain concentration and withstand distractions while attending to an internal body sense.

Given the range and number of studies which have used the EXP Scale or other measures of Focusing, it is clear that a useful research variable has been developed from first person process. Looked at all together the studies provide validity for the variable.

A startling discovery

The initial hypothesis tested, in using the EXP Scale, was that clients would increase in EXP level in the course of psychotherapy. However, much to the surprise and chagrin of the experimenters, the studies showed that clients who came to therapy already high in experiencing manner remained high and had a successful outcome, but that clients who began therapy in a low EXP manner did not significantly increase in EXP level during therapy and tended not to succeed. *A failure prognosis could be predicted as early as the second therapy session!* This posed an ethical dilemma. The finding showed a need for Focusing training and raised the question whether a high experiencing manner could be taught, thus reversing the failure prognosis.

A high experiencing manner (focusing) can be taught

This question has since been addressed in thirty nine studies which found that Focusing ability (EXP level)can be increased by training and by specific therapist interventions (Hendricks, 2002). For example, Durak *et al.* (1997) measured client EXP in two tape recorded therapy sessions before and in two sessions after focusing training. Eight therapists sent one or more clients who were then trained in Focusing by one of three trainers. The whole client group was higher on EXP after training. The studies indicate that some people who come into therapy without the ability to focus can be trained to do so and may become able to succeed in therapy.

In some of the studies the increase in EXP level or Focusing ability was not maintained after training. Sustaining a high EXP manner usually requires training and practice over months or years, depending on what level of proficiency is desired. In other studies, clients identified a number of factors that helped them focus: having a listener who refers to the Focuser's experiencing and helps the Focuser find a right distance from the problem, creating a safe space (Tamura, 1987; 1990), and 'trusting one's experiencing' and 'clearing a space' (Morikaya, 1997)

Client EXP level can be affected, by the Therapist EXP level.

Earlier in this article I gave examples of how the EXP level of therapist responses can support or can flatten the client's EXP level. This has been confirmed in the research. In a series of studies with fine grained analyses Sachse (1990) found that therapist 'processing proposals' can deepen or flatten subsequent client responses. He developed a Client Processing Scale and a Therapist Processing Scale, based on Gendlin's Experiencing theory. The higher stages on these scales represent Focusing. Sachse established reliabilities between .79 and .94. An initial study analyzing 1520 triplets (C-T-C statement units) from 152 clients at mid therapy found that clients deepened their process 70% of the time when the therapist made a deepening proposal and *flattened their process 73% of the time when the therapist made a flattening proposal*. These findings are corroborated by a number of similar studies.

The EXP/Focusing variable is just beginning to unfold its power. Related instruments have been developed for assessing the manner of experiencing in other contexts. For example a Clearing A Space Check List was developed (Grindler, 1991) to measure the ability to do the first step in Focusing The new instrument correlates with Experiencing Level at .70. It has been used in several studies with people who have cancer (Grindler, 1991, and Klagsbrun *et al.*, 2005). In the Grindler study experimenters used a standard training protocol to teach the process of Clearing a Space during six 90-minute weekly sessions. The purpose of the training was to experientially introduce each subject to the steps of this process and then to guide them through it each week. Results showed a significant decrease in depression and a significant improvement in body image for the treatment group when compared to the wait group.

In another example the EXP scale was adapted for use in rating EXP level in dreams (Hendricks, 1978). The concept of Dream Experiencing refers to the manner in which the events of dreams are explicated during the dream by the characters.[3] Dream EXP manner was found to be highly stable for individuals and to correlate positively with Witkin's Body Sophistication Scale (1962), a measure of waking psychological differentiation.

Many studies could benefit from including the EXP variable.

Training in Focusing for Anyone

Focusing instructions in six steps were developed to make the beginning of coming in contact with one's experiencing accessible to anyone, not just for clients and therapists. The book *Focusing* (Gendlin, 1981) has chapters explaining each step and has many examples. There are specific instructions for what to do in the case of typical

---

[3] Although EXP level is defined in a content-free way, it can be thought mistakenly that because an event is 'inner' that it would thereby be high in experiencing level. It is possible to confuse the high experiencing manner with 'internal' events, such as fantasy, dream or images. Events from both internal and external sources, can be experienced as a felt sense or as bare events.

difficulties. Since then, there has been much elaboration of different ways to teach Focusing. Any particular formulation for teaching is never the only 'right' one. The process of Focusing is always 'more' than any set of formulations. Once people know the Focusing process for themselves, they can train someone else, because they can see where another person gets stuck, and then they can create steps specific to that person. Ann Weiser Cornell, a linguist by background, has written *The Power of Focusing* (1996). This book and her student and teacher manuals (Cornell and McGavin, 2002) help many people learn Focusing. Robert Lee (2007) has developed twelve ways to find a felt sense. Many people have designed exercises to help with each aspect of the Focusing process. Instructions have been adapted for particular situations. For example, in Afghanistan, among many other innovations, Focusing has been taught with reference to the Rumi poem 'A Guest House'.

The process nature of Focusing allows people to not divulge content, but only indicate their process, e.g. 'Now I have a feeling in my stomach about the problem. Now I'm checking in my body whether the words that came are exactly right.' This has been important because disclosing problems is often not possible in many circumstances.

Focusing Proficiency

Focusing is a skill that requires development over time, and differs according to the practitioner With practice and training, one can expect to gain fluency, and become able to apply Focusing and its principles to an ever-broadening array of contexts. Many exactly differentiated nuances of the process have been articulated in three levels of proficiency. Below are proficiencies for levels 1 and 3 (see www.focusing.org for level 2).

Level 1 Focusing Proficiencies

- Can sense the body, be with it, from inside.
- Can get a 'felt sense,' a physical sensation that contains meaning and pertains to a particular situation, for example an issue in one's work, a creative project or a relationship.
- Can recognize how a felt sense differs from emotions.
- Can recognize when words or images have come directly from the felt sense.

- Is able to notice what would feel right to say from the felt sense of a particular situation.
- Knows when a decision regarding the situation 'sits right' and when it does not.
- Can name or describe the crux of a situation in a way that 'fits' the felt sense.
- Is able to recognize a distinct bodily knowing even when she/he has no words yet to describe it.

Stage 3 Focusing Proficiencies

- Is able to attend to a felt sense and allow many aspects of it to emerge.
- Often finds whole new fields or 'subtexts' emerging from a felt sense.
- Can let the subtexts inform a resulting decision on an issue.
- Can choose to wait for subtext changes before taking action on a particular situation.
- Recognizes new possibilities within a situation, which were not apparent from the original 'given facts'. New facts can be formulated.
- Can discover new questions arising from the felt sense of a situation, leading to a new gathering of information.
- Is able to make better decisions based on greater bodily knowledge.
- Finds an expanded bodily-sensed realm in which one can move between different 'places', clusters, and attitudes.
- Can choose to live from the intricacy which is now always accessible.
- Experiences a sense of reliable safety inside.

There are over 800 Certified Focusing teachers and Focusing-Oriented therapists in thirty-five countries. Most training towards certification takes two years and includes a weekly Focusing partnership for the whole two years. In addition there are numerous written, audio, and video materials.

Teaching Focusing in areas other than psychotherapy

Because Focusing (high EXP manner) is a specific carrying forward relation between words (images, gestures) and a felt sense, it can be introduced in almost any content area of human living. Focusing is used in many fields including medicine, education, business, furniture making, architecture and theory construction. I will briefly mention several applications and will give an example of each. The examples are instances of teaching Focusing. The ways of teaching are all different, but the reader can recognize the basic process of allowing words or images or gestures to arise freshly from a bodily felt sense.

Young children can Focus

There has been much work especially in The Netherlands and in Japan, on teaching children how to Focus. Sometimes a parent may teach the child. In classrooms the children may be taught focusing along with the teacher. I excerpt an example from Marta Stapert's book, *Focusing with Children* (2008) in which you can see the Focusing process with a six-year-old, being guided by her mother. Sophie illustrates a High EXP manner of process: She is able to turn her attention inside; locate a felt sense of her situation in her stomach; allow gestures and a metaphor to come. She draws a picture which emerges directly from her felt sense. With a subsequent felt shift and a smile, she says 'it is gone.' I will put the Focusing instructions in bold and my commentary in bold italics.

Story:

Sophie is thrilled to receive a bicycle for her sixth birthday and wants to bike to the park immediately. Her mother rides behind her. Sophie is having a great time. As she cycles she gets braver and starts to go faster. Her mother cautions: 'Watch out for the bend,' but it is already too late. Sophie can't slow herself down. She slips, falls, and scrapes her knee. Nearby, two girls watch without saying a word. Once at home, Sophie bursts into tears. Her mother does everything she can to comfort her. But Sophie keeps crying.

(Notice that mother has made her own assumption that Sophie is crying because her knee hurts We will see how different what comes is as Sophie focuses.)

Mother:Come here Sophie. Let me give your knee a big kiss. Shall we have some lemonade? . . . . .Maybe that bicycle is a little too big for you after all. Let me dry your tears. You were going fast . . . . .Did you hear me call out to you? You shouldn't cycle quite so fast anymore. Let's get a band-aid, shall we? We'll try again tomorrow and then you can take it a little bit slower.

But Sophie continues to sob. Then, her mother remembers what she learned in a course on focusing with children. She changes her approach and helps Sophie discover from within what the essence of the problem really is.

Mother: **Shall we listen inside together to hear what happened?**

Sophie: Yesss ...

Mother You took a really bad fall with your new bicycle, didn't you? You were just doing so well ... you dared to go fast ... and now you have a scraped knee. And it hurts.

Sophie: (*Continues to cry and sobs*) Yes ... yes ... yes ...

Mother: You also have to sob really badly. **Can you feel inside where that bad thing is?**

Sophie: *(Points to her stomach.)*

Mother: **Can you sit with it in a friendly way and ask what it feels like there?**

Sophie: It is in my stomach here ... really bad ... *(She grows quiet and attentive)* *(This is a felt sense)*

Mother: It is in your stomach ... **How is it there in your stomach?**

Sophie: It's all going around ... *(She moves her hands around)* around and around ... *(She is letting words and gestures come from the felt sense.)*

Mother: It just keeps going around inside ...

Sophie: Just like grabbing hands ... *(She makes a metaphor)*

Mother: Just like grabbing hands ... **If you sit still with that, do those grabbing hands and the feeling that goes with them have a story to tell you?**

Sophie: *(Sobbing loudly again now)* Yes, those big girls should not have stood there looking like that ... I'm sure they think I'm a stupid little kid ...

Mother: You hated that they were standing there looking ... they are bigger. And then you are afraid that they think you're small and stupid ... **Does that feeling have a color inside? Maybe you can close your eyes for a minute and wait for what comes ...**

Sophie: Yes ... red is coming ... and also something black ...

Mother: **Would you draw and color it? Your hand will know how it wants to put everything on the paper** ... It doesn't have to be beautiful ... Inside the feeling will know what it means ...

Hesitantly, Sophie starts with dark colors. Then the lines get stronger. The sobbing stops. She scratches fiercely, adding more lines and another color. She sighs deeply. Then she adds yellow and orange circles. She looks up at her mother and smiles.

Sophie: It's gone *(She has a felt shift with the typical body markers of a deep sigh and a smile.)*

Stapert's book includes chapters on Focusing with different age groups in schools, at home with parents, and in individual counseling. What does it tell us about consciousness, that Focusing can be done by a six-year-old? Children can consciously turn toward their body sense of a situation and make it a datum, a felt sense. They can allow words, images, gestures to come from it. What emerges carries forward what was sensed, and a shift is felt in the body as relief. The capacity to 'turn' on their sensed but not yet articulated experience is already present at six years. Young children can often access implicit functioning more easily than older children and adults, who need longer training. This finding further dispels the idea that children are in all ways less developed than adults.

Teaching Focusing to college students in creative writing classes

Sondra Perl is a professor of English at Herbert Lehmann College and founder of the New York City Writing Project. Her book *Felt Sense: Writing with the Body* (2004) includes a CD of her composing guidelines. I have excerpted two of her instructions to show how she teaches students to write from a felt sense. This is another example of specifying exact steps for teaching focusing in different contexts.

Perl invites the students first to write down what they *already know and have thought*, i.e. what is explicit. In the theory of experiencing, change, novelty, and creativity are possible when one begins from a felt sense – not from what is already explicit. She gives the students plenty of time to clear out the 'already thought' and become ready to attend to the implicit, and to let language come from it directly. The language she uses in this first instruction — 'associations' and 'parts' probably is deliberately not the language of Focusing.

> Now — taking a deep breath and settling comfortably into your chair — ask yourself, 'What are all the associations and parts I know about this topic? What can I say about it now?' Spend as long as you need writing down these responses. Perhaps it will be a sustained piece of freewriting or stream of consciousness, or perhaps separate bits, a long list, or notes to yourself.

Now she can have them take 'all of that' which they already know and put it aside. This brings them to an edge and helps the students find a felt sense of 'the whole topic' and then to pose Focusing questions to themselves.

Now having written for a while, interrupt yourself, set aside all the writing you've done, and take a fresh look at this topic or issue. Grab hold of the whole topic — not the bits and pieces — and ask yourself, 'What makes this topic interesting to me? What's important about this that I haven't said yet? What's the heart of this issue?' Wait quietly for a word, image, or phrase to arise from your 'felt sense' of the topic. Write whatever comes.

Take this word or image and use it. Ask yourself, 'What's this all about?' Describe the feeling, image, or word. As you write, let the 'felt sense' deepen. Where do you feel that 'felt sense'? In your head, stomach, forearms? Where in your body does it seem centered? Continue to ask yourself, 'Is this right? Am I getting closer? Am I saying it?' See if you can feel when you're on the right track. See if you can feel the shift or click inside when you get close, 'Oh yes, this says it.'

One of Perl's graduate students articulated the difference these guidelines made for her:

> ... ever since I've come to understand felt sense, I have a feeling of connectedness to my dissertation that I had lost ... it has to do with whose words I privilege in my own text. I had gotten to a point in my academic work in which I just tried to amass as much of other people's theories as possible because I didn't feel as if I myself had anything important to say about 'my author'. This even though I am one of about five people who really knows this author's work! I had been so indoctrinated with the idea that my work needed to reflect everyone else's that I no longer had a voice ... Writing the diss is still hard for me, but for the first time in years I am writing from a sense of centrality, my own. Everyone else's theory and criticism are fine, and they actually support a lot of what I want to say, but now find myself locating my message in my own sense — my felt sense — of what my author said, meant, implied, left out, etc. My experience of felt sense is more identifiable in personal and creative writing, yes, but I am using that experience to free my academic writing and make it what I hope is more creative and truer.

Thinking at the Edge (TAE)

After Focusing there is a second practice, coming from the model of explicating a felt sense. The graduate student quoted above is addressing what the practice of TAE places centrally — how to generate terms and make theory, starting from one's felt sense of knowing something but not being able to say it yet. The TAE protocol of instructions has fourteen steps (Gendlin & Hendricks, 2004). It makes three assumptions:

1. A person who is experienced in a field and knows Focusing may have a felt sense of some knowledge that cannot now be said in the usual phrases.

2. Letting linguistically unusual sentences come from the felt sense frees one from being trapped in the usual assumptions. This allows one to say something new.

3. Within such freshly generated sentences one can find and separate new terms which are internally related in a new pattern. This can be the starting point for a new kind of theory which is both logical and experiential.

TAE is a method for original thinking, 'original' meaning that thinking starts from implicit knowing and systematically uses the implicit in formulating each step. The terms then have internal or inherent interlocking relations, as well as the power of the external connections of logic. The example below is a tiny glimpse from the middle of the TAE process (Boukydis, 2004). It includes commentary by Kye Nelson, a Focusing trainer and TAE teacher. One can notice the odd use of language that characterizes a High Experiencing manner. I have bolded the words that point to the implicit knowing. In this exchange Gendlin is a TAE partner, listening, saying back, and writing down the exact new phrases and sentences as they come.

It is important that the TAE process be in an area where one has long experience and therefore a rich implicit 'knowing'. Boukydis, a psychologist, has spent thousands of hours with babies and mothers.

> Zack Boukydis: My felt sense is about the relationship between mothers and babies ... there's a certain way that inside of me for a long time I've kept saying ... there's **something missing** in all of these elegant theories.
>
> Gene Gendlin: In the territory between mothers and babies, and **there's something there** ... that is missing, in the theory
>
> Boukydis: It feels like the territory has got a lot of skid marks across a **very delicate sentient place. There are a lot of formulations that don't feel right, inside**.
>
> Gendlin: There's **something** painfully wrong about those.
>
> Boukydis: And then the critic says 'well, you think you can do better ...'
>
> Gendlin: Oh, well, the critic ... [both laugh]
>
> Boukydis: One of my sentences is ... 'When they are separate, mother and baby can still be... participating in the same body process.'
>
> Gendlin: When they are **separate**, they can still participate ... mother and baby can still participate in the **same body process.**
>
> ....

Boukydis: Then there's that ... turnaround question ... "What are human beings, such that they can be physically separate... and yet can still be working in the same body process?'...

Gendlin: They are the same body-living even if they are not physically in the same place, in contact.

Boukydis: Right. The first facet is the experience of parents who have prematurely born babies in special care in an isolette. The mothers tell me they have a body feeling of being separate from their baby, and yet, also they feel the life and death struggle of their baby.

Gendlin: They are ... physically ... in the same body process even though they are not in contact.

Boukydis: Right. It sounds so strange when I hear it, but ... it also sounds true.

Gendlin: It is what she experiences.

....

Boukydis: Yeah ... And ... **what's radical for me** ... as you said back the part about mother and the baby in the isolette ... [Pause] ... There is this tremendous yearning that the mother has to go and be with her baby, and to hold her baby or at least to touch her baby. But there's another way that the baby is also living the life process for the mother ... like, a lot of paradigms have the baby as dependent ... in some essential way ... the baby has ... as much effect.

Gendlin: The baby has as much effective power in carrying ... this single process forward. It's not just one way ...

Boukydis: [pause] ... **It still wants to say** the same body process ... I'm not even happy with the words, and yet that's the best I have, but ... **It still wants to say** the same body process.

Gendlin: The same body process.

Boukydis: Right. And um.

....

Gendlin: The current theories say that an infant isn't anything at all ... and gradually fills in. And you are saying that these are really two beings of the same order, and you are correcting this mistake.

Boukydis: And there's a lot, biologically, emotionally, historically, spiritually. They're biologically wired ... I'll stay on that level ... they're biologically made ... to be this way, or something.

Gendlin: Well, in TAE we would turn that around and say, the fact that they are this way tells us something new about biology and wiring.

Turning it around' is a basic move in TAE. This is the 'reversal.' Rather than saying something new only about mother and child and leaving the big words 'biologically wired' unchanged, the reversal lets Boukydis' point reformulate the entire field. If this turning around is not carried out, the new point will soon become impossible to articulate, because the old assumptions will destroy it. KN

We defend what we have to say here ... good ... but the minute we get to some other words, we are

Boukydis: ... [laughs]. And I want to protect it from the intellectual world that I live in, that says, 'Oh, I know what you're saying, it's like Sullivan said ... it's like Freud said ... it's like ...' And then I have to go away and ... two days later **it starts to come alive again**, and then I can try to begin to work with it ... I need to protect it.

....

Afterword: At the end of the transcript above, we were asking: 'What is a biology that could account for two human beings, though separate, who are living the same body process?' At the end of this session, I had little space for that question. It is now giving me a simple, spine-full stature in the world of ideas ... Now I have a way past where I have laid waste to my own thinking.

The importance of variables drawn from first person process

The implicit intricacy of experience, events, situations tends to be excluded from science, social structure, and human relations. TAE lets us speak and think about the world and ourselves in language and concepts that have our experiential intricacy built in, rather than with concepts which make us into only externally viewed objects. Concepts generated from a 'felt sense' have certain characteristics. Because they grow out of bodily sensing of implicit knowing, they retain their living organization, rather than violating it, as externally imposed concepts often do. In TAE new conceptual structures have the external relations of logic without losing their experienced internal connections. Such 'reflexive' concepts are essential. The experiential nature of what we want to think about needs to be built into the tools with which to think about it. Something like TAE is needed to create forms of language, theory and practices that take account of human experience.

When we help someone develop the capacity to pause and form a felt sense we increase the persons ability to think for him/herself, and not to be emotionally manipulated by ideologies and rhetoric.

The cross-cultural nature of Focusing

Focusing is practiced in cultures as diverse as those of Afghanistan, Japan and Chile. As the practice of Focusing deepens, the differences become clear between an emotional, culturally determined response and one which is from the wider sensing from which a carrying forward next step may come. We no longer just see 'a doctor', a 'bus driver', a 'fat' person, an Arab, a Jew. Rather than the role, or the general category, we see this totally unique person who is a vast intricacy never exhaustively described by any formulation or role. This shift rests on this new kind of process concept in which the carrying forward of the implicit creates emergent meaning. This kind of concept supports new ways of relating to the natural world and to other living creatures, including humans. When seeing oneself or another at this Focusing level, we become reluctant to act just from the cultural level in a way which would violate the particularness of *this* person.

Overcoming the rejection of first person process in studying consciousness

A 'felt sense' implies words (images, gestures) which will 'carry it forward' and thereby change the organism's implying into a next implying.[4] This model answers the question of the relation between subjective experience and the world. The explication model defines the body as *originally* a body–environment process, e.g. there are no lungs without air. Breathing IS the air-going-into-expanding-lungs. Usually, the body is thought of as what is physically within the skin. This generates the problem of the split between 'inner' and 'outer' and how to get the body and the environment together, and questions about the veracity of 'subjective experience' In this new kind of concept the body is *always already* an ongoing body-environment process. In humans a felt sense is how we are bodily living our situations. The world and the person are always already together. The many other ways to study living take place within this wider understanding.

The new kind of concept addresses the dilemma of wanting to study consciousness but ruling out the role of 'subjective' experience because of its unreliability. I have shown that verbalizations from felt

---

[4] This new kind of concept allowed Gendlin to develop a process theory of psychotherapy (Gendlin, 1964, 1996). In his philosophical book *A Process Model* (1997) he uses the carrying forward model to derive how human capacities emerge in an internal continuity from animals and plants. Current models have to assume that consciousness is somehow added on top, in the brain, but without the rest of the body. Using this new kind of concept Gendlin is able to *derive* motion, behavior, gesturing, perception, motivation, language and consciousness and to make many new distinctions.

experiencing can be reliably distinguished from other kinds, and that the Focusing process can help people access their experiencing through precise steps which can be learned. It has a wide range of sought after outcomes and applications. First person processes can become powerful and relevant variables which can add to our knowledge and which can generate teachable practices which help people.

To consider Focusing as an introverted internal process which is 'just subjective' is to deny that *our bodies are linguistic, situational, and interactive to begin with.* The living body is not just what is enclosed within the skin envelope. Our felt sense is OF our lived situations. It is our bodily sense of how all of 'this' situation is for us now. When our felt sense opens up, we say 'Oh, that is what this situation is for me.' It often implies steps of action. High experiencing shows something in so many different areas that we care about and across cultures because the Focusing steps allow one to find the door through which new, exactly relevant meanings emerge, regardless of content area. It is a basic human variable.

References

Bernick, N. and Oberlander, M.(1969), 'Effect of verbalization and two different modes of experiencing on pupil size', *Perception and Psychophysics*, **3**, pp. 327–39.

Boukydis, Z. (2004), 'Mothers and infants: One body process with equal initiative', *The Folio: A Journal for Focusing and Experiential Therapy*, **19** (1).

Cornell, Ann Weiser (1996), *The Power of Focusing* (Oakland, CA: New Harbinger Publications).

Cornell, Ann Weiser (2008), *Focusing Teacher's Manual* (Berkeley, CA: Focusing Resources, 2336 Bonar St., Berkeley, CA 94702) www.focusingresources.com

Cornell, A.W. and McGavin, B. (2002), *The Focusing Student's and Companion's Manual* (Berkeley, CA: Calluna Press).

Don, N.S. (1977), 'The transformation of conscious experience and its EEG correlates', *Journal of Altered States of Consciousness*, **3**, pp. 147–68.

Durak, G., Bernstein, R. & Gendlin, E.T. (1996), 'Effects of focusing training on therapy process and outcome', *The Folio: A Journal for Focusing and Experiential Therapy*, **15** (Fall/Winter), pp. 7–14.

Gendlin, E.T. (1962), *Experiencing and the Creation of Meaning: A Philosophical and Psychological Approach to the Subjective* (New York: Free Press of Glencoe).

Gendlin, E.T. & Berlin, J.I. (1961), 'Galvanic skin response correlates of different modes of experiencing', *Journal of Clinical Psychology*, **17** (1), pp. 73–77.

Gendlin, E.T., Beebe, III, J., Cassens, J., Klein, M. & Oberlander, M. (1968), 'Focusing ability in psychotherapy, personality, and creativity', in M.M. Shlien (Ed.), *Research in Psychotherapy: Vol. III* (Washington, DC: American Psychological Association), pp. 217–41.

Gendlin, E.T. (1996), *Focusing-Oriented Psychotherapy* (New York: Guilford Press).

Gendlin, E.T. (1997), *A Process Model* (New York: The Focusing Institute: www.focusing.org).

Gendlin, E.T. (1981), *Focusing* (New York: Bantam).
Gendlin, E.T. and Hendricks, M. (2004), 'Thinking at the edge (TAE) steps', *The Folio: A Journal for Focusing and Experiential Therapy*, **19** (1), pp. 12–24. Also available at: http://www.focusing.org/tae_steps.html
Goldman, R.N., Greenberg, L.S. & Pos, A. (2005), 'Depth of emotional experience and outcome', *Psychotherapy Research*, **15** (3), pp. 248–60.
Grindler Katonah, D. (1991), 'Focusing: An adjunct treatment for adaptive recovery from cancer',. Unpublished doctoral research, The Illinois School of Professional Psychology, Chicago, IL.
Hendricks, M. (1978), 'Experiencing level in dreams: An individual difference variable', *Psychotherapy: Theory, Research and Practice*, **15** (1), pp. 292–98.
Hendricks, M.N. (1986, May), 'Experiencing level as a therapeutic variable', *Person-Centered Review*, **1**, pp. 141–61.
Hendricks, M. (2002), 'Focusing-oriented/experiential psychotherapy: Research and practice', in D. Cain, D. and J. Seeman (Eds.) *Humanistic Psychotherapies: Handbook of Research and Practice* (Washington, DC: American Psychological Association), pp. 221–52.
Klagsbrun,J., Rappaport, L., Marcow-Speiser, V., Post, P., Stepakoff, S. & Karman, S. (2005), 'Focusing and expressive arts therapy as a complementary treatment for women with breast cancer', *Journal of Creativity and Mental Health*, **1** (1), pp. 107–37.
Klein, M.H., Mathieu, P.L., Gendlin, E.T., & Kiesler, D.J. (1969), *The Experiencing Scale: A Research and Training Manual* (Madison, WI: Wisconsin Psychiatric Institute).
Klein, M.H., Mathieu-Coughlan, P. & Kiesler, D.J. (1986), 'The Experiencing Scales' in *The Psychotherapeutic Process: A Research Handbook*, pp. 21–71.
Lambert, M.J., & Hill, C.E. (1994), 'Assessing psychotherapy outcomes and processes', in A. E. Bergin & S. L. Garfield (Eds.), *Handbook of Psychotherapy and Behavior Change*, p. 94 (New York: John Wiley & Sons, Inc.).
Lee, Robert (April 2007), '12 Avenues into Felt Sensing', Handout for workshops Available at www.focusingnow.com.
Lutgendorf, S.K., Antoni, M.H., Kumar, M. & Schneiderman, N. (1994), 'Changes in cognitive coping strategies predict EBV-antibody titre change following a stressor disclosure induction', *Journal of Psychosomatic Research*, **38**, pp. 63–78.
Miyaki, Maki (2008), 'Revising the Experiencing Scale', *Staying in Focus*, **VIII** (3); (New York: The Focusing Institute), pp. 3 & 5.
Morikawa, Y. (1997), 'Making practical the focusing manner of experiencing in everyday life: A consideration of factor analysis', *The Journal of Japanese Clinical Psychology*, **15** (1), pp. 58–65.
Oberhoff, R. (1990), 'The role of attention in experiential focusing', *Dissertation Abstracts International* (University Microfilms No. 9105629).
Perl, Sondra (2004), *Felt Sense: Writing with the Body* (Portsmith, NH: Boynton/Cook Publishers).
Perl, Sondra (no date), in *A Community of Writers: A Workshop Course in Writing* by Peter Elbow and Pat Belanoff, pp. 118–20, 124, 126–28.
Sachse, R (1990), 'Concrete interventions are crucial: The influence of the therapist's processing proposals on the client's intrapersonal exploration in client-centered therapy', in *Client-Centered and Experiential Psychotherapy in the Nineties*, pp. 295–308, (Leuven: Leuven University Press).
Tamura, R. (1987), 'Floatability: A focuser variable related to success in focusing', *The Japanese Journal of Humanistic Psychology*, **5**, pp. 83–87.

Tamura, R. (1990), 'The interrelation between the focuser-listener relationship and the focuser's floatability during focusing', *The Journal of Japanese Clinical Psychology*, **8** (1), pp. 16–25.

Witkin, H.A., Dyk, R.B., Patterson, H.F., Goodenough, D.R. & Karp.S. A. (1962), *Psychological Differentiation* (New York: John Wiley & Sons).

Zimring, F. (1990), 'Cognitive processes as a cause of psychotherapeutic change: self-initiated processes', in G. Lietaer, J. Rombauts, & R. Van Balen (Eds.), *Client-Centered and Experiential Psychotherapy in the Nineties*, pp. 361–80 (Leuven: Leuven University Press).

Zimring, F.M. & Balcombe, J. (1974), 'Cognitive operations in two measures of handling emotionally relevant material', *Psychotherapy: Theory, Research and Practice*, **11**(3), pp. 226–28.

Russell T. Hurlburt

Iteratively Apprehending Pristine Experience

Abstract: *Pristine experience is inner experience that is directly ongoing before it is disturbed by any attempt at apprehension; we live our lives immersed in our pristine experiences. I argue that an iterative method — one that successively approximates the desired result — facilitates the faithful apprehension of pristine experience. There are four main aspects of an iterative method: the refreshment by new experience; the improvement of the observations; the multiple perspectives on experience; and (perhaps most importantly) the open-beginningedness of the process. Because an iterative exploration of experience is open-beginninged, first interviews occupy a unique position in an iterative method. I comment on the transcript of a first interview, showing why and how an iterative procedure is desirable, if not necessary.*

Keywords:

Pristine experience, iterative method, inner experience, open-beginninged, Descriptive Experience Sampling, introspection, bracketing presuppositions

> *If a man will begin with certainties, he shall end in doubts, but if he will be content to begin with doubts, he shall end in certainties.*
>
> — Francis Bacon

This paper urges the advantages of using an iterative procedure faithfully to apprehend inner experience. Iterative procedures are common elsewhere: for example, preparing a series of drafts of a paper for publication, each draft an incremental improvement on the previous, is a widely accepted iterative procedure. Hurlburt and Akhter (2006) briefly discussed the desirability of iteration as a feature of Descriptive Experience Sampling; now I amplify and generalize that discussion.

Preliminary

By *inner experience* I mean anything that is 'directly present to' a person, anything that a person is 'directly aware' or '(reflexively) conscious' of, anything that is 'directly before the footlights of consciousness' at some given moment: thoughts, feelings, perceptions, tickles, seeings, and so on. I use the adjective *inner* to distinguish inner experience from other uses of the term experience (for example, a sentence such as 'I have 35 years experience exploring experience' is made much clearer by writing, 'I have 35 years experience exploring *inner* experience'), but I emphasize that my usage of inner experience includes perceptions of the external world, so long as they are directly before the footlights of consciousness. Some would prefer the term *conscious experience*, or *lived experience*, or merely *experience*. Hurlburt and Schwitzgebel (2007, p. 15) discussed the merits of these terms, concluding that there was no ideal. In this article, for the reasons described in Hurlburt & Schwitzgebel (2007), I will often use *experience* as a synonym for the more formal *inner experience*.

By *pristine* experience (Hurlburt & Akhter, 2006) we mean naturally occurring experience (or, more formally, inner experience) that is directly ongoing before it is disturbed by any attempt at apprehension or introspection. You go about your everyday life bathed in a stream of pristine experiences. We use 'pristine' in the same sense as we would say a forest is pristine—before the loggers clear-cut, before the Park Service installs the walkways and the signage, before the visitors leave their plastic bags and bottles. Pristine does not necessarily mean 'clean' or 'tranquil'; much of a pristine forest is mucky, bloody, brutal, and so on. A pristine forest is a forest as it freely existed before civilization altered it. Pristine experience is experience as it freely exists before it is altered by the act of trying to apprehend it.

It can be argued that pristine experience doesn't exist, but while such thoroughgoing skepticism is impossible to refute, it is hard to accept in the face of so much natural evidence (Hurlburt & Schwitzgebel, 2007). This paper accepts the existence of pristine experience and accepts that it may be desirable, useful, or interesting, at least in some circumstances, to apprehend it; that my pristine experience at one moment may be different from that at another; that the characteristics of my pristine experience may be different from the characteristics of yours (those arguments can be found in Hurlburt & Akhter, 2006; Hurlburt & Heavey, 2006; Hurlburt & Schwitzgebel, 2007). Our purpose here is therefore not to focus on pristine experience itself but on its *faithful apprehension*.

I use the term *apprehend* in two ways: the subject apprehends her own experience, and the interviewer apprehends the subject's experience. The subject's apprehension corresponds to Merriam-Webster's second definition of *apprehend*: 'to become aware of; perceive.' The subject apprehends by becoming aware of evanescent experience long enough to register or observe it. I prefer the term *apprehension* to *introspection* because introspection has a seeing-within connotation whereas apprehension more inclusively accepts that pristine experience may be sometimes seen, sometimes felt, sometimes heard, and so on, as well as being sometimes within and sometimes outside. The interviewer's apprehension corresponds to Merriam-Webster's third definition: 'to grasp with understanding.' The interviewer apprehends by understanding what the subject says about her experience, attempting to separate what is likely to be mistaken or distorted from what is likely to be a faithful account of the subject's experience. This paper is primarily concerned with the interviewer's apprehension; the subject's apprehension is a necessary intermediate step.

I accept that pristine experience may never be apprehended accurately by either subject or interviewer. *Accurate* means conforming exactly, and exact conformance is an unattainably (nirvana excepted) high standard: experience is always disturbed at least somewhat by the act of apprehending, and experience that is multi-dimensional or rich may be too complex to be apprehended in all its detail. We can aim at accurately apprehending pristine experience, but we will always fall short.

This paper is therefore about the *faithful* apprehension of experience rather than the unattainable ideal *accurate* apprehension of experience. By *faithful* I mean 'with fidelity'. Faithful implies unswerving adherence, not perfection; a *faithful* copy, for example, does not imply an exact copy but does imply adherence to the original in important ways. Whereas it is impossible to apprehend a complexly rich experience accurately, it may well be possible to apprehend it faithfully. A faithful apprehension will reflect the more important aspects of a rich experience while perhaps overlooking or distorting some minor details.

I accept that there are more and less faithful apprehensions of experience, just as there are higher and lower fidelity recordings of music.

There is, currently, no established measure of the fidelity of apprehension, in either the science of experience or music. But compare a Jascha Heifetz 1910 recording with a Heifetz 1970 recording and there will be no argument that the 1970 is of higher fidelity, but not as high as a modern recording. I therefore accept that, at least in broad strokes, we are acquainted with the notion of higher fidelity.

I use observe and observation the way those terms are frequently used in science: to apprehend carefully especially with attention to details. An observation here is an apprehension readied for scientific examination. Thus when I say that a subject observes her experience, I mean that she carefully apprehends her experience with the intention of describing it faithfully. I do not mean to imply that experience is separate from the experiencer, that experience can be observed as if it were an external object simply by turning one's attention inside.

This paper assumes that, currently, if a person (the 'interviewer') is to apprehend the inner experience of another person (the 'subject'), the privacy of inner experience requires that the subject will have to convey that experience in an 'interview.' If in the future it becomes possible to apprehend experience directly, this paper will become moot. 'Interviewer,' 'subject,' and 'interview' are intended to be construed broadly; an interview might, for example, include words, gestures, drawings, dancings, and so on.

I use *iterative* in the same way a mathematician uses it: a series of successive approximations leading to a satisfactorily close approximate solution. Suppose a mathematician uses an iterative method to determine the value of x when $f(x) = F$. She guesses an initial value x_1 and determines $f(x_1)$. If $f(x_1)$ is satisfactorily close to F, then she's done: x_1 is the desired solution. Otherwise, she uses this new information ($f(x_1)$) to make a second guess x_2 and then determines $f(x_2)$. If $f(x_2)$ is satisfactorily close to F, then she's done: x_2 is the desired solution. Otherwise she uses this new information ($f(x_2)$) to make a third guess x_3. If all goes well, x_{n+1} is a better guess than was x_n (that is, $f(x_{n+1})$ is closer to F than was $f(x_n)$), and eventually $f(x_m)$ will be close enough to F to consider x_m a satisfactory solution. Iteration is therefore not merely repetition; it requires refinement at each step. Iteration does not produce an exact result; it produces a satisfactory approximation.

This paper argues that an iterative process can lead to a more faithful apprehension of pristine experience. We begin by discussing the apprehension of pristine experience in a single interview and then across a series of iterative interviews. Then we examine a concrete example of the first interview in an iterative series.

A Single Interview

Suppose that at time *t* the subject undergoes a pristine experience, and at some later time a highly skilled interviewer attempts to apprehend that experience. The model shown in Figure 1 illustrates that the interviewer's initial apprehension of the subject's experience will arise partially from the pristine experience as conveyed by the subject (e.g., 'At time *t* I felt...'), but also from four other sources: 1. the subject's presuppositions (e.g., 'I *always* feel...,' '*Everyone* always feels...,' 'I presume you want to know how I felt...'); 2. the interviewer's own presuppositions (about the content that the subject begins to describe, about the subject, about the mask that the interviewer wants to display to the subject, about the interview process, etc.); 3. miscommunication (lack of vocabulary, failure of the interviewer to understand the subject's terminology, lack of understanding of the task, distraction, etc.); and 4. reconstructions that the subject has used to recall or otherwise reinvoke the pristine experience between time *t* and the interview. The first three of those (subject's and interviewer's presuppositions and miscommunication) are non-experiential impediments to the faithful apprehension of the pristine experience; the fourth (reconstruction) is an experience (or a series of experiences) that occurs at a time removed from the original pristine experience.

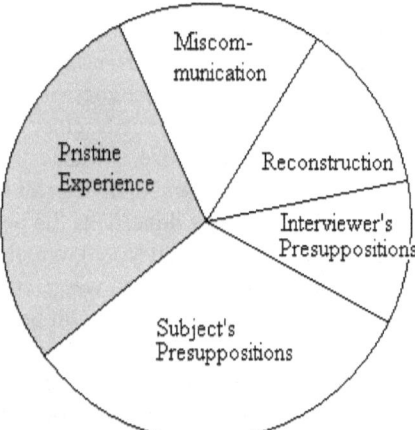

Beginning of Interview

Figure 1: Contributions to the interviewer's apprehension of the subject's experience at the beginning of the interview

There may well be other ways to slice this apprehensional pie. I use the pie-chart format only for its heuristic value; I don't presume to know the actual sizes of the slices in this pie; it is primarily the *change* in size of the slices within and across interviews that I wish to discuss. Figure 1 illustrates a highly skilled interviewer: the interviewer's presuppositions are shown to have a relatively small effect on apprehension.

Now suppose that over the course of the interview the interviewer attempts to refine his or her apprehension of the pristine experience. Clarifications will be requested (e.g., 'What did you mean when you said you felt...'), attempts to bracket presuppositions will be made ('Yes, I understand that you may *usually* feel..., but at time *t* did you....'), and so on. In responding to these requests, the subject will likely attempt, repeatedly, to reconstruct the original experience, either spontaneously or by explicit instruction (e.g., Petitmengin, 2006). Let's suppose that this interview is skillful, careful, and extensive, lasting, say, 15 minutes or an hour. Figure 2 illustrates the contributors to the interviewer's apprehension at the *end* of the interview.

If the interviewer is skilled, the influence of the non-experiential impediments can be reduced: some presuppositions of both subject and interviewer can be exposed and bracketed (Hurlburt & Heavey, 2006) and terminology can be refined and aligned. Figure 2 shows,

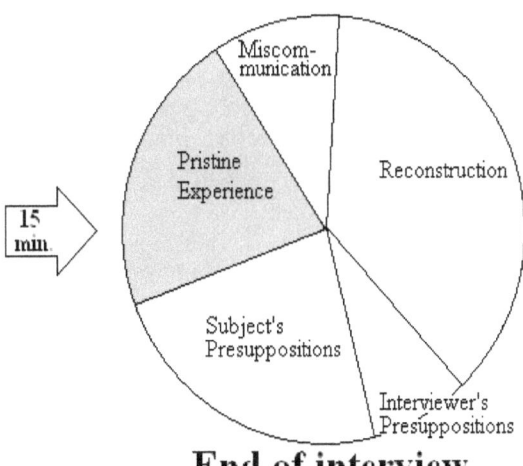

Figure 2: Contributions to the interviewer's apprehension at the end of the interview

therefore, that the relative contribution of those three aspects to the interviewer's apprehensions has been reduced compared to the beginning of the interview (Figure 1).

On the other hand, the interviewer's probing questions strongly encourage (explicitly or implicitly) the subject to try to reconstruct the pristine experience during the interview; the reconstruction slice is therefore substantially larger in Figure 2. The longer and the more intensive the interview, the more reconstructions.

The proportion that the original pristine experience contributes to the interviewer's apprehension is likely to be *less* at the end of the interview than at the beginning, because of the difficulty extricating the pristine experience from the reconstructions thereof. It is possible that the contribution of pristine experience will increase, but only if the reduction of presuppositions outweighs the effect of reconstruction.

Iterative Interviews

The preceding section concluded that the direct contribution of pristine experience to an interviewer's apprehension is likely to *decrease* across one interview as the reconstructed experiences increase. I now argue that an iterative series of interviews can increase the direct contribution of pristine experience and decrease (but not eliminate completely) the reliance on reconstruction.

There are four main aspects of an iterative method, all of which can contribute to the faithful apprehension of experience: 1. the refreshment by new experience; 2. the improvement of the apprehensions; 3. the multiple perspectives on experience; and (perhaps most importantly) 4. the open-beginningedness of the process. I will discuss these as separate aspects, but they are, in practice, synergistically interrelated.

Refreshment by new experience

Suppose that the interview illustrated in Figures 1 and 2 is the first in an iterative series of interviews. The second interview is illustrated in Figure 3. At some time after the first interview, the same subject undergoes a new pristine experience and is interviewed about it by the same interviewer. This is a fresh start. The pristine experience to be discussed in this second interview is not merely one more reconstructed experience overlaid onto the same original pristine experience — the new occurrence of a new pristine experience has the potential to refresh the entire process from the beginning.

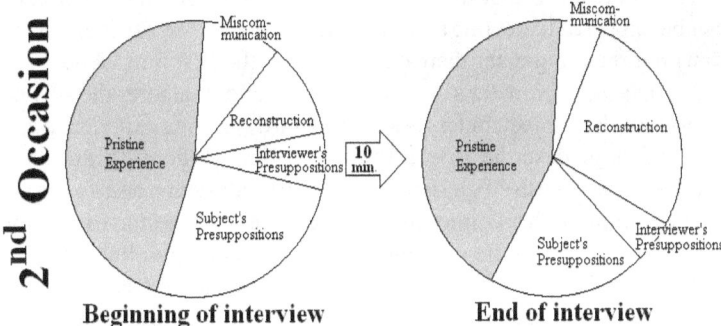

Figure 3: Contributions to the interviewer's apprehension at the beginning and end of the second interview

The sources of the interviewer's apprehension of the subject's experience at the beginning of the second interview are illustrated in the left side of Figure 3. Whatever progress was made during the first interview in reducing the non-experiential impediments (bracketing the influences of the subject's and interviewer's presuppositions, clarifying communication) is likely to be at least to some degree maintained. Thus these three slices are shown to be roughly the same at the beginning of the second interview as they were at the *end* of the first interview (Figure 2). The necessity for reconstruction between the new pristine experience and the second interview should be no greater than between the first pristine experience and the *beginning* of the first interview (the reconstruction slice in the left side of Figure 3 is about the same as in Figure 1). The result is that the relative contribution of the new pristine experience at the beginning of the second interview is greater than it was at the beginning of the original interview.

The right-hand side of Figure 3 illustrates the end of the second interview. The second interview is likely to be more efficient and probably shorter (let's say '10 minutes' instead of '15 minutes') because of the progress made in bracketing-presuppositions and communication—no need to do that again. Reconstruction still occurs during the second interview, but because the interview is shorter, it is likely that there will be fewer reconstructed experiences than in the first interview. The second interview may make further progress on bracketing presuppositions and clarifying communication.

The net result is that the direct contribution of pristine experience can be expected to decline across the second interview (as it did in the first) but remain greater than at any point in the first interview.

N^{th} occasion. Now let's suppose that at some time after the second interview, the subject undergoes a new (third) pristine experience and undertakes to describe it in a third interview (Figure 4), and then another new (fourth) experience and fourth interview, and so on. At the beginning of the nth interview, the relative contribution of pristine experience is the whole pie minus the non-experiential impediments (presuppositions and miscommunication) minus the reconstructed experience. The sizes of the non-experiential impediment slices at the beginning of the nth interview are likely to be roughly the same as those at the *end* of the $(n-1)^{st}$ interview, because the progress participants made in the $(n-1)^{st}$ interview is likely to be maintained. However, the size of the reconstruction slice is similar to that at the *beginning* of the $(n-1)^{st}$ interview, because each interview starts fresh with a new pristine experience. (Actually, the size of reconstruction slice may lessen across occasions; see below.)

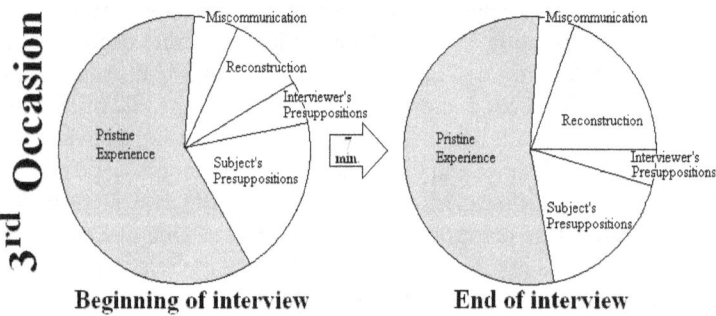

Figure 4: Contributions to the interviewer's apprehension at the beginning and end of the 3rd interview

To the extent that genuine progress is made in the bracketing of the subject's and/or the interviewer's presuppositions and/or the clarifying of communication, the relative contribution of the pristine experience at step n will be greater than at step $(n-1)$. This improvement is made possible by the refreshment of each interview by an always new pristine experience, the starting over and over again with new pristine experience at each step.

To summarize, the direct contribution of pristine experience is likely to *decrease within each interview* because the influence of reconstructions during the interview is likely to outpace the bracketing of presuppositions, even if genuine progress is made in bracketing presuppositions and clarifying communication. However, if genuine progress is made in bracketing presuppositions and clarifying communication, the direct contribution of pristine experience is likely to *increase across interviews* because of the refreshment by the new pristine experience at each step.

I make no claim that the non-experiential impediments can be eliminated completely — presuppositions are stubborn. I therefore do not claim that pristine experience can be apprehended with absolute accuracy. I do claim that genuine skill at bracketing presuppositions can lead, across interviews, to a more and more faithful apprehension of pristine experience.

Improvement of the apprehensions

We have seen that each step in the iterative process can be refreshed by new pristine experience and therefore the relative contribution of pristine experience can increase across interviews. Now we notice that, beyond this increase in contribution, each iterative step can improve the quality of the apprehensions of the pristine experience themselves. That is, not only can the pristine experience slice of the pie increase in size, the slice itself can become of higher quality, for six main reasons: 1. practice may refine the observational skill; 2. practice may improve interview skill; 3. iteration allows the synergy of refining observation and improving interviews; 4. iteration may make the observer more prepared to observe; 5. iteration may lessen the need for reconstructions; and 6. iteration may improve the fidelity of reconstructions.

Practice in observing. Any subject's first observation of a pristine experience is likely to be of low quality: the subject doesn't skillfully know what experience is and what it is not, doesn't skillfully know the difference between observation and theorizing, doesn't have an appreciation or skills for holding presuppositions at bay, and so on. The first interview, skillfully conducted, may incrementally improve some or all of those skills, allowing the subject to become more skillful at the time of the second observation. This incremental refinement of observational skill may obtain at each occasion.

Practice in being interviewed. Because the subject has little practice in carefully describing inner experience, the first interview is itself likely to be quite rudimentary, making only relatively crude distinctions about what was and was not apprehended and crude characterizations of the pristine experience. At each subsequent occasion, those distinctions and characterizations can become incrementally refined.

Synergy of observation and interview. Not only may practice improve observation skills and interview skills, the improvement in those skills interact synergistically. If the nth interview provides an incremental improvement in the skill of bracketing presuppositions about experience, that bracketing skill may carry over to the $(n + 1)^{st}$ *observation* of pristine experience. Presuppositions blind, amplify, or otherwise distort, and to the extent that subjects learned to bracket them in the first interview, the second observation may be less distorted. But the $(n + 1)^{st}$ observation serves as the starting point for the $(n + 1)^{st}$ interview, and the improved quality of that observation can lead to an improved ability of the *interview* to focus more directly on the characteristics of the subject's own particular experiences, more able to bracket the subject's own particular presuppositions. That can make the $(n + 1)^{st}$ interview more effective than was the nth interview, not merely because of the practice effect but because the improved observational input. This improvement in the $(n + 1)^{st}$ interview can lead to an improved quality of the $(n + 2)^{nd}$ observation, which can lead to a better $(n + 2)^{nd}$ interview, which can lead to an improved quality of the $(n + 3)^{rd}$ observation, and so on.

Readiness to observe. Pristine experience always comes 'out of the blue,' is unanticipated, more or less surprising. The practice gained in early observations and early interviews may help the observer become more prepared, more poised, more ready to observe a subsequent pristine experience when it occurs. As a result, the subject may well be quicker and more effective at apprehending the subsequent pristine experiences. This increased readiness to observe is separable from the skill of observation in the same way that a news photographer's learning to carry a camera that is prepared (what lens is likely to be useful here? what film?) is separable from skill of composing the photograph. The skilled photographer's readiness makes her more likely to be able to deploy her composition skill when the emergent situation occurs.

Lessening reconstructions. The subject acquires, over the course of the iterative interviews, an understanding of the kinds of questions the interviewer might ask, the kinds of features experience might have, and so on. As a result, the subject becomes more and more able, *at the time of the occurrence of the pristine experience*, to make contemporaneous observations that require less and less reconstruction. Thus the reconstruction slice of the pie may decrease across interviews.

Improvement of reconstructions. The sixth aspect of the subjects' successive skill acquisition is that subjects may iteratively learn the skill of conforming their reconstructions more and more closely to their pristine experiences. Reconstructing experience is a skill like any other skill, and the practice of that skill can lead to improvement (e.g., learning how to take better contemporaneous notes about the experience, and how to refer to those notes effectively when reconstructing). If the reconstructions are more faithful, then apprehensions (which rest on both the original pristine experience and reconstructed experience) may mirror pristine experience with higher fidelity.

But not necessarily. The foregoing has assumed a skilled interviewer; in particular, it has assumed that the interviewer is effective at bracketing his own and helping the subject bracket her presuppositions. Without such skill, iteration can lead to the *amplification* of presuppositions: the subject or the interviewer may start to develop a theory about the subject's experience based on early observations, and that theory then can inform and distort future reports. If presuppositions increase, fidelity of apprehension of pristine experience decreases.

Multiple perspectives on experience

Pristine experience at any moment is determined by the characteristics of the subject, by the features of the environment, and many other factors. Suppose a subject describes her pristine experience on a series of occasions. On the first occasion her pristine experience is $X + A$; at the second occasion her pristine experience is $X + B$; at the third occasion her pristine experience is $X + C$; and so on. X could be said to be a salient feature of the subject's experience. For example, on the first occasion, Sally is simultaneously smelling pizza and recalling a scene from *Schindler's List*; on the second occasion she is smelling the sea breeze and worrying about the stock market; the third occasion she is smelling the dog's fur and contemplating a move in chess.

There are two ways that an iterative method aids in the faithful apprehension of X. First, at the outset, neither the interviewer nor the subject needs to know that X even *exists*, much less that it is a salient feature of experience, and even less what are the essential features of X (Sally needn't know, prior to the interviews, that she frequently pays attention to smells in the environment). If X is a salient feature of the subject's experience, it will *emerge* from a series of careful examinations of pristine experience. On the first occasion, the recollection of *Schindler's List* was no more and no less an important feature of Sally's pristine experience than was the smelling of pizza. But *across occasions*, X (the smelling) occurs again and again, and will therefore be naturally recognized as salient, whereas the nonrecurring features (*Schindler's List*, stock market, chess) will therefore naturally be recognized as incidental and not salient. Thus the multiply refreshed instances of pristine experience allow the more central features to emerge, unbidden, as salient.

Second, each fresh encounter with pristine experience is a view from a somewhat different direction, highlighting experience from a new perspective on each occasion. The first occasion highlights smelling from the concrete perspective of *pizza*; the second highlights smelling from the concretely different perspective of *the sea breeze*; the third highlights smelling from the yet again concretely different perspective of *fur*. The features of the experience of smelling can be discovered by triangulating from the several vantage points.

Thus iteration allows both for the emergence of salient phenomena and for the elaboration of phenomena once they emerge. Both those characteristics taken together can, across occasions, allow a greater clarity of apprehension of the central features of pristine experience.

Open-beginninged probes

Presuppositions about experience are a primary, if not *the* primary, impediment to faithful apprehension of experience (Hurlburt & Heavey, 2006). Presuppositions can be held by the subject or by the interviewer (or, worse, both), and they blind or otherwise distort the apprehension of experience.

One of the most insidious but frequent presuppositions is the presumption that people have the kind of experience that the interviewer seeks. Interviewers interested in images, for example, frequently ask subjects to form an image and then to answer questions about it, without leaving adequate space for the possibility that the subject never actually formed an image. That procedure can have very negative consequences for an investigation: the results are an inextricable aggregate of responses by those subjects who have images and those who don't have images but answer the questions anyway.

There is an alternative: Use only open-beginninged probes (Hurlburt & Heavey, 2006, ch. 8; Hurlburt & Schwitzgebel, 2007) about experience.

Open-*ended* probes are 'designed to permit spontaneous and unguided responses' (Merriam-Webster), but it is only the *end* of the response that is 'spontaneous and unguided' — the beginning is entirely specified by the probe. 'Tell me about your image' is an open-*ended* probe, but it nearly always produces talk that *begins* 'My image was…,' even in subjects who do not create images in such situations. Such talk may be a plausible characterization of 'my imagery' that has nothing at all to do with my experience.

An open-*beginninged* probe is one that leaves *both* the beginning and the end of the response spontaneous and unguided. There is, as far as I know, only one open-beginninged question about experience: 'What, if anything, was in your experience at the moment?' Hurlburt and Heavey (2006) called this the 'one legitimate question' about experience. But calling this the one legitimate question is not to say that this precise wording is the best or only instantiation. On the contrary, it is desirable to be deliberately inconsistent (Heavey & Hurlburt, 2009; cf. Hurlburt & Schwitzgebel, 2007, p. 15) in the framing of this and other questions and let the iterative process do the work of sharpening the meaning. Deliberate inconsistency means using a variety of versions of this question ('What is your experience at the moment?' 'Right then, what were you aware of?' 'What if anything presented itself before the footlights of consciousness right then?' etc.), each with its own advantages and disadvantages. If those questions aim (each imperfectly) at pristine experience, and pristine experience is a robust phenomenon, then pristine experience will (iteratively) emerge, free from the specific influence of any specific version of the question. If there is not a robust phenomenon, no amount of care in crafting the question will help.

A genuinely open-beginninged probe adumbrates the general arena (experience or lack thereof) but provides no specification of alternatives and no pre-training, because either may limit the potential beginning of a subject's reports. The genuinely open-beginninged probe simultaneously conveys (explicitly or implicitly) all the following: I don't know what are the features of your experience; I don't want to speculate about some potential aspect of your experience because then you may 'go looking for' that aspect; I'm interested in whatever presents itself directly to you, whatever is before the footlights of your consciousness; Maybe there is nothing in your experience; Maybe your experience is different from anything I have previously encountered; I don't know what is in your experience so I can't tell you what to look for; If thinking is in your experience, I'd like us to talk about thinking; But if you're not experiencing thinking, then I don't want to talk about thinking; If you're feeling something I'd like us to talk about that, but if not, not; Same for seeings, tickles, hunger pangs, hearings; I'd like us to talk about whatever you *actually* experience out of the welter of possibilities that you *might* experience; I emphasize that I don't know what you experience; Maybe you will be able to perform this task, maybe you won't — either way is fine with me because I'll probably learn something either way; If you can report your experience, fine, but if you can't, fine as well; Maybe you'll find it easy, maybe you'll find it difficult at first and then it will become easy, maybe you will find it always difficult, maybe you will find it impossible — any of that is OK with me; I'm sincerely interested in your experience, whatever that is, including nothing; I'm interested in our talking honestly about your experience, including that this task is difficult or impossible if that's the way it is; Some people can do it easily, some find it difficult or impossible, and either is OK with me; Perhaps together we will be able to apprehend faithfully your experience, and if so, that would be good; But if not, that would be good, too; I want you to observe your experience; I don't want you to guess about it, or theorize about it; I want you to describe exactly what you directly observe; I don't want you to explain it or speculate about it.

(And if that is genuine, of course, there can be no hint of 'I'm really interested in images, so let's talk about images'; no hint of 'I need to get a publication out of this'; no hint of promotion, tenure, or merit considerations; no hint of 'I don't have time'.)

Obviously an interviewer can't say all that at once — it would overwhelm. But an interviewer can consistently convey that every time, and eventually, across occasions, *iteratively*, the subject will get the message: The interviewer really does want to hear about the details of my experience, whatever those details happen to be or not be. But that can happen only if the investigation is genuinely open-beginninged. Sooner or later, any un-genuineness will bleed through.

Open-beginning probes are designed to be nebulous and ambiguous, designed to create a level playing field when approached from any direction, thus allowing subjects to penetrate their own experience on their own terms. Any other approach favors one thing over other things and therefore distorts the process. In some ways an open-beginninged probe is similar to applying gesso to a canvas prior to painting. The gesso has no relationship at all to what you will paint; you don't plan, at the end of the painting, to see the gesso; applying the gesso is a temporal distraction, seems to waste time you'd rather spend painting. But the gesso, once applied, allows your artistry to flourish: the oil doesn't bleed into the canvas, the colors stay purer, the imperfections of the cloth disappear, and so on.

Even if the interviewer's probes are genuinely open-beginninged, the subject will likely not initially believe them to be open-beginninged. The investigation operates in a context of psychological and philosophical studies, almost all of which are manipulative and goal-verification oriented, if not downright deceptive. There is little historical context for the genuine appreciation or apprehension of pristine experience. It is naïve to expect that a one-shot open-beginninged conveyance, no matter how sincere or eloquent, can overcome that context. A series of open-beginninged probes delivered in an arena where the subject can test the intention and veracity of the interviewer *for him- or herself* may be able to overcome the context, but that can happen only across occasions.

Pre-training about what might be observed is inimical. Asking open-beginninged questions is an inefficient approach — as inefficient as possible, one might say. But if the aim is a faithful apprehension of experience, there is, as far as I have been able to see, no alternative, because pre-training about potential observations is *inimical* to the faithful apprehension of pristine experience. Because pre-training takes place before concrete observations have been made, pre-training must be about abstract concepts: pre-training defines a concept, teaches how to recognize that concept, teaches what to do about that concept. But *concepts are not experiences*. If the object is to apprehend pristine experience, then non-experiential aspects are to be avoided. It is often useful, after the fact, to determine whether some particular pristine experience can be considered an instance of a concept, but the order must be to apprehend pristine experience first and to make abstract determination second. Otherwise the concept pollutes the experience.

For example, Hurlburt, Heavey, and Bensaheb (this issue) describe the concept of sensory awareness, saying that it is a frequently occurring characteristic of inner experience that is usually overlooked by subjects and interviewers. But Hurlburt, Heavey, and Bensaheb *should not* (and in fact did not) pre-train subjects about the potential existence and characteristics of sensory awareness; subjects' descriptions of sensory awareness emerged unbidden.

Suppose you pre-train subjects on the characteristics of sensory awareness (or some other aspect of experience) and then ask them to apprehend their pristine experience. To the extent that subjects paid attention to and were impacted by the pre-training, the pre-training will have three undesirable effects: (a) distraction, (b) selective sensitization, and (c) leading. (a) Distraction: When they should be engaged in the direct observation-of-pristine-experience task, they will instead (at least in part) be engaged in a conceptual task: they will be rehearsing the definition of sensory awareness, recalling what was said in the pre-training about sensory awareness, and so on. That conceptual focus distracts from, if not obliterates entirely, the direct observation of pristine experience. (b) Selective sensitization: Subjects will approach the apprehending-pristine-experience task sensitized to the possibility of sensory awareness, and therefore selectively *de*sensitized to other potential aspects of experience. The attempt at apprehending pristine experience is no longer a level playing field but is tilted in the direction of sensory awareness and away from other potential aspects. (c) Leading. Any report that the subject provides that sounds like sensory awareness is now quite possibly the result of having been led to sensory awareness by the (explicit or implied) pre-training suggestion of the interviewer.

Suppose a subject says: 'I was driving. I know this sounds weird, but I wasn't paying any attention at all to my driving. My entire focus was on the particular yellow color of the yellow line; it was like I was drawn to the color of it. I guess my driving was happening on auto-pilot.' If this was given as a 'free-range' report, that is, by a subject who has *not* been pre-trained about sensory awareness, and particularly because it was advanced with some misgivings ('sounds weird'), this apprehension of pristine experience is quite believable. But if the subject had been pre-trained in sensory awareness, instructed that sometimes people are 'immersed in the experience of a particular sensory aspect of his or her external or internal environment without particular regard for the instrumental aim or perceptual objectness' (Hurlburt *et al.*, 2009 this issue), then the same report may well be merely a reflection of the training. As a result, pre-training should *increase* the skepticism about the possibility of apprehending pristine experience. This pre-training dilemma presents itself not only for sensory awareness but for *all* features of experience. Every pre-training reifies some presupposition about what will or won't be found in experience. It is impossible to provide pre-training that keeps a level playing field for reports of all sorts of inner experience.

An open-beginninged probe avoids that dilemma. If sensory awareness is indeed a characteristic of a subject's inner experience, it will emerge from a series of pristine experiences faithfully apprehended even if (or especially if) no pre-training has been given (it will become the X of the 'Multiple Perspectives on Experience' section above). The price for reducing the dilemma is the inefficiency and discomfort

— open-beginningedness often is initially uncomfortable for both subject and interviewer because it involves genuinely acknowledging ignorance.

Fortunately, in our Descriptive Experience Sampling studies (see below), we have found that the open-beginninged approach is not as inefficient as it might appear. Most people apparently can, within two or three interviews, become adequately skillful in apprehending their experience. In fact, what appears to be an inefficient procedure may be not only the most direct path, but perhaps the only path to faithful apprehension.

Open-beginningedness is inextricably related to an iterative process. It's likely to be a waste to ask an open-beginninged question in a single interview: it requires one occasion to clarify what the beginning might be, and then another occasion to reap the benefits of that clarification. And it's likely to be a waste to conduct an iterative process that is not open-beginninged; the improvements brought about by iteration will then be built on a substantially impure foundation.

Synergistically interrelated

For analytical purposes, I have separated out refreshment by new experience, improvement of the apprehensions, triangulation of the observations, and the open-beginninged process, but these are all synergistically interrelated. Refreshment by new experience results in improvement of the apprehensions; but improvement of the apprehensions also increases the refreshingness of new experience. Refreshment by the new experience is what makes an open-beginninged process possible, but the open-beginning process improves the observations, which increases the refreshingness of the new experience. And so on. All these features work in concert to potentiate each other and may lead to the high fidelity apprehension of pristine experience.

A First Interview

First interviews occupy a unique position in an iterative (and therefore open-beginninged) investigation: they have to start nowhere, say nothing, and head some unknown where — head with as little interference as possible in the direction of some yet to be discovered experience. I now comment on a word-for-word transcript of the beginning of a typical first Descriptive Experience Sampling (DES; Hurlburt, 1990, 1993, 1997; Hurlburt & Akhter, 2006; Hurlburt & Heavey, 2006; Hurlburt & Schwitzgebel, 2007) interview. I use DES as an example because (a) it is the method with which I have the most practice and (b) DES is designed to be a fully iterative method.

This interview was conducted by Nellie Mihelic (a graduate student training in the DES method, called NM in the transcript) and me (RTH) with 'Joshua Thomas' (JT), a subject who was recruited as a guinea pig for Nellie's DES training. Prior to the interview, we knew nothing about Joshua other than that he was a student in an introductory psychology class who volunteered for this study as a course requirement. Prior to this interview, Joshua had been given a random beeper and given a 45-minute instruction in DES (see Hurlburt & Heavey, 2006, Ch. 6, for typical instructions): he was to wear the beeper in his everyday natural environments until it beeped six times; at each random beep he was to pay attention to the experience that was ongoing at the last undisturbed moment before the beep began and then, immediately, to jot down notes about his experience in a notebook that we provided. The first beep occurred on September 21 at 2:14:38 pm. The first interview (the following morning) was videotaped for training purposes; we join the interview 30 seconds into the recording, during which time the camcorder was set up and adjusted, small talk exchanged, and so on. We superscript each conversational turn for ease of reference.

[0:30]

Nellie Mihelic:[1] Joshua, when did you collect your beeps?

Joshua Thomas:[2] Yesterday between about 2:30 and 5:30 or 6.

NM:[3]   And did you collect all six?

JT:[4]   Yes. Except for the last one. I kind of rushed it. I pretended there was a beep. I just want to be honest.

NM:[5]   [inaudible] OK. And the other, the first five, they were all beeps?

JT:[6]   Um hm.

NM:[7]   OK.

JT:[8]   I don't know if that ruins anything for you guys, but...

[1:00]

RTH:[9]   Well, let's see when we get there.

JT:[10]   Alright. [laughs]

Subjects do not follow one-shot instructions

In JT's instruction session, which had lasted about 45 minutes, we had emphasized, re-emphasized, given verbal descriptions, used visual aids, and employed metaphors all aimed at raising JT's appreciation for the importance of the exact moment of the beep. That instruction was delivered with substantial skill and sensitivity to JT's level of understanding. Despite that effort, he still simulated a beep. This kind of imperviousness to instruction is not peculiar to JT; most subjects have preconceived notions about what is important to a study and what is not, and pre-training has difficulty penetrating those preconceptions.

This failure to follow instructions is not the result of naiveté. To the contrary, very sophisticated DES subjects (consciousness scientists, for example) often fail to follow important basic instructions. One basic reason that iterative training is necessary is that subjects often don't follow the instructions given on one occasion.

Note that at RTH[9] I don't say it's OK to pretend a beep (which it is not; Hurlburt & Heavey, 2006), but I also don't say that it is not OK. JT has just demonstrated (by allowing himself to pretend the beep in the first place) that he is currently incapable of understanding why such a pretending is not OK. I'm confident that this understanding will naturally arise in him later in the interview when he discovers the difference in his ability to describe a beeped experience and a non-beeped experience. Thus the iterative nature of DES allows his failure to follow instructions to be a valuable training experience *for the next occasion*.

That JT volunteered his pretending augurs well for the future: it demonstrates that he is motivated (even though he is currently failing) to apprehend his experience faithfully.

NM:[11]   Well, why don't you tell us what was in your experience at beep 1.

JT:[12]   Beep 1. [pause] Ah, well, I guess I could tell you what was happening right before. I was actually learning how to drive stick shift and I had the earpiece in my ear and then I just got out of the car 'cause the cops pulled up, and like 'What are you doin?' And my friend said, 'Well, I'm teaching him how to drive stick.' So I got out of the car and I was thinking, 'It still hasn't beeped yet' and it beeped. And I was also thinking that, um, I wanted to drive on the street to get some gas for my friend's car.

Subjects (initially) don't know what a moment is

We had, in the initial instructions, tried to convey to JT the 'flashbulb' brevity of a moment, but JT, like most subjects, didn't grasp that and refers instead to a whole series of moments: the cops pulling up; the cops asking 'What are you doin?'; the friend's reply; JT's thinking about the beeper; JT's thinking he wants to drive on the street; JT's thinking about getting gas. JT's pristine experience is doubtless quite different from one of those moments to the next. We have found it impossible to convey, before sampling has been attempted, the brevity of a moment as we intend it; an iterative procedure is necessary to refine the subject's initial (mis)understanding of the moment.

[2:00]

NM:[13]   OK. So, I know you gave me some background there, so if you can help me clarify. Right when the beep went off, what was in your experience?

JT:[14]   Um. What do you mean, in my experience? [sounds puzzled] What was I thinking?

Subjects (initially) don't know what experience is

JT's puzzlement is a typical and necessary first step of an open-beginninged iterative procedure. We had said in the initial instructions that experience was anything that is occurring directly before the footlights of his consciousness at the moment of the beep, but that instruction is apparently (and not surprisingly) difficult for him. Evident here is JT's presupposition that *thinking* is the primary feature of experience or the primary goal of the study; sooner or later we will have to disabuse him of that notion.

NM:[15]   Whatever was in your awareness or in your experience right at the moment of the beep. That could be....

JT:[16]   Well, I was standing like right at the hood of my friend's car, and, and then I was just thinking, it still hasn't beeped yet. And I actually said that out loud, too, to my friend, 'cause I had told him about the experiment. And it beeped.

NM:[17]   OK. Um, so the beep came right after you had said, 'It still hasn't beeped yet'?

JT:[18]   [laughs] Yeah, like, pretty much. [laughs]

Subjects (initially) don't know how to describe experience

The JT[18] 'Yeah' seems to be an agreement with Nellie's NM[17] characterization of his experience. But JT[18] is what DES calls a 'subjunctified' response (Hurlburt & Akhter, 2006; Hurlburt & Heavey, 2006; Hurlburt & Schwitzgebel, 2007): the subjunctifiers ('like, pretty much') indicate Nellie's NM[17] summary is probably *not* what actually was ongoing in JT's experience at the moment of the beep, or is at best a loose approximation thereof.

JT's willingness to go along with loose approximations is quite typical of most subjects on their first attempt at describing experience. It requires an iterative procedure to refine JT's understanding that a faithful description requires reporting the specific details, not an approximation.

[3:00]

NM:[19] [laughs] And did you, um, you said that you said that out loud, but then, before, you also said you were thinking it? Was it both? One or the other?

JT:[20] It was both, pretty much. Is that normal? I don't know. [laughs nervously]

Subjects (initially) may be reluctant to describe experience

JT, like nearly all others, has never had the opportunity or occasion to expose his moments of private experience. This makes it likely that he will be reluctant to reveal his private experience on the first day. When he discovers that the interviewers are sensitive and skillful, he will likely drop that reluctance, but that will require more than one occasion.

RTH:[21] Yes. That's normal.

JT:[22] I'm the kind of person that says what they think, usually, so...

Subjects (initially) don't distinguish between apprehension and theorizing

As evidenced by 'I'm the kind of person' and 'usually,' JT[22] is a statement about a theoretical presupposition about himself, *not* a statement about a direct apprehension of his experience. Our aim is to get a faithful apprehension of JT's experience, so eventually, iteratively, we will have to convey to him that we are *not* interested in his self-theorizings.

We had told him that in the pre-training, but that instruction (as expected) was not effective.

RTH:[23] I would like to clear up the 'pretty much' part, because I'm not exactly sure what you mean by that. So, first off, let me get the sequence right. So you had been driving, you stopped driving — did the cops pull you over while you were driving? Or were you ...

JT:[24] Well, we were driving in the Thomas & Mack [a basketball arena] parking lot, it was like a whole empty parking lot, and I had just parked the car and the cop came over. And my window was rolled down, and my friend was in the passenger seat of his car, ...

RTH:[25] But that was all before the beep, and then you....

JT:[26] Um hm. It was all leading up to the beep.

RTH:[27] OK. And then you got out of the car and moved to the front of the car, ...

JT:[28] Yeah.

RTH:[29] ... next to the hood of the car, and then you say out loud [questioningly], 'It still hasn't beeped yet'? You say that to your friend? Or is that, or was that before....

[4:30]

JT:[30] I said that like, I said that out loud, because that was what I was thinking.

RTH:[31] OK. And when you said 'because that was what I was thinking,' are you separately thinking, 'I'm thinking this hasn't beeped yet,' and *then* I say, 'This hasn't beeped yet!' er, [uncertainly] 'Still hasn't beeped yet'?

JT:[32] Yeah.

RTH:[33] And where does the beep come exactly in that sequence, as best you can say?

JT:[34] Like right after I said 'yet' it beeped.

RTH:[35] OK. So the sequence is something like, *thinking* this thing hasn't beeped yet, and then *saying* 'It still hasn't beeped yet,' beep! Is that right?

JT:[36] Yeah. Exactly.

RTH:[37] OK. Cool.

Subjects (initially) don't know what the moment of the beep is

In the initial instruction, we had given JT considerable training about the importance of the moment of the beep. We had stressed that experience was fleeting and momentary, and apprehending experience would therefore require being very careful to note exactly where the beep occurs. But it is clear that that training did not 'take'; we are about three minutes into this interview, pressing to ascertain with some precision where the moment of the beep had occurred in the stream of JT's experience. RTH[35] summarizes, and JT[36] assents, but I'm quite skeptical of the veracity of this summary. JT wasn't prepared, *at the time of the first beep*, to note with precision where in his stream of experiences the beep occurred.

JT is entirely typical in this regard. Regardless of how often we say in the necessarily abstract initial instruction, 'We want to know the exact microsecond of the beep,' only the very rare subject actually understands this.

Now, however, as a result of the concrete conversation RTH[23-37], JT *does* probably have a clear idea of what is meant by 'the moment of the beep' and its importance. He will be far better at observing the precise moment of the beep when he wears the beeper next time. But that is the result of the concretely literal iterative training, not the initial abstract instruction.

Note carefully that even though the conversation RTH[23-37] appears to be my attempt to determine when the beep occurred in the stream of experience that was ongoing at 2:14:38 pm September 21, that is really not my aim. Instead, I am attempting here to improve, iteratively, his ability to apprehend the moment of the beep *on future occasions*. He was not a skilled observer at 2:14:38 pm September 21, and I completely accept that, and so am highly skeptical of his accounts of that experience. It's *tomorrow's* experience that I am primarily interested in here, not *yesterday's*.

> [Here I omit 30 seconds of training conversation between me and Nellie that would distract us from our present purpose.]

RTH:[38] So, so far I've understood you to be saying, I first of all *thought* this thing hasn't beeped yet, and then I *said* it. Now is that really the case? That... Some people would say that what really happened was that it was both at the same time, and some people say, well I just said it so I *must* have been thinking it, so I want to be as explicit about that as we can be.

[5:00]

JT:[39]   Well, OK. In that case it could have been I said it and it must have been what I was thinking.

RTH:[40]   OK. So there's no really separate thought, then? ...

JT:[41]   I don't think so.

RTH:[42]   ... as far as you know at the moment?

JT:[43]   As far as I know.

Subjects (initially) don't bracket presuppositions

All iterative interviews are a balance of backward looking (ascertaining what was in pristine experience on some past occasion) and forward looking (skill building for future occasions). In first interviews, this balance is predominately forward looking iterative improvement; in later interviews, the balance shifts toward the backward-looking data gathering.

Here, my aim is to level the playing field about what I take to be JT's presupposition about a sequence in inner experience: first think, then say. I don't *disbelieve* his report about this sequence; I am *skeptical* about it, and those are two very different things. I would be delighted to discover that his sequence actually is first think, then say. But I would be equally delighted to disabuse him of this presupposition if presupposition it is. So my aim here is forward looking: I raise the question about his presupposition so that the *next* occasion's interview may shed light on it.

Some might object that I am leading JT in the direction of my presuppositional theory about thinking/saying and away from his presupposition, but I disagree. First, I don't have a theory of thinking/saying — I don't care whether there is an experienced thought before an utterance or not. Second, it is JT's own comments, not my presuppositions, that lead me to this speculation about his presupposition. His utterance at JT[22] ('I'm the kind of person that says what they think, usually') is a general statement about something he presumes about himself, not a description of a particular experience; thus this statement was *his* announcement of the potential existence of *his* presupposition. It is my (iterative) obligation to try to level the playing field for JT with respect to his own presuppositions. That is not a presupposition on my part; that is proficiency at hearing JT's actual talk and expertise at helping him improve his faithful observation skills.

Such skill building *must be* iterative, and could not possibly have been performed before JT's participation in this interview, for six reasons: 1. Prior to this interview, we had no way of knowing that JT had (perhaps) this thinking-and-saying presupposition; 2. Even if we had clairvoyantly known about his thinking-and-saying presupposition, a pre-training conversation about it would have had to have been abstract. Now, by contrast, JT has a specific, real-in-his-own-life example of what is meant by a distinction between thinking-and-saying and just saying; 3. He is innately, personally involved in the process: the question stems from his own concrete behavior and his own inability to answer my questions; 4. I have demonstrated that I, as a real individual, am interested in JT's, as a real individual, getting it right about his own experience, demonstrated that I am willing to work at it; demonstrated that I have some skill in this regard. He can't just blow it off as mere boilerplate about the quality of science; 5. Had I tried to make this distinction in the abstract before it raised itself in JT's own samples, it would have focused JT on abstractions, not on the attempt to be faithful to his own experience; and 6. presuppositions are mini-delusions, and attempting to argue someone out of his delusions is generally futile.

> [Here I omit 30 seconds of training conversation between me and Nellie that would distract us from our present purpose.]

RTH:[44] So you're standing at the hood of the car, the cops are around....

JT:[45] The cops had left.

RTH:[46] The cops had left. And so you're saying to your friend, 'It hasn't beeped yet.' Are those the exact words?

JT:[47] Yes.

RTH:[48] 'It still hasn't beeped yet.' And is anything else in your awareness other than the saying of those words?

JT:[49] Well. I know you showed me that whole slide [an illustration of the concept of the moment of the beep that we used in his pretraining] on, like, whenever the different situations leading up to the beep, but right before I was thinking it still hasn't beeped yet, I don't know if that's pertinent, but I was thinking that I could drive on the street to get my friend some gas.

RTH:[50] OK. But that was before the beep? That was like...

JT:[51] That was before.... It still hasn't beeped yet.

RTH:[52] And is that still present to you or has that come and gone? So the sequence is, the cops came, the cops go, I want to drive on the street, now I say to my friend it still hasn't beeped yet, and then it beeps, like separate links in a chain of sausages, one thing and then another thing and then another thing? Or do these things overlap?

JT:[53] I'm pretty sure it's still in the back of my mind, the driving on the street, and then I was just thinking it still hasn't beeped yet and I say it out loud, and then it beeps. But, I don't know, like the beep kind of like interrupted my thought process, y'know.

[7:00]

RTH:[54] Right.

JT:[55] It's really hard to narrow it down. It really throws you off.

RTH:[56] OK. I agree with all that. But this is only the first beep, and you're probably going to get somewhat better at that, or maybe you won't. But most people do get a little better at it as they get accustomed to what the beep...

JT:[57] Conditioning!

RTH:[58] I would think of it as sort of a practice, that after a while you figure out, Well, *that* is what the beep is! and it doesn't startle you as much. That's probably conditioning, if you like.

Subjects (initially) don't observe skillfully

'I'm pretty sure' and 'I don't know' (at JT[53]) and 'It's really hard to narrow it down. It really throws you off' (at JT[55]) indicate that JT thinks he is not adept at apprehending his experience, and I agree with that. Most people are not very good at apprehending their experience on their first sampling occasion. So subjects need support, and I try to provide it. But note that even while supporting, I allow the subject ('or maybe you won't' at RTH[56]) the opportunity to advance an alternative that differs from my expectation and permission not to be a 'good subject.' Both are parts of the open-beginningedness of the process.

RTH:[59]   So now I'm a little bit confused. A bit ago I thought there was no thought that was before the speaking. But now it seems like maybe there is a thought that it still hasn't beeped yet, that's before the speaking.

JT:[60]   Well, there must have been. Maybe it was a thought at the same time as I was saying it, you know. Maybe I was thinking that it still hasn't beeped and then I say that out loud, 'It still hasn't beeped yet' (snaps fingers simulating beep).

[8:00]

RTH:[61]   OK. And that's fine with me. I'm not trying to talk you into or out of what's in your experience.

JT:[62]   Right.

RTH:[63]   What I'm trying to do is to say that we are interested in that fine of a distinction. If you're saying 'it still hasn't beeped yet,' and as part of your experience you're also thinking that separately from the saying of it, we would like to know about that. But we don't want to just *presume* that that's the way it is, because we're trying to find out the way it *really* is. So we're ... and so we're happy with you're saying, if it's true, 'I was just saying out loud, 'It still hasn't beeped yet'. And that expressed myself. But I didn't really have a thought first.' That's possible. And it's also possible, 'Well I thought to myself, Hm, this still hasn't beeped yet, and then said, 'It still hasn't beeped yet'.' And it's also possible that, 'While I'm saying 'it still hasn't beeped yet', I also am separately thinking, in my experience, that it still hasn't beeped yet. All those things are possible. And we're trying to figure out, what's that like for you? ...

Distinctions are made when and where distinctions are important

The repetition and the fine distinctions at RTH[59-63] are possible *only* because JT has a personal stake in the discussion. This discussion is squarely on his turf, and he knows it. It fascinates him because it is *his*. It would have been impossible to have a discussion this precise before JT had himself struggled to try to make the distinction.

I'm not attempting to argue JT out of his mini-delusion; I'm trying, with him, to understand exactly what he meant about a particular pristine experience. JT himself indicated that there is a fissure in his presuppositional structure: he himself is not certain that there was a thought before a speaking (he uses the subjunctifier 'pretty much' twice in his opening description of his experience). We express a sincere interest in what he is saying, including a sincere appreciation for his qualifying expressions. We are trying to understand what he is telling us. As a result, we never attack, so he doesn't have to defend.

But I re-emphasize that this conversation is primarily aimed at skill building for *tomorrow's* sampling, *not* at trying to figure out *yesterday's* experience. Yesterday he didn't have adequate observational skill to support the kinds of distinctions we are raising.

RTH:[64] ... And I think we told you when we talked to you last week that we didn't expect you to know what this was going to be like until we've done it. And this is an example of that. You had no way of knowing that we were going to be interested in that fine a detail of what your experience is like. And nobody does. There's no way that you can know that until after we've had this kind of conversation. So basically, the first sampling day or two is our trying to convey to you, We really want to know about the microscopic details of what's in your experience, as best you can report it. It could be that you can say, 'You guys are asking me questions that are way too difficult for me to answer! My experience isn't like that! I can't make that distinction.' That would be fine, too. But we want to get sort of right up to that point, where we can take you as far as you are willing to go, or can go, or your experiences can take us, about what your experience is like.

[10:15]

JT:[65]   Alright. I'll try my best.

RTH:[66] That's what we're here for...

Iterative training is inherently frustrating

We don't tell subjects what they are to look for but then ask detailed questions about it. That is frustrating but is unavoidable because the alternative would be worse: We *do* tell subjects what they are to look for and then feign 'discovery' when they report it.

So we get to the end of the first interview without collecting any reports that are believable. It appears that all we have done is to point out to JT his inadequacy, that we have done nothing of positive value. But that's not true. He *was* an inadequate observer of his experience, and we have demonstrated our will at speaking the truth about his inadequacy. We have demonstrated that we are skillful at understanding what he is saying and what he is not saying, and skillful at knowing the difference between apprehension and speculation, between truth and plausibility. We have demonstrated that we are supportive of him and non-judgmental. We have demonstrated that we are sincerely interested in obtaining faithful reports about experience. All that is really quite a lot. Even though it does not get us believable reports today, it sets the stage for obtaining believable reports *tomorrow*.

The fact is that JT (like most first-time subjects) was *not* ready to observe—he didn't have the skill, wasn't prepared, didn't accept that we really were interested in what was really in his pristine experience, didn't know what experience was, didn't really trust us to take him seriously, didn't understand how brief a moment is and how much pristine experience may change from one moment to the next, didn't really know the difference between apprehending and theorizing/speculating, didn't really adequately distinguish between what was truly apprehended and what was plausibly present. So yesterday his original pristine experience came and went, was apprehended in a low-fidelity way, mixed with presupposition and self-presentation. *No amount of interviewing, no matter how skilled, could have reversed that.* Next time, however, he can, perhaps, do better. And the time after that, better still.

Discussion

This paper has drawn three main conclusions: 1. in any interview, an interviewer's apprehension of a subject's pristine experience arises from conflated contributions of pristine experience and reconstructed experience diminished by non-experiential impediments (subject's and interviewer's presuppositions, miscommunication); 2. regardless of skill, within-occasion interviewing is likely to *decrease* the direct contribution of pristine experience (because of the increase in the contribution of reconstructed experience); and 3. skillful across-occasion 'iterative' interviewing may, incrementally on successive occasions, *increase* the direct contribution of pristine experience (and decrease the contribution of reconstructed experience).

An apprehension that arises from a conflation of pristine and reconstructed experience may well be quite similar to an apprehension that might arise from pristine experience alone. A reconstructed experience is, after all, itself an experience; the subject may well have intended the reconstructed experience to mirror the pristine experience; and the reconstructed experience was created by the same bag of bones and neurons that created the pristine experience. To the extent that the reconstructed experience is similar to the pristine experience, the interviewer's apprehension of (pristine and reconstructed) experience at end of an interview can more faithfully mirror the subject's pristine experience than was possible at the beginning of the interview (the combined contribution of the pristine and the reconstructed experiences in Figure 2 is larger than in Figure 1). However, Hurlburt and Akhter (2006) argued that it is unwise to assume similarity between reconstructed and pristine experience — after all, the situations are much different (interview vs. the original), subjects may not have been skilled observers at the time of the pristine experience and so may not know what they are trying to reconstruct, and the reconstructions may reflect presuppositions as much or more than the pristine experience. At present, the science of experience has no effective way of determining in what kinds of situations and for what kinds of experiences the reliance on reconstructed experience is useful.

Some non-recurrent experiences cannot possibly be directly subjected to an iterative procedure (the experience at the moment of impact of survivors of the World Trade Center, for an extreme example, cannot be iterated). But science could iteratively influence the apprehension of even such never-to-be-repeated events by training iteratively a large number of subjects. A few of those individuals may subsequently undergo some non-recurrent event, and therefore might be more prepared to apprehend experience during it. At present, the science of experience does not know whether such a strategy is worth the effort.

I have argued that these features of iterative interviews may lead to higher fidelity apprehensions: 1. refreshment by pristine experience; 2. commitment to bracketing presuppositions; 3. practice in observing; 4. practice in being interviewed; 5. readiness to observe pristine experience; 6. reducing the need for reconstructions; 7. improving the fidelity of reconstructions; 8. multiple perspectives on experience; and 9. open beginning. A science of experience should examine which of these features is important in what situations. For example, clinical interviews could be said to be iterative: the therapist gets to know the client better on each occasion. But clinical interviews have no procedure designed to assist in the bracketing of presuppositions by either therapist or client. Armchair observation can be said to be iterative — always trying to improve the observation of experience — but armchair observation is not about pristine experience: observation occurs only after a self-initiated intention to observe (Hurlburt & Schwitzgebel, 2007). The Experience Sampling Method (ESM; e.g. Csikszentmihalyi & Larson, 1987) uses beepers to trigger subjects to fill out questionnaires about the experience that was occurring when beeped. Those repetitions could be called iterative, but the use of a pre-constructed Experience Sampling Form at each beep eliminates the possibility of bracketing presuppositions from one observation to the next, and ESM typically trains subjects in the use of the form on only one occasion. Descriptive Experience Sampling incorporates all the iterative features described in this paper, but perhaps that slows the method down too much to be useful in science. At present, the science of experience does not know which features of iteration are useful in which circumstances.

I have observed that iteration does not always or automatically increase the contribution of pristine experience; that the beneficial effect of iteration depends on interviewer skill, particularly the skill of bracketing presuppositions. At present, the science of experience does not expend much effort training its practitioners in the bracketing of presuppositions.

I have argued that iteration can increase fidelity, not that it leads to complete accuracy. At present, the science of experience has not worked out a method to measure the fidelity of an observation.

At present, most empirical studies in the science of experience rely on one-occasion, non-iterative observations. The analysis in this paper suggests that such reliance is problematic.

Consciousness science can be said to be caught in the crossfire between those who think experience is easy to apprehend (and therefore attempt to do so without much concern for methodological niceties) and those who think experience is impossible to apprehend (and therefore eschew the attempt altogether; Hurlburt & Heavey, 2004). Iterating the observing of experience/interview sequence may improve the apprehension of experience and thus reduce the crossfire.

References

Csikszentmihalyi, M. & Larson, R. (1987), 'Validity and reliability of the experience-sampling method', *Journal of Nervous and Mental Disease*, **175**, pp. 526–36.

Heavey, C.L. & Hurlburt, R.T. (2009), 'Descriptive Experience Sampling: Exploring moments of inner experience', in press, *Qualitative Research in Psychology*.

Hurlburt, R.T. (1990), *Sampling Normal and Schizophrenic Inner Experience* (New York: Plenum).

Hurlburt, R.T. (1993), *Sampling Inner Experience In Disturbed Affect* (New York: Plenum).

Hurlburt, R.T. (1997), 'Randomly sampling thinking in the natural environment', *Journal of Consulting and Clinical Psychology*, **65**, pp. 941–49.

Hurlburt, R.T. & Akhter, S.A. (2006), 'The Descriptive Experience Sampling method', *Phenomenology and the Cognitive Sciences*, **5**, pp. 271–301.

Hurlburt, R.T. & Heavey, C.L. (2002), 'Interobserver reliability of Descriptive Experience Sampling', *Cognitive Therapy and Research*, **26**, pp. 135–42.

Hurlburt, RT. & Heavey, C.L. (2004), 'To beep or not to beep: Obtaining accurate reports about awareness', *Journal of Consciousness Studies*, **11** (7–8), pp. 113–28.

Hurlburt, R.T. & Heavey, C.L. (2006), *Exploring Inner Experience: The Descriptive Experience Sampling Method* (Amsterdam: John Benjamins).

Hurlburt, R.T. Heavey, C.L. & Bensaheb, A. (2009, this issue). Sensory awareness.

Hurlburt, R.T. & Schwitzgebel, E. (2007), *Describing Inner Experience?* (Cambridge, MA: MIT Press).

Petitmengin, C. (2006), 'Describing one's subjective experience in the second person: An interview method for the science of consciousness', *Phenomenology and the Cognitive Sciences*, **5**, pp. 229–69.

Jane Mathison and Paul Tosey

Exploring Moments of Knowing

Neuro-Linguistic Programming and enquiry into inner landscapes

Abstract: *This article is an account of reflections drawn from a total of four explicitation interviews (Vermersch, 1994), with two people. The article has both methodological and substantive purposes.*

Methodologically, we explain the contribution of Neuro-Linguistic Programming (NLP) in the elicitation of first person accounts through guided introspection. Aspects of NLP have been used by both Vermersch (1994) and Petitmengin-Peugeot (1999) as means for exploring people's inner worlds. We further elucidate NLP as a set of tools for researchers, emphasising the distinctions these enable researchers to make within the structure of consciousness. As the nature of NLP's methodological contribution to the field of Psychophenomenology (Vermersch, 1996, Maurel, 2008) has been little articulated, this represents an original feature of this article.

Substantively, we show how the application of these tools has generated insights into the fine experiential detail of what we term 'moments of knowing'. First, our data suggest that suspension and Epoche, which manifested themselves as unrecognised, or pre-reflective moments of understanding for the participants, may be part of everyday 'knowing'. Second, consciousness appears to be multidimensional. In particular it appears that it may be helpful to distinguish between different dimensions of awareness that may be involved when exploring an inner landscape. Third, we consider the apparently transformative effect of the explicitation interview for one of these participants, which emphasises that the interview is an active exploration. Our findings question established views of transformative learning, which hitherto have regarded 'critical reflection' as the central process involved in transformative learning (Mezirow, 1990, 1991, 2003).

Keywords

Explicitation Interview, Guided introspection, Inner landscapes, Neuro-linguistic Programming, Transformative Learning,

Introduction

No matter how sophisticated the methodologies of rational-empirical science become, they remain inherently vulnerable so long as the study and understanding of the human experience upon which they are based remain primitive. (Hartelius, 2007, p. 25)

Depraz *et al.* (2002)) suggests that phenomenological inquiries into awareness and conscious experience are needed to support a new generation of cognitive science in which cognition itself is perceived as an aspect of embodied action, in Varela's words, as a 'history of structural coupling that brings forth a world' (Varela *et al.*, 1993, p. 206). Varela proposed that cognition should no longer be thought of as separated from embodied knowing, but recognised as rooted in a corporeal existence that engenders meaning (Varela, 1997; Weber, 2002). The emerging science of Neuro-phenomenology (Varela, 1996; Lutz, 2002; Lutz and Thompson, 2003) is predicated on the belief that a marriage between an individual's introspectively arrived at data, and findings using instruments such as a fMRI scanners, may generate new ways of understanding aspects of consciousness. For instance, Petitmengin (Petitmengin *et al.*, 2007) reports on how she used the explicitation interview in association with the analysis of neuronal synchronization with people suffering epileptic seizures to enable them to become aware of the subtle bodily changes that heralded the onset of a seizure.

Guided by the belief that the developing sciences of consciousness needed to include 'first person, subjective experience as an explicit and active component' (Varela and Shear, 2000, p. 2), the challenge to researchers is to investigate subjective experience through returning to 'the things themselves', where the object that is being studied is given 'in flesh and blood' (Depraz *et al.*, 2002, p. 177). This means developing ways of exploring the dimensions of subjective experience which Petitmengin proposes unfold 'below the threshold of consciousness' (Petitmengin, 2006, p. 230).

This raises certain methodological issues. What is valid knowledge when it relies on introspectively arrived at information? Overgaard *et al.* (2008) have reviewed a number of different first person methodologies. They stress that their findings, which engage with introspectively arrived at data, are epistemologically distinct from the kind of knowledge derived through applying the third person perspective which dominates the more 'acceptably scientific' paradigm.

Vermersch makes the point that introspection as a means of investigating ways of knowing has for too long been denigrated and that ignoring its potential leads to 'an extremely impoverished subjectivity' (Vermersch, 1999, p. 27). He also believes that the ignoring of first person data by traditional cognitive psychology is producing an incomplete psychology and an inherent blindness to the significance of the dimension of subjective experience gained through introspection (Vermersch, 2004).

Depraz *et al.* (2002, p. 82) suggest an elegant solution to any confusion that might arise about the legitimacy of either first or third person perspectives; their view is that there are varieties of validation, just as there are varieties of points of view. Using three perceptual positions (those of first, second and third person) as essentially complementary and unable to stand alone confers validity to the material. The introduction of a second person position, as 'an exchange between situated individuals focusing on a specific experiential content developed from a first person position.' (Depraz *et al.*, 2002, p. 81) adds to the richness of the data.

Psychophenomenology has been developed as a methodology that employs the explicitation interview (Vermersch, 1994) as a protocol for venturing into the territory of embodied knowing, by eliciting first person data obtained through introspection. In summary, the explicitation interview explores a short segment of experience (perhaps lasting only a few seconds) by reassociating the interviewee into that experience and then eliciting an increasingly fine-grained description of its various sensory details (Vermersch, 1994). In order to do this, it employs specific forms of question that direct the interviewee's attention to that evoked experience.

The role of the guide, or mediator in this interview, is perceived as essential to psychophenomenological inquiry: 'It is easier with a companion, even when you are gifted or already an expert', (Vermersch, 1994). Depraz *et al.* (2002) encourage 'the use of expert external mediators who know how to guide description, without leading it', (Depraz *et al.*, 2002, p 74). Language forms a bridge between an individual's verbal descriptions of his or her inner worlds, and the guide's developing understanding of the features of the other's unfolding landscape. Understanding the architecture of this bridge, as it were, becomes as important as gaining insights into the complexity of what may unfold. This is where NLP may be illuminative.

This article considers how tools derived from Neuro-Linguistic Programming (NLP) play a significant role in this process. NLP has not only influenced the development of the explicitation interview to date, but also can further refine this process. Vermersch (1994) and Petitmengin (Petitmengin-Peugeot, 1999) both draw on NLP sources in their texts and bibliographies.

The discussion is illustrated with data from explicitation interviews with two participants conducted by the first author. The interviews came about partly by chance, when the first author's (JM) desire to practice explicitation to explore other people's experiences of their inner processes met with relevant opportunities. One participant, S, is a 29-year old doctoral student studying photographing a Japanese dance form called Butoh. S approached us because she had been seeking the opportunity to be interviewed in this way to enable her to understand better, for the purposes of her research, her experience of knowing the moment when to photograph the dancers. The other participant, X, an academic, was interested in gaining experiential knowledge of the explicitation interview as a potential research methodology. In his case the interview focused on his experience of insight.

Both participants gave their consent to be interviewed, and for the use of the data in academic publications; as stressed by Vermersch (1994), assent is part of an ethical contract between the guide and the interior voyager. The explicitation interviews were carried out by the first author. The second author conducted a further interview (not an explicitation interview) with the first participant in order to assist her to reflect on what she had learnt from the explicitation interviews. All interviews were recorded digitally then transcribed, two by one of the participants, and one by the first author. Quotations in the text below are verbatim. What role did NLP play in these explorations?

Neuro-linguistic Programming (NLP)

NLP (Bandler and Grinder, 1975) emerged in the 1970s, at the same time as Cognitive Linguistics (Evans and Green, 2006). These fields both take as a starting point the belief that syntactical language patterns reveal and mirror the processes involved in conceptualising and sense making (Evans and Green 2006, p. 5). In NLP these syntactical structures are treated as if they have an epistemological dimension; they are an active medium for generating understanding. Fauconnier (1997, p. 40) sums up this approach: 'The natural-language sentence is a set of (underspecified) instructions for cognitive constructions at many different levels.'

There are, however, important differences between the two. NLP draws on the linguistic tradition of Chomsky, Sapir and Whorf. It is informed by the cybernetics of Gregory Bateson (1973, 1979) and his circle, and is imbued with the philosophy of the constructivist school (Von Foerster, 1973), having also drawn on many contemporary developments at the Palo Alto School of Mental Research (Watzlawick *et al.*, 1967; Watzlawick, 1990). It also considers the sensory realm to be an important aspect of sense making. Its founders, Bandler and Grinder, seem then (in the late 1970s) to have deliberately taken NLP out of what they perceived as the confines of academia, making it into a commercial venture accessible to all who could pay the training fees.

Whilst there are various criticisms that can be levelled at this field (Tosey & Mathison, 2009), these should not distract attention from the pragmatic tools that NLP offers for investigating conscious experience and taking people deeper into introspective realms. Thus NLP can be, and has been (Petitmengin-Peugeot, 1999; Petitmengin, 2006), used as a tool for psychophenomenological inquiry and the exploration of people's experience of what Depraz *et al.* (2002) have called pre-reflective layers of consciousness.

The tools that NLP offers fall into two main categories. One is its approach to language; the other is from its insights into the non-verbal dimensions of consciousness.

Language

A guide to the language tools on which NLP is based was initially published in *The Structure of Magic I and II*, (Bandler and Grinder, 1975, Grinder and Bandler, 1976). This work resulted from their study of Virginia Satir's and Fritz Perls' use of questions and language patterns with their patients. Further developments followed from their work analysing and modelling the communication patterns of the psychiatrist and hypnotherapist Milton Erickson (Bandler and Grinder, 1975A).

NLP is not unique in its approach to language; as noted; cognitive linguistics too is based on the same premise. Where NLP differs is that it encourages a pragmatic, 'hands on' approach; users need to have been trained in it, or have had extensive practice, and there is emphasis on the application of these tools in everyday contexts by professionals and lay people. Cognitive linguistics, on the other hand, has remained a strictly academic (though complementary) field. NLP was derived from studying people who were considered excellent in their field then replicating their language and behaviours to test whether this achieved the same results in others (Tosey & Mathison, 2009). The main method used in Cognitive Linguistics on the other hand has been to validate theories through introspection (Evans and Green, 2006).

NLP provides two main insights into language that can be applied in phenomenological research. One is the notion that the syntax of a statement can both reveal, as well as elicit, certain aspects of the inner architecture of sense making. This is the basis of the core NLP language model, known as the 'meta-model' (Bandler and Grinder, 1975). Such insights guide a researcher to elicit further information about an interviewee's experience. We have also used this as a basis for analysing transcripts of interviews and identifying personal changes that subtle syntactical alterations reveal (Tosey *et al.*, 2005).

The other is the concept of the 'trans-derivational search' (Bandler and Grinder, 1975A, p. 220), which refers to the phenomenon whereby questions direct people to search internally. Bandler and Grinder were struck by Milton Erickson's language patterns; he often used apparently vague suggestions, phrases, and unspecific abstract words when guiding his patients in trance. Whereas in their initial work Bandler and Grinder had focused on designing questions that elicited further information about people's meaning making, they observed that Erickson used language patterns in a way that left the listener to make sense of his utterances, at the same time setting directions for introspective searching. In phenomenological research, this means that any question will direct an interviewee's attention in particular directions. Carefully crafted statements or questions, skilfully applied, can therefore facilitate an introspective journey by purposely directing attention to dimensions of awareness that may previously have appeared inaccessible. For instance, people usually respond differently to the different suggestions, '*Notice the tension in your shoulders*'; and '*You can notice wherever there is any tension in your body*'. In effect these distinguish between levels of abstraction in language — the first is a directive to attend to a specified feeling in the shoulders, whereas the second has a more artful vagueness that elicits internal searching so that individuals discover for themselves wherever such tension may be. The ability to make this distinction is extremely useful to the interviewer, both when listening to people's language patterns, and guiding someone on an introspective journey.

The sensory realm

NLP also addresses the dimension of the senses - not, as described in traditional physiology, as receptors and responders to certain bandwidths in the electromagnetic spectrum beamed in from the external world, but as actively involved in creating an experienced reality. Many NLP texts address how the senses are used internally to create an inner landscape of images, sounds, feelings, tastes, smells, movement and other sensations (e.g. Bandler & Grinder, 1979). In NLP training, participants learn how to investigate the way they represent events in their lives in the various sensory modalities — in other words, through internal pictures, sounds, feelings, smells and tastes. In her research into consciousness, Petitmengin refers to this dimension as sensorial and emotional (Petitmengin-Peugeot, 1999, p 46). She suggests that it underlies all cognitive processing (Petitmengin, 2007). What do people see, hear, and/or feel as they remember, say, that special day on the beach, or visit to an art gallery? Using NLP terminology, what internal representations (Dilts and Delozier, 2000) do people make as they plan, fantasize or daydream? How does this pre-reflective, sensorial dimension unfold temporally?

Developments in cognitive psychology linked to findings in neuro-biology (Barsalou, 1999; Barsalou *et al.*, 2003; Barsalou, 2008, Pecher *et al.*, 2004) also support the notion that our concepts are not just platonic abstractions, but are actively grounded in the world of the senses. That is, they make use of what NLP terms 'internal representations'. Furthermore, it is now assumed that the same neural state that underlies perception and action also underlies conceptual representations (Pecher *et al.*, 2004, p. 167).

This raises some ontological puzzles. The term 'internal representation', much used in NLP, may imply that our nervous systems present us with a copy of what is 'out there'. Varela, Thomson and Rosch, (1993) on the other hand, perceive this domain of the senses rather as creating and enacting what we consider to be 'real'. There is a distinction between the ontological position that we 're-present' an external reality of some kind, and the one that holds that we create, embody and enact the world we live in. Varela (1997, p. 81) resolves this dichotomy, proposing that we bring the world into being, and that autopoesis and cognition are characteristics of living beings, (Maturana and Varela, 1998). This puzzle is not addressed as such in the NLP literature; we believe that it is a significant lack, and an aspect of the utilitarian approach embedded in most of the practice of NLP (Tosey and Mathison, 2009).

NLP also suggests that internal sensory modes are reflected in a person's language. Certain types of words are classed as 'sensory predicates'. Such words refer to a particular sensory modality; 'seeing' is classed as visual, 'it sounds like' would be considered as an auditory sensory predicate, and so on. It is part of NLP practice to listen for such words, in case they reveal that the speaker is paying attention to information presenting in that particular modality.

Significantly, NLP extends familiarisation with this world of internal representations by making more finely grained distinctions in each of the sensory modes. These finer distinctions are called 'sub-modalities', (Bandler and MacDonald, 1988; Faulkner, 1999), because they are subsidiary to the main sensory modalities. They address questions like: are the internal images in colour? What kinds of colour? Are they two dimensional or three dimensional? Where, if there are sounds associated with this particular representation, do they seem to be coming from? What is the apparent location of the representation? What are the differences at this sub-modality level between the memory of a pleasant and an unpleasant experience? Developing awareness of these dimensions is impossible without introspection. To access such information from others needs sensitive and skilful facilitation to guide the interviewee through their inner world.

Applying NLP to Phenomenological Enquiry

Association and evocation; turning attention inwards

Guided introspection begins with evoking an act of awareness (Depraz *et al.*, 2002). This involved both a turning inwards, and a period of waiting, of suspension, of letting 'it' come: 'This is the only way you can change the way you pay attention to your own lived experience' (Depraz *et al.*, 2002, p. 25). Importantly, in the explicitation interview it is essential that the guide enables the interviewee to become 'associated' with that experience. In NLP terms, someone is 'associated' when he or she has accessed the physiological state associated with a remembered experience as if it were happening to them now. Vermersch refers to this state as being in 'evocation'.

An early task of the guide is therefore to facilitate the person undergoing the elicitation interview to reassociate with a chosen experience. It can be useful to encourage the emergence of the memory at the sensory level, to invite them to become aware of what is happening to them physically when in the state of association or evocation. To achieve this, the guide may use specific language patterns, and match the rhythm of speaking with the participant's breathing. For example, with our second participant, who had asked to explore an experience of insight, I (JM) began as follows:

J.   ...so can you think of a time, or allow a time to emerge in your memory, when you had an insight ... into whatever it was ...

His first reply, which is typical of a third person perspective (Depraz *et al.*, 2002, p. 80), shows he is not in evocation.

X.   [...] I guess my perceptions are coloured in a way by academic understanding of what I mean by insight. I tend to think of it in theoretical and conceptual terms. [...] When invited to give an example of my own insights it's a little more difficult. Let me think, let me think, let me think.

Now there was a long silence. I suggested:

J.   Just let it come by itself.

After a long pause, he said 'I'm driving a car'.

This suggestion *just let it come by itself* is loaded with examples of a pattern found in the NLP language model called *presuppositions*. A presupposition implies 'the existence of some condition, state or feeling' (Battino and South 2005, p. 82). Such information, transmitted through presuppositions, is thought to bypass the conscious mind; presuppositions usually do not immediately engage the participant's rational analytical faculties. Among the presuppositions here are that 'it' (whatever that is) has an existence, that it can emerge, and that it will, without further effort, and the apparently innocent word *just* implies ease and spontaneity.

Depraz *et al.* (2003, p. 31) stress that in the basic cycle of phenomenological inquiry 'you have to change from voluntarily turning your attention from the exterior to the interior to simply accepting and listening ... you go from "looking for something" to "letting something come to you," to "letting something be revealed"'. There was a deliberate intention, on the part of the interviewer, to enable this by using carefully crafted guiding language.

X's comment 'I'm driving a car' was indicative that he was now in evocation, immersed in the sensory realm of this particular memory. We were ready for the next phase of the journey.

Eliciting the details of sensory experience

This section illustrates how questions can be used to elicit detailed descriptions of sensory experience.

Example 1

Our first participant, who wished to develop greater insights into how she photographed the Butoh dancers, had asked to explore how she had decided that a particular suggested location was 'interesting' while others were not. She began by talking about a discussion with her partner. As she evoked the memory of this conversation, I (JM) asked:

J.   OK, can you slow the film down, and just hear him suggesting the options ... really slow it down. How do you know they are 'not interesting'?

The question first directs her to slow the unfolding of the remembered event, then to begin the transderivational search for the sensory evidence leading to the judgement 'interesting'.

S.   I think they didn't feel challenging.

I note that the sensory predicate 'feel' is used. This may be an indication of a bodily sensation which could be the physically experienced correlate of 'challenging' and which might be worth exploring. The next question is designed to elicit how she has made distinctions between the two classes of experience, 'challenging' and 'not challenging'. I mirror back the sensory predicate 'feel' used in her response, to maintain her awareness on embodied sensations.

J.   OK, so they didn't *feel* challenging. [...] So what's the difference for you between challenging and not challenging?

S.   Well if I look at one of the suggestions which was to do it somewhere on the street in front of some building, it just felt very easy to just go there, to show up.

Here she indicates that after making a visual image (*if I look*) of the suggested location, she attends to a bodily sensations; (*it just felt very easy*). I confirm this by repeating back to her the last sensory predicate (feel) that she used.

J.   You felt?

S.   Yes.

Example 2

During the course of the explicitation interview with our second participant, X reported what he experienced just after he had the insight.

X.   What happened then was the feeling of sliding out of control was just replaced by calmness, stillness.

I noticed that the words 'calmness' and 'stillness' are what are termed in the NLP meta-model 'nominalisations'; that is, abstractions from which the original actions have been deleted. Also deleted are the sensory or embodied experiences linked to these particular words. Depraz *et al.* (2002) warn against ignoring the distinctions between description and interpretation (p. 93). The interviewer's task is to enable the participant to recover this missing sensory detail, at what Vermersch calls a more finely grained level of density, and to direct the person's attention to the embodied experience linked to the words. Therefore my question aims to enable X to uncover the embodied correlates of 'calmness' and 'stillness'.

J.   How did you know it was calmness, stillness?

X.   Because there was no movement, it was as though above my head there was space that went on forever.

The question 'how do you know' is another example of the deliberate use of presuppositions. Specifically, the question '*how did you know it was calmness, stillness?*' presupposes both that these existed for X as experiences, and that it was possible for X to identify how he knew he experienced them. This question, in effect, sent him on a transderivational search for the embodied correlates of 'calmness' and 'stillness'.

X's abstract words therefore begin to be translated into a more precise description of his experience of an embodied sensation of space, having size, location and extension (the words 'it was as though' also warn the interviewer that this description may be verging on the metaphorical, which could open up other directions for inquiry). What could be the significance of such a metaphor? What role might it be playing in his sense making?

Here the awareness of nominalisations, and the processes that lead to them, was useful to the guide. Bandler and Grinder's metamodel (1975) was influenced by Noam Chomsky, who held that in all languaging, information was deleted. Questions based on the meta-model enable the questioner to help the interviewee recover such deletions, as well as other underlying dynamics such as distortions and generalisations. In this case, there was a bodily sensation which underlay the nominalisation. This lends credence to the increasing recognition that cognition is rooted in the sensorial and corporeal realms (Wilson, 2002).

Calibration

The skills of observing and listening are as important when guiding an introspective journey as awareness of language patterns. In the interview with the Butoh photographer, for example, I (JM) had noticed tension in her shoulders as she described photographing dancers on a staircase at a London Underground station. When inviting her to evoke this event, I deliberately used sensory predicates relating to feeling and vision, deliberately mirroring the ones she used most often.

J. Just allow yourself to experience that feeling, being in your body, observing what's happening through your eyes, through your hands, with your feet...

After a pause, she replied:

S. I can clearly see the camera in front of my eyes

Here she tells me that she is attending to internal visual information, but I notice her shoulders tensing. I continue guiding her evocation, consciously using Ericksonian language patterns.

J. ... and what sort of tension there is in your shoulders and how it makes you feel...

S. I can feel that I use muscles, I can feel that my body is made of muscles.

Initially this did not appear significant. However, in the de-briefing interview (with PT) she realised that the explicitation process had made her more aware of the whole dimension of her physicality and how it was involved in her creativity. She identified this as a profound, qualitative change in her awareness, apparently stemming from a subtle observation in the initial interview.

When guiding an interior journey, one is evoking altered states of consciousness. The guide needs to be able to observe, listen and be aware of the slightest physical changes that indicate a possible change in the person's state. Awareness can swing between our 'external' and 'internal' worlds; Overgaard et al. (2008) cite Antrobus's (1966) findings of a continual shifting of attention between external tasks and 'interior' thought content that may be unrelated to external events.

Marti (2003) suggests that one of the most important contributions that NLP has made to the study of altered states is precise 'calibration' by an observer. In this, Grinder and Bandler were influenced chiefly by Milton Erickson's legendary ability (Grinder et al., 1977) to discriminate very fine changes in people that to the 'normal' observer would be either insignificant or non-existent. According to Marti, calibration forms the basis for the 'objectification of subjectivity'[1] (Marti, 2003, p. 116).

In NLP training, people are encouraged to develop the skills of recognising external signs that indicate when a person is in a particular state, and when it changes. This can go as far as training people to distinguish very small (and usually ignored) changes in breathing, skin colour, muscular tension, lip size, corneal shape, even heart rate, when people are lying or telling the truth. Some trainers go so far as to challenge practitioners to observe and list physical differences in someone when they are engaged in imagining, or interiorly visualising, being surrounded entirely by a red colour, and how their non-verbal signs differ when they are imagining being completely surrounded by green.

Among the possibilities for calibration, a controversial hypothesis of NLP is that the direction in which people's eyes move indicates which sensory modality they are attending to internally. A defocused gaze may indicate attention to a representation experienced in more than one modality.[2] It is interesting, therefore, that both Vermersch (1994) and Petitmengin (2006) have emphasised the importance of observing the changes in, and movements of people's eyes when they attend inwardly, and encourages guides to question their significance. Do they look away, perhaps indicating inward attention? What is this person's posture when in evocation? How is it different? Where do

---

[1] Author's translation. *La calibration fonde ainsi l'objectivation de la subjectivité.*

[2] We are grateful to Professor Monique Esser for this observation.

they direct their gaze when searching? Sometimes people's eyes dart about as if they were trying to locate a feature they had not noticed before in a familiar landscape (Vermersch, 1994).

What NLP brings to the psychophenomenological exploration of inner landscapes is a refinement of our understanding of the effects of syntax on sense making, an awareness that we operate a complex inner world of sensory experience which can be investigated through careful and respectful guidance, that altered states have physiological correlates which can be identified and tracked, and that the dimensions of our consciousness manifest themselves at different levels of complexity or granularity. NLP has transformed itself from its early emphasis on the pursuit of excellence and self-improvement, to a tool which is increasingly being used in the exploration of inner space. In the following section we aim to make this more explicit with examples drawn from the explicitation interviews.

The Internal Dynamic of the Structure of Experience

We now turn from describing the ways in which NLP can be used in the explicitation interview, to a discussion of themes that have emerged from our analysis of these interviews. These concern:

- Epoche
- Dimensions of awareness
- Emergence
- Transformative learning

Epoche: suspension and emergence

Of particular and unexpected interest in both our interviews was the description of the moments in which knowing arose. Our two participants experienced emergent moments of knowing through an enhanced awareness of the physical correlates of their verbal descriptions. Both reported experiencing a kind of suspension, from which their respective forms of knowing emerged. Although we would not seek to generalise from the explicitation interviews of only two participants, in both these cases such moments had a structure which appeared to be similar to that of Epoche, occurring as precursors to the emergence of an insight or a decision which was then felt to be significant by participants. Thus Depraz *et al.* (2002) propose that Epoche is naturally completed by an intuition that crystallises for the subject, and which serves as strong internal evidence (p. 63).

Our participant S, the photographer, wanted to find out the finer aspects of how she decided that one suggested location for a photographic session could appear 'interesting' and another not. What could it be that made 'interesting' different to 'not interesting' in her interior world? In part of the explicitation interview she explores how she came to choose the National Gallery as an 'interesting' location.

S. [...] I thought about National Gallery (sic).

J. How did you know that you were thinking about National Gallery?

S. That was again the image.

J. (...) what were you doing in terms of images to choose the National Gallery?

S. I don't know. I feel it just came.

As she said this, she pointed to her chest with her hands. I wondered what exploring this physical correlate to her thought of the 'National Gallery' might reveal. I suggested that she go back in time to just before the 'interesting' happened. I was curious to find out more about her experience of how 'it' came.

J. Can you go back to that time, and just be there in that situation when you were whatever it was that you were doing. (...) slow it down and go backwards to just before.

There was a pause, then she said:

S. It was like a sudden hit.

J. What happened before the sudden hit?

S. I think I was waiting for something to be ... (pause)

J. Go back to the waiting; go back to that sense of waiting. What were you paying attention to?

S. I think it was like the whole body was one. So there wasn't any part of my body that was waiting. It wasn't empty, it wasn't waiting for emptiness to be fulfilled, my whole body was there. It was more waiting to be influenced in a way so that something happens to it. I don't know how to explain it. (Pauses) Before I was saying that there was emptiness, here there isn't a hole, [...]. *And it's something that waits to happen without knowing to which part of the body it will happen.* (Authors' emphasis).

I realised at one point that her state of evocation was becoming less intense, perhaps because we had been using the past tense. The next question was designed to deepen evocation, to invite her to be aware of the unfolding of time. I deliberately switched to the present tense.

J. So as you're in that state and your body's waiting, what else is happening?

S. I think it's just waiting, but without any pressure that something needs to happen which wouldn't feel true.

J. OK, so just stay with that feeling. And just move on in your own time, slowly, as it's appropriate to you, to the time when that realisation happened.

Then she described two images coming to her. One was *a very old small tiny old frame*. The other was more difficult to describe; it seemed to be letters making the words National Gallery. She was aware of them sequentially. Later she said she thought that each image had appeared at the same time, but she was only aware of one, and then the other.

What is interesting here is that the images seemed to emerge for her from this 'waiting' for something to unfold that would 'feel true'. Our second participant reported an experience that has a similar quality, just before his insight happened:

> It's like suspended animation, it kind of just stops. Before, it's a puzzle, thinking. This kind of 'what does it mean?' and then, just for a very brief moment, it's almost like you're suspended [...] like someone has pressed the pause button on a DVD. It stops.

Both our participants described experiencing a state of waiting, of feeling suspended, and in which time appeared to stop. In each case this was a component of their sense of knowing; a precursor to a realisation which was both experienced as true and meaningful. We note that Petitmengin has reported that many of her participants experienced 'being "open" enough to let the unexpected come' (Petitmengin-Peugeot, 1999, p. 67).

These findings would appear consistent with a view of Epoche as a natural movement in the dynamics of awareness, part of an emergent, embodied knowing that is the fruit of suspending existing understanding. Such an act of awareness is thought to consist of three main stages (Depraz *et al.*, 2002). These are suspension, redirection of attention, and letting go. Hartelius (2007) has criticised Depraz *et al.*'s concept of Epoche as too abstract and obscure, doubting that it can serve as a foundation for a method of inquiry, as it lacks epistemic validity. We found, using the explicitation interview, that our data supports Depraz *et al.*'s contention that there is a structure and sequence to Epoche, which can be elicited through introspection. This makes it more empirically verifiable. We suggest that it may be part of the process of emergent, embodied, knowing.

Johnson (1987) and his co-author George Lakoff (Lakoff and Johnson, 1999) propose that a new paradigm in cognitive science recognises that our conceptual system is grounded in, neurally makes use of, and is crucially shaped by our perceptual and motor systems (p. 555). Gendlin (1999) believes that we should approach knowing, and understanding knowing, through the body, because sensing is prior to verbal expression and explanation. He developed a technique enabling people to access their own physical precursors to thought, known as 'focusing', or bodily explicitation. Lethin (2002) suggests that consciousness is based on the individual's sense of agency. It includes intentionality which partly originates in the activity of the sensory-motor system of the body's muscle spindles, and is thus embodied. Hartelius (2007) proposes a protocol for the development of a first person methodology based on somatics. Gendlin (2008) adds that the corporeal can contain information which is not, (or not yet), possible to put into words. Vermersch (2008) agrees, suggesting that 'the body becomes the possible source of information which integrates the totality of the actively available data'[3] (author's translation). To access this level of information, Vermersch suggests that it is necessary to learn to become more aware of bodily responses as a rich source of further insights, using Gendlin's technique of focusing.

These tentative findings raise further questions. What are the dynamics of embodied knowledge? How can we find out more about emergence? What are the implications for the development of an epistemology that takes into account this different kind of knowing? What do we now know about how we know that we know? What methodological issues are raised? Might we be touching on a tangible, empirically verifiable distinction between the cognitivist, and the

---

[3] Il devient la source possible d'une information intégrant la totalité des données actives disponibles. (p 39).

embodied, enacted approaches to consciousness studies (Varela *et al.*, 1993)? Traditional cognitivism is predicated on the idea that consciousness is 'programmable', using images from computers and information processing as the underlying explanatory metaphor system. The embodied, enacted approach understands consciousness as complex and embodied, in which the act of knowing is essentially emergent (Varela *et al.*, 1993). Insights from more such psychophenomenological inner journeys, one of whose vehicles is the explicitation interview, may enable more of such distinctions to be mapped with greater precision.

Dimensions of awareness

Maps are represented by different scales, the larger the scale, the less detailed the map. One of the aims of Psychophenomenology is to uncover information at ever greater magnification, so that more finely grained distinctions emerge which are not 'there' in the larger scale map.

One of the aims of Vermersch's explicitation interview is for participants to become aware of increasingly more finely grained distinctions in their inner landscapes. As anticipated, we noticed that both our participants became conscious of features which appeared to be at different levels of granularity (or magnification), almost as if there were different strata to experience in these sensorial dimension. However we also noticed qualitative shifts in the type of awareness involved. That is, the interviews did not consist of a uni-dimensional focusing of a microscope on either finer or broader detail; there were also different dimensions of experience which could metaphorically be examined through lenses of different magnifications.

From our data we can identify potentially three different dimensions of awareness. Each of these may be viewed at different levels of magnification, and/or tracked through different time scales (again at different levels of granularity ranging from microsecond to several minutes). Petitmengin (2006) stresses the importance of tracking the structure of an experience as it develops through time, as well as emphasising the complexity of the process. Knowing more about these kinds of structure may be useful to interviewers, who can then choose to direct the participant in different directions (metaphorically speaking).

Objects and events in inner landscapes

Once the participant's attention has been guided away from the external world to their inner world, one dimension of awareness involves a description of the objects and events of that inner world, such as the contents of a remembered experience. Both our participants were able to describe the features of the evoked experience — what they saw, heard and felt when they were associated into the state of evocation.

For example, when participant X revealed that he was driving a car. I (JM) questioned him about what he was now aware of.

J. You're driving a car. OK, so as you're driving a car, can you just notice what's happening around you?

X. Yeah, the trees are flashing by at the edge of my vision, the road ahead is clear, it's a narrow winding road which I know very well, so I'm able to focus on a conversation, on the subject, drive the car safely, and I'm aware of the person here (points to his left) and nobody in the back.

The participant may then be asked to describe the finer detail of the sensory modalities, including the submodalities, of the features identified. The narrow winding road, for example, may have a colour, a texture, and a more specific size and location. These are details, as it were, at a higher magnification or degree of granularity.

Experiencing the inner landscape

This is a different type of awareness because it switches X's attention from the content of the landscape to an aspect of how he is experiencing it. In the interview with X, I (JM) sought to create this shift of awareness by asking a question of the form 'how do you know?'. This is a classic NLP question (Bandler and Grinder, 1975) which is fundamentally epistemological in that it directs the person's attention to what, in their internal world, enabled them to conclude that they know. The question that arises here is, does the process of knowing reduce itself to the criteria of experiencing certain internal sensations which 'tell' us to know that we know? This is an area for further investigation.

It is likely that the participant will become more 'deeply' associated and inward looking when they attend to these kinds of internal sensations. The next questions I asked was:

J. How do you know you are aware of that person there?

X. Sensing their presence, really, angled towards me a little, my head is slightly turned to the left because I'm trying to project my voice that way, against the engine noise, eyes on the road ahead.

The next question was intended to focus attention on that 'sensing' of the presence of the other person.

J. What is the sensing of the presence like?

X. Like? What's it like? Mmmmhh, (a pause, perhaps indicating a trans-derivational search). It's kind of like a sense of puzzlement, and a sense of anticipation. [...] The sense of puzzlement is stronger.

In this instance this question elicited the nominalisations — 'puzzlement' and 'anticipation' — which are abstractions. The information I (JM) now wants needs to be not only more detailed but also physically rooted so as to reveal more of its underlying embodied structure. I realise that I need to change the question, and proceed on the assumption that 'puzzlement' will have a physical, bodily location.

J. Can we stay with the sense of puzzlement?

X. Mmmh

J. Where is the sense of puzzlement located?

X. In my head.

J. Is it anywhere else?

This produces another long pause. Then he tells me *the place is in the head, the neck and the upper part of the abdomen, the chest, and this is where the space is, this is where the puzzlement space is, here* (pointing to his chest).

One of the things that intrigued us most when reflecting on transcripts of the explicitation interviews was the difficulty our participants had with describing what they were experiencing at certain points. Rather than being able to give finer sensory detail, their descriptions began to introduce symbols and metaphors.

For example, when X was describing the physical location in his body of what he experienced as the 'puzzlement space' which happened before his experience of suspension and the emergence of insight, I asked:

J. Tell me more about that space, if you like.

X. It feels like an empty vessel.

What was this mysterious vessel? Was it a symbol that carried potential new meaning? Or a metaphor introduced because X could not find adequate words to describe the sense of emptiness? Petitmengin (2006, p. 238) has pointed out that we lack a descriptive vocabulary for the features that are emerging in such psychophenomenological explorations.

When I questioned X further about his awareness at the stage of the emergence of the image of the empty vessel, he replied:

> There are two levels of awareness I think for me now, the physical, strong physical awareness that I'm touching, (touching his desk with his hands) but there's another awareness which is inside, an inner awareness of this image. [...] it's me and I'm empty.

Making distinctions between metaphor and symbol is a challenging task, especially when they are part of people's descriptions of their interior journeys. Lakoff and Johnson (1980) proposed that all our conceptual thought and ways of explaining were based on metaphor. In essence, a metaphor enables one to seek to explain something in terms of another conceptual domain. Lakoff and Johnson (2003) proposed that we 'systematically used inference patterns from one conceptual domain about another conceptual domain' (Lakoff and Johnson, 2003, p. 246). They emphasise that the source domains for our conceptual metaphors come from embodied experience. Was X's 'empty vessel' a metaphor, a way of describing his experience at that moment? Or was it a symbol?

In Jungian terms, a symbol seems to be an image that apparently arises spontaneously, sometimes bearing with it new insights (Jung, 1982). Symbols are 'expressions of a content not yet consciously recognised, or conceptually formulated', which arises from the unconscious (Jung, 1982, p. 104). Petitmengin (2006, p. 240) proposes that symbols can act as pointers to feelings which 'isolate it from the flow of experience'. S's image *of a very old tiny old frame* coming to her had more of the quality of a symbol; emergent, illuminative, spontaneous, and bringing with it new insights that showed her a way forward. These are reflections from a second person point of view. This is a tentative exploration of an area which could yield rich findings through further psychophenomenological research, before we achieve more precise and detailed information of the relationships between these language structures, and the pre-reflective layers of our subjective experience.

Emergence

The third dimension of awareness occurs when new events and connections start to happen spontaneously in the interior world. We have described elsewhere (Mathison and Tosey, 2008) how, when being coached in dressage, the spontaneous emergence and physical experience of the image of a sailing ship with its spinnaker fully extended in the wind apparently re-organised the rider's whole body in the saddle. That image was accompanied by an unexpected, inexplicable and strong physical sensation.

Exploring inner landscapes, and ways of knowing, may generate the emergence of symbols. An awareness of this dimension, and its possible significance, and the complexity of distinguishing between metaphors and symbolic content, is one of the challenges for researchers in this field.

Transformative learning.

Finally, we consider how the data from these interviews, and specifically the way that exploration of awareness and embodied experience led to suspension and new insight, might challenge established notions of transformative learning (Mezirow, 1990; 1991; 2003). In our view, those notions over-emphasise and possibly reify the role of 'critical reflection' in the process of learning. Instead, the explicitation process would appear to highlight the significance of mindful awareness as a process from which learning may emerge.

Transformative learning proposes that people who experience some form of crisis in their lives can, through engaging in critical reflection, profoundly change their meaning schemes. 'Critical reflection' has not, to our knowledge, been specified satisfactorily in sensory terms. Van Woerkem (2008) believes that the term reflection is ill defined in the literature. It is thought to involve people in an examination of their own presuppositions and beliefs, or declarative knowledge, through critiquing the presuppositions on which these were built. Mezirow (2003) states that such critical reflection requires an understanding of the nature of reasons, logic, methods and justification.

A brief overview of some commentators on transformative learning demonstrates the dominance of third person, theoretical perspectives in its discourse. Atherton (2005) has criticised Mezirow, doubting that reflection alone leads automatically to a change in meaning schemes. Cranton and Roy (2003) suggest that the many theories about transformative learning should be thought of as reflecting different aspects of the process. Duerr *et al.* (2003) criticise Mezirow for his over-emphasis on the epistemic dimensions of reflection, and his minimal attention to the emotional and the spiritual. Most recently Kitchenham (2008) has reviewed the development of Mezirow's theory and includes a typology of his views on reflection.

None of these sources, however, make reference to embodied knowledge or the notion of exploring the sensory, many layered landscape of a learner's inner world. These conceptions of reflection are surely inadequate to meet the challenges of the new approach to understanding knowing, one that is embodied, emergent, self organised and enacted (Depraz *et al.*, 2003). The current paradigm of transformative learning is mired in constructivism and cognitivism, seemingly taking no account of developments in the field of consciousness studies.

We have mentioned that we explored the effects on one of our participants of having undergone three very intensive explicitation interviews through a further, reflective interview conducted by the second author. The participant revealed there that she had undergone significant shifts in her perceptions of herself as an embodied being as the result of the explicitation process. These changes resemble those described in the literature of transformative learning.

For example, as with our article on experiencing learning during riding lessons (Mathison and Tosey, 2008), S underwent a change in her awareness of her body. In the follow up (non explicitation) interview with PT, she described these:

> I think the biggest revelation was when [...] she asked me whether I was a dancer, and I said no no no, my body is not my medium .[...] I can't use my body. [...] Then when we did the interview it appeared that actually my consciousness during the act of photography is fully on my body; this was the biggest revelation for me, [...] It was the opposite to what I was claiming [...] realising that it works in a completely different way.

S reported other changes. She had previously participated in workshops in Butoh dancing where she had felt inept. After the explicitation interview, when she became so much more aware of her own embodiment, she found she understood dancing differently, and was able to make sense through her body, of the instructors' suggestions. Previously she had been unable to link these teachers' directives to her sensory experience. This is similar to the riding coach M, (Mathison and Tosey, 2008) whose frustration with the BHS technical terms[4] led her to explore the complexities of riding anew, and thus gain a different understanding of horse and rider.

S's awareness of her own complexity also changed: *you realise how much more is happening inside you than you are aware of*. This went hand in hand with an alteration of her understanding of the creative process, which in turn had such an impact that it led her to alter the research question she was addressing for her doctoral studies.

She also reported developing a greater belief in her own body's signals when photographing, trusting it 'to know when to click'. Now she looked at her own photos differently; seeing more in them. When taking photos, 'I feel more free, and not so desperate to catch the image because I suspect, I know I trust that there is something more happening'.

In contrast to the prevailing notions in the literature, we propose that transformative learning may be viewed as an embodied and enacted process, powered by an increased awareness and embodied mindfulness. Mezirow and his school also stress the catalytic role of personal crisis in initiating transformation. With our participants it seems enough to be curious about one's own deeper processes, and willing to explore them, their arising, and their embodiment with a child's sense of wonder.

While the explicitation interview does not set out to produce transformative learning, Vermersch certainly comments that 'working in this way inevitably produces collateral changes which were neither necessarily wanted nor controlled'[5] (Vermersch, 2008, p 40). This leads us to wonder whether the power and potential of the process of explicitation have been underestimated, particularly when coupled with the use of the metamodel as a tool for inquiry, and linking the transderivational search with allowing for the unfolding of awareness and providing space for the emergence of knowing.

Summary and concluding reflections

In this article we have illustrated the methodological applications of NLP to the exploration of consciousness through the explicitation

---

[4] British Horse Society.

[5] Author's (JM) translation. (*Travailler de cette manière produit inévitablement des changements 'collatéraux' non voulus et non contrôlés.*)

interview, and given some examples. The tools that NLP offers fall into two main categories. One is its approach to language; the other is from its insights into the non-verbal dimensions of consciousness. Drawing on data from explicitation interviews with two people, we have shown how NLP can assist with the evocation of experience, with the elicitation of sensory detail, and with calibration of the interviewee's responses.

We then turned to substantive themes from our analysis. Here we discussed how suspension and Epoche seem to be integral to the emergence of a new awareness. We reflected on qualitatively different dimensions of awareness apparent from the explicitation interviews, and suggested that further effort to map the structures of inner experiencing may be of service to interviewers. This is still a terra incognita of enacted knowing and mindful awareness

Finally we suggested that, in contrast to the established views in the literature, transformative learning, whether it be about a personal act of creation, or the complex, emergent quality of an individual's insight, is unpredictable, embodied, and emergent. The symbolic may also be a significant dimension. This offers an alternative to the cognitivistic emphasis of Mezirow's school of transformative learning, which appears to ignore the richness of embodied knowing and the complexities of our interior worlds.

Acknowledgments

We would like to acknowledge the following people who read our manuscript and whose comments helped us to develop our thinking and challenged us to clarify it on a number of issues: Claire Petitmengin, Monique Esser and Pierre Vermersch.

References

Atherton, J. (2005), 'Critical Reflection' http://www.learningandteaching.info/learning/critical1.htm accessed 26/09/2007

Bandler, R., Grinder, J. (1975), *The Structure of Magic I, A Book About Language and Therapy* (Palo Alto, CA: Science and Behaviour Books, Inc.).

Bandler, R., Grinder, J. (1975A), *Patterns of the Hypnotic Techniques of Milton H. Erickson, M.D. Vol 1* (Cupertino, CA: Meta Publications).

Bandler, R., Grinder, J. (1979), *Frogs into Princes: Neuro-Linguistic Programming*, ed. Steve Andreas (Moab, UT: Real People Press).

Bandler, R., MacDonald, W. (1988), *An Insider's Guide to Sub-Modalities* (Cupertino, CA: Meta Publications).

Barsalou, L.W. (1999) 'Perceptual symbol systems', *Behavioral and Brain Sciences*, **22**, pp. 577–600.

Barsalou, LW. (2008), 'Grounded cognition', *Annual Review of Psychology*, **59**, pp. 1–21.

Barsalou, L.W., Kyle Simmonds, W., Barbey, A.K., Wilson, C.D. (2003), 'Grounding conceptual knowledge in modality specific systems', *Trends in Cognitive Sciences*, **7**(2), pp. 84–91.

Bateson, G. (1973), *Steps to an Ecology of Mind: Collected Essays in Anthropology, Psychiatry, Evolution and Epistemology* (Granada and London: Paladin).

Bateson G. (1979), *Mind and Nature* (Glasgow: Fontana Collins).

Battino, R., South, T.L. (2005), *Ericksonian Approaches, A Comprehensive Manual* 2nd Edition (Wales: Crown House Publishing).

Berger, J.G. (2004), 'Dancing on the threshold of meaning: Recognising and understanding the growing edge', *Journal of Transformative Education*, **2**(4), pp. 336–51.

Bowers, J. (2005), 'Is transformative learning the Trojan Horse of western globalisation?', *Journal of Transformative Education*, **1**(3), pp. 245–63.

Brookfield, S. (2003), 'Putting the critical back into critical pedagogy: A commentary on the Path of Dissent', *Journal of Transformative Education*, **1**(2), pp. 141–49.

Cohen, J.B. (2004), 'Late for school: Stories of transformation in an adult education program', *Journal of Transformative Education*, **2**(3), pp 242–52.

Cranton, P. and Roy, M. (2003), 'When the bottom falls out of the bucket: Towards a holistic perspective on transformative learning', *Journal of Transformative Education*, **1**(2), pp. 86–98.

Depraz, N., Varela, F.J., Vermersch, P. (2003), *On Becoming Aware: A pragmatics of experiencing* (Amsterdam & Philadelphia: John Benjamins).

Dilts, R., DeLozier, J. (2000), *Encyclopedia of Systemic NLP and NLP New Coding* (Capitola, CA: Meta Publications).

Duerr, M., Zajonc, A., Dana, D. (2003), 'Survey of transformative and the spiritual dimensions of higher education', *Journal of Transformative Learning*, **1**(3), pp. 177–211.

Esser, M. (2004), *La Programmation Neuro-linguistique en Debat: Repères cliniques, scientifiques et philosophiques* (Paris: L'Harmattan).

Evans, V., Green, M. (2006), *Cognitive Linguistics: An Introduction* (Edinburgh: Edinburgh University Press).

Fauconnier, G, (1997), *Mappings in Thought and Language* (Cambridge: Cambridge University Press).

Faulkner, C. (1999), *Sub-modalities: An Insider's View of Your Mind* (Lakewood, CO: NLP Comprehensive).

Gendlin, E.T. (1999), 'A new model', in *The View from Within: First person approaches to the study of consciousness*, ed. F.J. Varela and J. Shear, pp. 232–37 (Exeter: Imprint Academic).

Gendlin, E.T. (2008), 'La primauté du corps et non la primauté de la perception: comment le corps connaît la situation et la philosophie', *Expliciter, le journal de l'association GREX*, **74**, pp. 41–47.

Grinder, J., Bandler, R. (1976), *The Structure of Magic II: A Book about Communication and Change* (Palo Alto, CA: Science and Behavior Books, Inc.).

Grinder, J, DeLozier, J. Bandler, R. (1977), *Patterns of the Hypnotic Techniques of Milton H. Erickson, M.D. Vol II* (Capitola, CA: Meta Publications).

Hartelius, G. (2007), 'Quantitative somatic phenomenology: Towards an epistemology of subjective experience', *Journal of Consciousness Studies*, **14**(12), pp. 24–56.

Illeris, K. (2004), 'Transformative learning in the perspective of a comprehensive learning theory', *Journal of Transformative Education*, **2**(2), pp. 79–89.

Johnson, M. (1987), *The Body in the Mind: The Bodily Basis of Meaning, Imagination and Reason* (Chicago & London: University of Chicago Press).

Jung, C.G. (1982), *Dreams*, trans. R.F.C. Hull (London: Routledge, ARK Paperbacks).

Kitchenham, A. (2008), 'The evolution of John Mezirow's transformative learning theory', *Journal of Transformative Education*, **6**(2), pp 104–23.
Korzybski, A. (1958), *Science and Sanity: An Introduction to non-Aristotelian Systems and General Semantics* (Lakeville, CT: The International Non-Aristotelian Library Publishing Company, the Institute of General Semantics).
Lakoff, G., Johnson, M. (1980), *Metaphors We Live By* (Chicago and London: University of Chicago Press).
Lakoff,G., Johnson, M. (1999), *Philosophy in the Flesh: The embodied mind and its challenge to western thought* (New York: Basic Books).
Lakoff, G., Johnson, M. (2003), 'Afterword', in *Metaphors We Live By*, pp. 243–74 (Chicago and London: University of Chicago Press).
Lethin, A. (2002), 'How do we embody intentionality?', *Journal of Consciousness Studies*, **9**(8), pp. 36–44.
Lutz, A. (2002), 'Towards a neurophenomenology as an account of generative passages: A first empirical case study', *Phenomenology and the Cognitive Sciences*, **1**, pp. 133–67.
Lutz, A., Thompson, E. (2003), 'Neuro-phenomenology: Integrating subjective experience and brain dynamics in the neuroscience of consciousness', *Journal of Consciousness Studies*, **10**(9–10), pp. 31–52.
Marti, C. (2003), 'PNL et Scientificité', in M. Esser (Ed) *La Programmation Neuro-linguistique en Débat*, pp. 103–30 (Paris: L'Harmattan).
Mathison, J., Tosey, P. (2008), 'Riding into transformative learning', *Journal of Consciousness Studies*, **15**(2) pp. 67–88.
Maturana, H.R.., Varela, F.J. (1998), *The Tree of Knowledge: The Biological Roots of Human Understanding* Revised Edition (Boston and London: Shambhala).
McLendon, T. L. (1989), *The Wild Days: NLP 1972–1981* (Cupertino, CA: Meta Publications).
McWhinney, W., Markos, L. (2003), 'Transformative education across the threshold', *Journal of Transformative Education*, **1**(1), pp. 16–37.
Maurel, M. (2008), 'La Psycho-phénomenologie, Théorie de l'Explicitation', *Expliciter*, **77**, pp 1–29.
Mezirow, J. (1990), 'Conclusion: Towards transformative learning and emancipatory education' in *Fostering Critical Reflection in Adulthood*, ed. J. Mezirow and Associates (San Francisco & Oxford: Jossey Bass Publishers).
Mezirow, J. (1991), *Transformative Dimension of Adult Learning* (San Francisco & Oxford: Jossey Bass Publishers).
Mezirow, J. (2003), 'Transformative learning as discourse', *Journal of Transformative Education*, **1**(1), pp. 58–63.
Overgaard, M., Gallagher, S., Zöega-Ramsøy, Z. (2008), 'An integration of first person methodologies in cognitive science', *Journal of Consciousness Studies*, **15**(5), pp. 100–20.
Pecher,D., Zeelenberg, R., Barsalou, L.W. (2004), 'Sensorimotor simulations underlie conceptual representations: Modality-specific effects of prior activation', *Psychonomic Bulletin and Review*, **11**(1), pp. 164–67.
Petitmengin-Peugeot, C. (1999), 'The intuitive experience', in *The View from Within: First person approaches to the study of consciousness*, ed. F.J. Varela and J. Shear, pp. 43–78 (Exeter: Imprint Academic).
Petitmengin, C. (2006), 'Describing subjective experience in the second person', *Phenomenology and the Cognitive Sciences*, **5**, pp. 229–69.
Petitmengin C., (2007), 'Towards the source of thought: The gestural and transmodal dimension of lived experience', *Journal of Consciousness Studies*, **14** (3), pp. 54–82.

Petitmengin C., Navarro V., Le Van Quyen M. (2007), 'Anticipating seizure: Pre-reflective experience at the center of neuro-phenomenology', *Consciousness and Cognition*, **16**, pp. 746–64.

Russell, B. (1996), *Introduction to Mathematical Philosophy* (London and New York: Routledge, Taylor and Francis Group).

Simmons, W.K., Pecher, D., Hamann, S.B., Zeelenberg,R., Barsalou, L.W. (2003), 'fMRI evidence for modality specific processing of conceptual knowledge on six modalities'. http://userwww.service.emory.edu/~barsalou/Papers/CNS_2003_Poster_2003_Poster.pdf accessed 18/11/08.

Tosey, P., Mathison, J., Michelli, D. (2005), 'Mapping transformative learning: The potential of NLP', *Journal of Transformative Education*, **3**(2), pp. 140–67.

Tosey, P., Mathison, J. (2008), 'Do organisations learn? Some implications for HRD of Bateson's levels of learning', *Human Resource Development Review*, **7**(1), pp. 3–12.

Tosey, P., Mathison, J. (2009), *Neuro-linguistic Programming: A critical appreciation* (London: Palgrave MacMillan).

Van Woerkom, M. (2008), 'Critical reflection and related higher-level conceptualizations of learning: Realistic or idealistic?', *Human Resources Development Review*, **7**(1), pp. 3–12.

Varela, F.J. (1996), 'Neurophenomenology', *Journal of Consciousness Studies*, **3**(4), pp. 330–49.

Varela, F. (1997), 'Patterns of life: Inter-twining identity and cognition', *Brain and Cognition*, **34**, pp. 72–87.

Varela, F., Shear, J. (2000), 'First person methodologies, what, why how?', in *The View from Within: First person approaches to the study of consciousness*, ed. F.J. Varela and J. Shear (Exeter: Imprint Academic).

Varela, F.J., Thompson, E., Rosch, E. (1993), *The Embodied Mind: Cognitive Science and Human Experience* (Cambridge, MA & London: MIT Press).

Vermersch, P. (1994), *L'Entretien D'Éxplicitation* (Issy-les- Moulineaux:EDF Editeur).

Vermersch, P. (1996), 'Pour une Psychophénomenologie', *Expliciter*, **13**, pp. 1–16.

Vermersch, P. (1999), 'Introspection as practice', *Journal of Consciousness Studies*, **6**(2–3), pp. 17–42.

Vermersch, P. (1999A), 'Pour une Psychologe phénoménologique', *Psychologie Francaise*, **44**(10), pp. 7–19.

Vermersch, P. (2008), 'Introduction à la lecture de l'article de Endlin: "La primauté du corps et non la primauté de la perception"', *Expiciter*, **74** (March), p. 40.

Von Foerster, H. (1973), 'On constructing reality', in *Environmental Design Research Vol II*, ed. F.E. Preiser, pp. 25–48 (New York: Spartan Books).

Walker, W. (2004), *Abenteuer Kommunikation: Bateson, Perls, Satir, Erickson und die Anfänge des Neurolinguistisches Programmierens (NLP) 4 Auflage* (Stuttgart:Klett-Cotta).

Watzlawick, P., Beavin-Bavelas, J., Jackson, D.D. (1967), *Pragmatics of Human Communication: A Study of Interactional Patterns and Paradoxes* (New York & London: W.W. Norton & Company, Inc.).

Watzlawick, P. (1990), *Muenchausen's Pigtail, or Psychotherapy and 'Reality': Essays and Lectures* (New York & London: W.W. Norton & Co.).

Weber, A. (2002), 'The "Surplus of Meaning": Biosemiotic aspects in Francisco J. Varela's philosophy of cognition', *Cybernetics and Human Knowing*, **9**(2), pp. 11–30.

Wilson, M. (2002), 'Six views of embodied cognition', *Psychonomic Bulletin and Review*, **9**(4), pp. 625–36.

Connirae Andreas and Tamara Andreas

Aligning Perceptual Positions
A new distinction in NLP[1]

Abstract: *This article describes and refines an experiential distinction which has been highlighted by neuro-linguistic programming (NLP), perceptual positions. When you are imagining a past or future scene, you may perceive it (usually pre-reflectively) from three different viewpoints or perceptual positions. If you are looking at the world from your own point of view, through your own eyes, you are in the first perceptual position. If you are looking at the scene through another person's eyes, appreciating the other person's point of view, you are in the second position. If you are seeing the world from an outside point of view, as an independent observer, you are in the third position. NLP highlighted the fact that our feelings change dramatically according to the perceptual position we adopt. Through a concrete example, Connirae Andreas shows that this distinction does not only concern visual perceptions, but also auditory and kinaesthetic perceptions. She also shows that our visual, auditory and kinaesthetic perceptions may be split in different perceptual positions at the same time, and that this misalignment may cause difficulties. Learning to 'align' our perceptual positions brings us greater wholeness, enables us to become more integrated.*

Editors' Introduction

We have chosen to reproduce this article by Connirae and Tamara Andreas in this special issue dedicated to first person methods,

---

[1] First published in *Anchor Point*, Feb. 1991 (Vol. 5, N° 2), with minor edits April 2006.
© Connirae Andreas and Tamara Andreas

because it illustrates several important aspects of first person investigation at the same time: the structured character of lived experience, its pre-reflective character, and the usefulness of becoming aware of one's pre-reflective experience. The article also exemplifies interview techniques enabling a person to elicit his/her pre-reflective experience.

First, 'perceptual positions' are a striking example of the generic structure of lived experience. Whatever its contents are, and whatever its mode is (visual, auditory or kinaesthetic), a perception is experienced from a given position, a given 'viewpoint' that neuro-linguistic programming (NLP) calls 'perceptual position' — a position which does not necessarily correspond to the localization of our sensory organs. This is the case for a present perception as well as for the evocation of a past perception or the imagination of a future perception. This perceptual position may take different values that NLP calls 'self', 'other' and 'observer'.[2] Moreover — and this is the discovery of Connirae Andreas — at a given moment our perceptual position may differ from one sensory modality to the other: for example, I can be in 'self' position in the visual mode, and in 'other' position in the auditory mode. In other words, my 'viewpoint', my 'listeningpoint' and my 'feelingpoint' may differ. The perceptual position is therefore a generic experiential variable, which could be represented as a matrix for a given instant of experience, and as a three dimensional matrix if we consider its evolution in time. The importance of this structure is especially obvious in the processes of communication and especially the empathetic process which consists in adopting the 'other' viewpoint. But this structure may also play an important role, which has attracted less attention up to now, in some other cognitive processes.

Secondly, perceptual positions are a striking example of pre-reflective dimension of lived experience. It is rare for novices being asked to describe their lived experience to spontaneously give indications of their perceptual position, it is rare that they are reflectively conscious of it. It is even rarer that they are reflectively conscious of the variations of this position in time, and of the differences of position according to the sensory modes at a given instant. Yet this dimension of experience is always there for each of us, it determines the quality, the 'what it feels like' of our experience, the way we interact with the world, and probably the performance of some of our

---

[2] Dilts also speaks of 1st, 2nd and 3rd perceptual position (e.g. in Dilts, 1998, p. 48). Gallagher introduces slightly different descriptive categories: first-person-egocentric perspective, third-person-egocentric perspective, first person and third person allocentric perspective (Gallagher, 2003a).

cognitive processes. But a specific support is necessary so that we can acquire a reflective consciousness of it. Such a support enables us to become aware of very fine variations of our perceptual positions, even within a given position and sensorial mode. For example, in 'self' position, the bodily zone that is perceived as the centre of visual attention may move subtly from the eyes toward the back of the skull, or even slightly outside of the head. Or the zone that is perceived as the centre of kinaesthetic attention may move down from the chest toward the belly.

Third, this example illustrates the usefulness of becoming aware of one's pre-reflective experience. Becoming aware of our perceptual positions and of the possibility we have to shift from one position to another enables us to learn how to adapt our position according to the circumstances, instead of being 'stuck' in one position. For example, phobic people may be trained to remember the traumatic event as an 'observer', resulting in more resourceful feelings. The authors discuss how becoming aware of the position differences according to the sensory modes permits even subtler adjustments, consisting in 'aligning' our perceptual positions at a given moment on a given position. To take an example related to our preoccupations in this volume: in the context of an explicitation interview, it is important for the interviewer to be acutely conscious of his/her own perceptual position at a given instant and to know how to shift flexibly from one position to another. As far as the interviewee is concerned, in order to enter into contact with his experience and describe it, it is essential for his different perceptual modes to be aligned in 'self' position,[3] and for the interviewer to know how to lead him into this position.

Finally, the interview which is the basis of the following article exemplifies elicitation techniques used in NLP (as well as in some other first person methods). The reader will note the importance of 'calibration' (Mathison, this issue), that is the capacity of the interviewer to observe closely his interlocutor's physiological reactions as well as the pre-reflective gestures accompanying his words (or substituted for his words), and the way the interviewer uses these observations in his prompts in order to help the subject to become reflectively aware of his experience and to refine his description.

We thank Connirae Andreas for permitting us to reproduce this article here.

---

[3] The so-called 'evocation state' (Vermersch, this issue; Petitmengin & Bitbol, this issue) or 'association state' (Mathison, this issue) which enables someone to come into contact with a past experience in order to describe it, corresponds to an aligned 'self' perceptual position.

Aligning Perceptual Positions: A new distinction in NLP

'Perceptual Positions' has been an important and useful distinction in neuro-linguistic programming (NLP), one that can be used to enhance our flexibility, wisdom and resourcefulness. There are three major perceptual positions:

SELF position is experiencing the world from my own position: I see and hear other people and the world around me from my own point of view, have my own feelings, etc. This is also called association.

OTHER position is experiencing the world literally from some other person's position. If I remember a conversation with a friend, I recall it as him, seeing and hearing events from his viewpoint, feeling his body feelings, etc.

OBSERVER position means experiencing the world from the outside, as an observer. If I do this, I literally observe myself and whatever situation I am in from the outside, as if seeing someone else. This is also called dissociation.

Brilliant people in many disciplines are able to shift their perceptual position flexibly, and this is a basis for their special skills. Most Practitioner Trainings include training in shifting from one position to another.

Many limitations have been usefully described as being 'stuck' in one perceptual position. A phobia, for example, arises from being 'stuck' in Self position. Phobics plunge right back into a terrible memory and panic. The phobia technique trains people to experience the traumatic event as an Observer. At the other extreme, people can be described as so dissociated into an Observer position that they no longer experience their own lives.

Co-dependence has been described as being 'stuck' in Other position. Co-dependents report feeling the feelings of another person intensely.

While I (Connirae) have always found the perceptual positions model tremendously useful, I noticed several of my own experiences just didn't fit with the model. This led me to develop a new way of thinking about perceptual positions that has produced fascinating results.

We've all had the experience of asking someone to step out of an experience and dissociate into Observer position, and heard them say, 'I can't do it; I still feel the feelings.' From the Basic Perceptual

Positions model, we could describe this as, 'They fell back into the experience', or 'They couldn't get out of the experience'.

One day, as I was doing an NLP process, I noticed that as I stepped out of the experience, into the Observer position, I felt my own feelings more strongly. Clearly, I wasn't 'falling back into it', or even 'taking my feelings with me'. I was feeling my feelings much more intensely when I was watching myself from the outside. I thought, 'That's strange', and stepped back and forth several times, to be sure.

I began thinking, 'What if it's not that limitations arise out of being stuck in one perceptual position? What if limitations actually arise out of our representational systems[4] being split in different perceptual positions at the same time?' For example, as I experience an event, I could be seeing out of my own eyes (Self position); I could be feeing the feelings of the other person (Other position); and I could be hearing an internal voice making comments from the outside (Observer position). In this example, each of my three representational systems would be in a different perceptual position.

This new way of thinking gives rise to a new model for what to do: *The goal now becomes what I decided to call 'aligning perceptual positions'. This means having all three major representational systems in the same perceptual position, at the same time.*

This sounds rather obvious — we might think it would be commonplace to have our vision, hearing, and feelings in the same perceptual position at the same time. However, in considerable research to date, *we have found no one who has their perceptual positions fully aligned in situations of difficulty.* And while aligning perceptual positions doesn't magically turn every difficulty into a wonderful event, it does get consistent, significant shifts toward resourcefulness. Sometimes it clears up relationship problems quite dramatically, and sometimes it makes the crucial difference in whether another NLP pattern works or not. Thinking about our experiences in this way brings into awareness misalignments that were not obvious to us with the old model.

One NLP Practitioner who had been through many perceptual positions exercises reported that this process finally allowed him to be completely in Self position. 'Before this, I felt like I was trying to get into Self position, but I couldn't stay there. I automatically moved out,' he said. When he aligned his Self Position, he felt a strong physiological flushing — a rush of heat — that let him know he was really in his own experience and feeling it. Another Practitioner reported having 'boundaries issues' where she found herself falling into other

---

[4] In NLP 'representational systems' are sensory modalities (Note of the Editor).

people's feelings. After aligning her perceptual positions, she reported that this work had made more difference for her than any other work she had done with 'boundaries'. It is worth noting that some have experienced perceptual shifts as striking as regaining hearing loss, recovering peripheral vision, and improving vision, after using this process.

The transcribed example that follows provides a demonstration of the alignment process. More complete information and examples are available in the references section at the end of this article.

1. Eliciting Perceptual Position Misalignment

The first thing Connirae does with Bob is find out how he naturally experiences the situation, before any changes are made. She will use this information for the alignment later in the process.

Visual:

> Connirae: Think of an unresourceful situation that involves you and one other person. When you think of this situation, first notice what you see.
> Bob: Visually, it's my perspective.
> Connirae: NLP-trained people tend to give a label for which perspective it is, but we want to gather more detailed information. It turns out that our first impression of what we are doing is usually not precisely it. So, Bob, tell me exactly what you see. Where is the other person?
> Bob: I'm seeing out of my own eyes. The other person is to the side (gesturing to his left).
> Connirae: All right. This next question may sound a little strange, and that's okay. Check to find out if you are seeing exactly out of your eyes, or if it's as if your eyes have shifted slightly. Notice if your visual perspective is even slightly dislocated in any direction from your eyes — in front, behind, to one side, above, or below.
> Bob: I'm looking from a little to my right (gesturing slightly to the right of his eyes and higher than eye level).
> Connirae: OK. And are you looking from eye level, or is it higher or lower?
> Bob: Actually, I think I'm looking from a little higher than eye level.
> Connirae: Great. That matches your gestures. So, visually you are looking from a place between Self and Observer positions.

(Note: In Self position, we are looking out of our own eyes. When we look from Observer position, we are watching both Self and Other interacting, from a position outside of either Self or Other. Bob's viewpoint is just a bit to the right of Self position, so while it is not in Self position, it is far from a true Observer position.)

Auditory:

> Connirae: Now let's find out about what you hear. What sounds are you aware of when you think of the situation?
> Bob: I'm aware of the dialogue.
> Connirae: And where are you listening from?
> Bob: It's as if I'm listening from way over there. (He gestures in front and to the right, about 15 feet away.)
> Connirae: Do you hear what's actually going on, or is it some commentary about the situation?
> Bob: Both.
> Connirae: Tell me a couple of sample sentences of the commentary you're hearing.
> Bob: 'I'm really stupid. I can't believe this.'
> Connirae: And where is the commentary voice coming from?
> Bob: Around my head (gesturing close to his head, in a semicircle around the back and sides).
> Connirae: OK. So the commentary voice is coming from around your head, using the pronoun 'I', and you're listening from fifteen feet out to the side. Your voice is almost in Self position, and your ears are in Observer.

(Note: When Bob gestured to where he was listening from, he indicated a spot where an Observer might stand to observe the situation from the outside. However, his commentary voice is very close to his own throat, which is where a Self position voice would be speaking from.)

Kinesthetic:

> Connirae: Now let's find out about the kinesthetic system. Notice whose feelings you have, and where they are located.
> Bob: They feel like they're my feelings (gesturing to the centre of his chest).
> Connirae: Are they right in the centre, or are they slightly dislocated?
> Bob: Right in the middle.
> Connirae: So, feelings are in Self position.

2. Aligning Observer Position

Connirae: The next step is to align the Perceptual Positions. We can align either Self or Observer Position first. With you, I'm inclined to align Observer position first, because you already have much of your awareness there, and because Self position looks quite unpleasant right now (Bob nods emphatically).

Visual:

Connirae: I'll be inviting you to make some changes, and you can notice what happens in your experience when you do that. We'll start with Visual. Sometimes aligning one system allows other systems to change automatically.

First, let this whole scenario swing around (gesturing in a half-circle) so that you see Bob and the other person interacting out there in front of you. ... Now you are in Observer Position, watching Bob and the other person. Make it so that both Bob and the other person are exactly the same distance from you as the Observer. You can also let these people move to eye level. (Bob's breathing, expression, and colour change considerably.)

(To Audience, with a smile)
In NLP, one of the skills we develop as practitioners is called 'sensory acuity', which means when someone's inner experience shifts, a trained observer will notice 'subtle' external shifts.

Bob, what happened in your experience as you played around with that?

Bob: Most of the feelings drop out! There's a lot more clarity, a lot more sense of perspective and distance. It's more egalitarian.

Connirae: That makes sense. Before, more than half of the available information was missing.

(To the group)
While Bob was looking at the situation from outside his body, the viewpoint was so close that he couldn't really see himself clearly. Without that, he couldn't see the communication loop between himself and the other person clearly, either.

Auditory:

Connirae: Now that we've done the visual part, let's check the auditory, and find out if that's already done or if we still need to do more. As you look at them over there, notice whether your ears came over here also, and have already rejoined your body as the Observer.

Bob: Yes, I'm hearing from here now.

(When we make one change toward alignment, such as seeing both people at eye level, or equidistant, frequently other changes toward alignment just happen. As Connirae continues, she is sensitive to the fact that Bob's voices may already by more aligned. She continues to invite alignment wherever it has not yet occurred.)

Connirae: Great. Now, do you still have the commentary voice that was around your head? The one that said 'I'm really stupid. I can't believe this'?

Bob: It's different.

Connirae: Okay. Where is the voice that's commenting now?

Bob: It's coming from in front of me. (Bob's gesture indicates that the voice is talking from about 2 feet in front of him.)

Connirae: The ideal location of the Observer voice works slightly differently for different people. Usually it comes from inside our body, as the Observer. So, Bob, let's find out if this will be useful for you. What happens if the voice commenting on the conversation comes from your throat as the Observer? ... (Connirae gestures where the voice was, and moves her hand to indicate where the voice will go. She gives Bob a moment to notice what this shift is like.) Which do you like better?... What we want is a clean Observer voice that allows you to take in data the most resourcefully.

Bob: This whole thing is so unfamiliar, I'm not sure. It's so different to have the sound coming from my throat!

Connirae: So, you can experiment with that a little more, and as it becomes more familiar, notice which way works better for you.

Bob: I think it's better from inside (he gestures toward his throat).

Connirae: And Bob, you can make sure this Observer voice is also using Observer pronouns. Rather than saying 'I' and 'you', this voice will say 'he', 'she', and 'they'. 'They are doing this, she this, he that,' etc.

(Connirae allows time for Bob to listen to his voice stating observations using 'he', 'she', 'they', etc.)

Kinesthetic:

Connirae: Now we'll do the kinesthetic part. As you look at them, equidistant from you, at eye level, and your internal voice is describing the situation using 'he, she, they' pronouns, notice what feelings you have. Do you have any feelings left that really belong to one of the two people over there?

Bob: A little bit.

Connirae: Whose feelings are they?

Bob: Bob's.

Connirae: OK. (joking) Now, Bob might start being annoyed if you run around with his feelings! So just notice where in your body you have any remnant of his feelings. And when you're ready, let those feelings go back to him, over there. Schhoop! ... (Connirae adds sounds effect as she gestures from where the feelings have been, toward the Bob out in front.) And notice what Observer feelings fill in place.

Bob: The word 'vacuum' comes to mind.

Connirae: Is that resourceful for you, or are there some other feelings that would be more resourceful, while being neutral Observer feelings?

Bob: I think I want something a little more resourceful.

Connirae: So you can let that feeling fill in now, and your unconscious mind can be a guide in what kind of feelings begin to radiate and fill in, ... with something more resourceful ... (Bob gains more skin colour and looks more resourceful.) Your unconscious mind has already noticed that this is unfamiliar, and that's wonderful, because that's the news of difference, and this is certainly different from what you were experiencing before. So your unconscious can mark this out, and already begin experimenting with just where and when you will be automatically taking this position in the future, so that what was unfamiliar becomes very familiar, an automatic resource to you.

Bob: It just said, 'Be sure to have the flexibility to bounce back and forth between positions.'

Connirae: That's wise, and that's what we're getting to next. It's good for our unconscious to know that a clean Observer position is available to us as a resource. Having this can make it easier to align the Self position, because we know we can get back to Observer position whenever we want to. It's a position of safety and comfort we can go to at any time.

3. Aligning Self Position

Now we'll align the Self position. First notice what it's like when you step into Self position. Notice what's different from before. ... Are you seeing out of your own eyes?

Bob: I'm seeing exactly out of my eyes now.

Connirae: Is there any difference in how you see the other person from Self position now?

Bob: They're much clearer, and they're right in front of me.

Connirae: Good. Often the other person is clearer after aligning Observer position. Check your voice now, in this position. Do you have any internal dialogue?

Bob: I just hear the conversation. I hear the other person on the outside and me responding.

Connirae: Are you hearing from your own ears, already?

Bob: Yes. ... This is all very unfamiliar!

Connirae: And that's fine. ... Now I want to be sure you have the choice of having internal dialogue in this position. So, notice what happens if you say on the inside, 'I feel this. I think this. I want this.'

Bob: The voice is coming from my chest (speaking softly, smiling slightly). And some very powerful feelings come with it (gesturing across his whole torso, Bob's body is more relaxed than earlier, and has more skin colour).

Connirae: Good. And this looks different from before. In Self position, the voice is inside the body, from the chest/throat area, and uses 'I' pronouns.

Kinesthetic:

Connirae: Check to be sure you have your own feelings, inside your body.

Bob: Yes.

Connirae: Is there any difference in the quality of your feelings now, compared to before we aligned these positions?

Bob: Yes, a dramatic difference! I have an awareness of my body, going out into my arms and legs, that wasn't there before.

Connirae: Great. Now pop back into Observer position, and notice if anything is different in Observer position now that you have been in an aligned Self position ...

Bob: Yes, the main difference is that Bob's voice in the interaction sounds very different.

4. Other Position

Connirae: OK. Now that we've aligned Self and Observer positions, it is possible to go into Other position and gather uncontaminated data. Before aligning Self and Observer positions, it's very difficult if not impossible, to gather clean data about the Other. If we aren't cleanly sorted ourselves, we tend to carry bits of ourselves into the Other Position and strongly colour what we learn about the other person.

For this exercise, when we step into Other position, we won't align it, we will just discover what we find there. The reason we aren't aligning it is that we are primarily discovering what we can learn about that person and their experience. Most likely they are not aligned in this situation, just as we weren't. Often the other person is not in a very resourceful state, so you don't need to stay there very long — just long enough to get a sense of what it's like.

To make this easy, you can just let the situation swing around and pop into the other person, looking out at Bob.

Bob: That's really different. As her, I feel confused. That's kind of a revelation to me.

Connirae: Good ... And ... we need to remember that this is still a hallucination — a guess. It's our experience of being them, not their experience of being them. The more we align our perceptual positions, the more accurate our guesses become.

So, now you can let the scene rotate again, so that you move back into Observer position ... and then back into Self.

5. Discussion

Becoming aligned is different for each person. Once Bob's Observer position was aligned, his Self position was automatically aligned. Usually, it's still necessary to align each representational system in Self position: to invite the person to move the viewpoint into exactly their own eyes, to invite the voice to come exactly from their own throat, the listening to come exactly into the ears, feelings to be centered in the body, etc.

We've found many interesting ways people can be misaligned. In one of our workshops, a man named Dan noticed that his point of view moved in a circle around his eyes. When he discovered this, he said, 'Oh, that's so interesting! That really fits, because I've never wanted to let anyone pin me down.'

Joseph was seeing himself from the outside, while having his own feelings of being observed. As you can imagine, he reported feeling self-conscious.

Sometimes misaligned perceptual positions make if difficult for other NLP interventions to work. One participant reported that this made sense out of why submodalities changes hadn't worked for him. He said, 'I could change all the submodalities, but it didn't change my feelings. When I realized my feelings were out to the side, and I moved them back into me, the submodality changes had an impact.'

Rebecca, who was NLP-trained, discovered that when she took Observer position, she was looking straight at the Other person directly in front of her, but her Self was way off to the left side. After she aligned this position, moving her Self and the Other to be centered in front of her as Observer, she commented: 'Now I can see much more how my behaviour impacts the situation. Before I thought I was peripheral and it was just the other person who mattered. I realize I've done all the NLP dissociation processes that way, so I didn't get the full benefit.' Rebecca used the word 'peripheral' to describe how she thought of her potential for impact; it turned out that this was a direct expression of where she had seen herself in her inner picture.

Our inner sensing configuration is always a reflection of how we experience ourselves and interact with our world. It is a direct expression of our many beliefs about ourselves and others. As such it gives us a powerful window to notice and transform aspects of our experience to become more resourceful and whole as human beings.

Some of us trained in NLP may have spontaneously done a few of these kinds of interventions before. However, thinking of it in this new way — that it's about aligning our inner experience including all of our representational system — means I notice things I never would have noticed before. Practitioners, Master Practitioners and Trainers who were already experienced with perceptual positions are also reporting this.

A useful mindset when exploring aligning perceptual positions is to assume that whatever inner configuration we are now using, we originally developed as a solution to something. It was our being's best wisdom in a difficult situation. For instance, when someone is part inside and part outside of their body, it may have been an attempt to dissociate from an overwhelming situation when they were so young they didn't have the ability to fully dissociate. Whatever we are currently doing originally served some useful intent. Aligning the perceptual positions offers another choice that will 'stick' whenever it is a better solution. We invite you to explore this model gently, with respect for any objections and full attention to ecology. The process lives up to its potential when we have an attitude of curiosity and discovery, noticing what happens when we allow our configuration to be aligned. We can trust our being to keep any arrangement that is, for us, a 'better solution'.

This article is just a brief introduction. This method can actually be taken to quite a bit of depth — the process of alignment can continue. One of my workshop participants who was an experienced meditator, commented that he experienced the method as a direct way of accessing the kind of 'clean' and empty state that he reached through meditation. In this brief demonstration with Bob, I aligned the most obvious things. With 'advanced' use, we find more subtleties to align. There are more criteria for alignment, unique ways to work with people who have different configurations, ways to honor ecological considerations within the process, etc. (See reference materials below and trainings for more information.)

With exploration, this method can be used as a practice that brings about greater wholeness as human beings. We become literally more integrated. Some methods help us get particular outcomes in our lives that we have decided we want — for example we might want to be confident when asking someone on a date, or motivated to finish a project. In contrast, this method assists us in becoming more whole human beings. We become more aligned — and then discover what we and our world are like. We may find that we want different things — our goals might be different than when our inner world was out of alignment.

References

NLP

Andreas, C. and Andreas, S. (1989), *Heart of the Mind* (Real People Press).
Andreas, C. and Andreas, S. (1996), *Core Transformation Trainer Materials Packet* (Real People Press).
Andreas, C. and Andreas, T. (forthcoming), *Coming Home to Yourself* (Real People Press).
Bateson, G. (1979), *Mind and Nature* (Dutton).
Dilts R. (1998), *Modeling with NLP* (Capitola, CA: Meta publications).
Grinder J. and Delozier J. (1987), *Turtles All the Way Down* (Grinder, DeLozier and Associates).

Other references on perceptual positions

Gallagher, S. (2003a), 'Phenomenology and experiential design', *Journal of Consciousness Studies*, **10** (9–10), pp. 85–99.
Gallagher, S. (2003b), 'Complexities in the first-person perspective: comments on Zahavi's *Self-Awareness and Alterity*', *Research in Phenomenology*, **32**, pp. 238–48.
Nigro, G. and Neisser, U. (1983), 'Point of view in personal memories', *Cognitive Psychology*, **15**, pp. 467–82.

Audio and video resources

Demonstrations and workshops on aligning perceptual positions are available on CD and DVD from NLP Comprehensive (nlpco.com) and from Real People Press (realpeoplepress.com).

Russell T. Hurlburt, Christopher L. Heavey & Arva Bensaheb

Sensory Awareness

Abstract: *Sensory awareness — the direct focus on some specific sensory aspect of the body or outer or inner environment — is a frequently occurring yet rarely recognized phenomenon of inner experience. It is a distinct, complete phenomenon; it is not merely, for example, an aspect of a perception. Sensory awareness is one of the five most common forms of inner experience, according to our results (the other four: inner speech, inner seeing, feelings, and unsymbolized thinking). Despite its high frequency, many people do not notice its appearance nor recognize its theoretical import. We describe sensory awareness and distinguish it from other aspects of experience. We give examples and discuss how it appears when moments of inner experience are examined carefully. We note that there are large individual differences in the observed frequency of sensory awareness and consider its relationship to mental health and other aspects of psychological functioning.*

Keywords

Sensory awareness; Descriptive Experience Sampling; phenomenal consciousness; inner experience

Sensory Awareness

Careful examination of momentary experience will reveal moments such as the following:

Example 1:
Andrew is dialing his cell phone. At the moment, he is just 'zeroed in' on the shiny blueness of the brushed

aluminum phone case. He is not, at that moment, paying attention to the number he is dialing; his experience has momentarily left that task (which continues as if on autopilot) to be absorbed in the shiny blueness.

Example 2:
Betty is in conversation with her friend Wendy, and as Wendy speaks, Betty takes a sip of Dr. Pepper. At that moment, Betty is drawn to the coldness of the liquid as it moves through her throat. Wendy continues to talk, but Wendy's voice is not part of Betty's experience; Betty is focused on the coldness in her throat.

Example 3:
Carol's friend Candy is telling Carol how to log into a computer web site. Carol is paying attention to the sweetly longish *a* sound in Candy's slight drawl; at that moment, Carol is not paying attention to what Candy is saying about the log-in procedure.

Example 4:
Damian is checking out at the grocery store, and at the moment is noticing a twinge in the back of his neck — a slight stabbing sensation. He is in the act of putting three candy bars on the conveyer, but at that moment he is not at all noticing candy bars, the checker's activity, or anything else in his environment — his attention is occupied by the neck sensation.

These examples represent a common phenomenon that we have found frequently in the inner experience of the hundreds of people whom we have examined over the last several decades. Each example involves the individual's being immersed in the experience of a particular sensory aspect of his or her external or internal environment without particular regard for the instrumental aim or perceptually complete-objectness. We have called such phenomena 'sensory awareness' (Hurlburt, 1990; 1993; 1997; Hurlburt & Heavey, 2001; 2002; 2006). In example 1, Andrew's momentary interest is not instrumental: he's dialing but he's attending to the shiny-blueness, not the dialing. And his momentary interest is not in the complete object: he is drawn not to the *phone*, which happens to be shiny-blue, but to the *shiny-blueness*, which happens to be of the phone.

Heavey and Hurlburt (2008; Hurlburt & Heavey, 2002) showed that sensory awareness is a feature of roughly one quarter of all apprehended moments of waking experience, and thus appears to be one of the five most common features of everyday inner experience (the other four: inner speech, inner seeing, feelings, and unsymbolized thinking). Despite the prevalence of sensory awareness it remains little discussed within the consciousness literature.

Sensory awareness is certainly nothing new or unusual: almost everyone can notice a shiny blueness, feel the coldness of an iced drink, hear a feature of a friend's voice, or feel a muscle twinge. What is extraordinary, and what needs to be taken seriously by consciousness science, is that some people may experience such sensory awareness at nearly all their waking moments (Heavey & Hurlburt, 2008), others may experience it at almost none, and others may experience it frequently but not always.

This paper describes not only the sensory awareness phenomenon but also its manner of appearing, a necessity because of the nature of the phenomenon. Sensory awareness becomes an interesting phenomenon only when it is explored as it naturally occurs in natural environments, as part of pristine experience (Hurlburt, 2009, this issue; Hurlburt & Akhter, 2006). In the laboratory, it is easy to contrive situations where subjects *always* report sensory phenomena and other situations where subjects *never* report sensory phenomena. If individual differences are important, we will have to use a method that allows those differences to emerge and to be observant about how they emerge.

The Appearing of Sensory Awareness

The examples above are typical products of investigations using the Descriptive Experience Sampling (DES) method, a method aimed at exploring inner experience in natural environments (Hurlburt, 1990, 1993; Hurlburt & Akhter, 2006; Hurlburt & Heavey, 2006; Hurlburt & Schwitzgebel, 2007). Briefly, DES gives a subject a beeper that is carried into the subject's natural environments. At the beeper's random beep, the subject is to pay attention to the experience that was ongoing at the last undisturbed moment before the beep began and then, immediately, to jot down notes about that experience. Within 24 hours, the DES investigator interviews the subject about the (typically six) sampled moments from that day. Then the sample/interview procedure is repeated (iterated; see Hurlburt, this issue) for several (typically three) more sampling days. The adequacy of the DES procedure has been discussed by Hurlburt (1993; 1997), Hurlburt and Heavey (2002; 2006), and Hurlburt and Schwitzgebel (2007).

Example 5:

> Here is a typical example of the manner in which sensory awareness appears in a DES interview. This verbatim (but slightly edited to remove redundancies and irrelevancies) transcript is from a second-sampling-day interview conducted with 'Ephraim' by Arva Bensaheb, who begins by asking Ephraim to describe his experience at the fifth beep:

Ephraim: [laughs nervously] At the moment of the beep I'm eating clam chowder with a relatively large spoon. And at the moment of the beep I'm pushing ... I had ... I had put the spoon [laughs sheepishly] laying on the top surface of the soup, and I was pushing down slightly, feeling the resistance of it, and then watching the soup spill over the edges really slowly, and watching [laughs sheepishly] the way that it cascaded over the edges of the spoon and filled it up. [scratches head in apparent resignation] I'd done this quite a few times already, but it was still very fun [smiles sheepishly] — I ate the whole bowl of soup that way. But I was definitely ... the things that stuck out in my mind were the resistance of having to push the spoon down, and the way that — particularly because it's clam chowder — it's [laughs sheepishly] going over the edge: it was like you could see it, the path that it took over the edge, and how it didn't fill, like, symmetrically. Like one part would go over faster, rather than just like going in, in a slowly collapsing circle. It was more of like an amoeba shape [sighs resignedly] getting smaller. [smiles nervously] At this point there ... I know as a fact of the universe there was music in the background, but I wasn't ... it wasn't there ... any more.

Arva: So right at the moment of the beep you are aware of this resistance of the spoon against the soup...

E: Um hm.

A: ... and watching the soup spill into the spoon asymmetrically.

E: [nods affirmatively, nervously]

A: Anything else [laughs] in your experience at the moment of the beep? ...

SENSORY AWARENESS 235

E: [shakes head negatively, resignedly]

A: ... The music, you said, was there.

E: Yeah ... I know it was on, but it wasn't ... I wasn't listening to it. I was just really intent on the shape and watching the way that it moved over the spoon. [pauses, shakes head in resigned sheepishness] That's about it.

A: And this resistance ... Does it make sense to ask you, like, where you were feeling this resistance? Like, I don't know, if you were holding the spoon, was it in your arm, or in your hand, or ...

E: I felt the resistance in the end of the spoon, like the spoon part of the spoon. Like I don't even know if that makes sense, but ...

A: The spoon meaning not the handle, ...

E: Not in the handle, yeah...

A: ... the scoopy part. [laughs]

E: [laughs] Yes, in the scoopy part of the spoon. That's where I perceived the resistance, not in my fingers or in my hand. [shakes head in resignation] Just kind of weird.

A: And what is this feeling/sensation? Can you describe it any further?

E: Resistance. Like soft, like, I don't know, it's hard to explain, because it's like [laughs sheepishly] you have to be kind of gentle with how hard you push on the spoon, but the more ... like it builds up [laughs sheepishly]. You have to push the spoon [laughs embarrassedly] rather gently, but in order to do it gently enough the resistance actually feels pretty great, to the point where once the end of the spoon finally gets right below the surface of the soup, you can feel it just go away, like there was a *ton* of resistance, but [smiles sheepishly] it's probably not that much resistance. But just the carefulness of it made it seem that way.

A: So was there like a different degree of resistance, by any chance? I don't know if this makes sense, but, like, at the moment of the beep, and I don't know how much the

>
> beep caught, but it seems like there's more resistance and then the spoon goes in and resistance is less, and …. Is there a change, or anything like that, in your experience, or is it just the initial …
>
> E: Hm. [nods quizzically] I would say that what I was experiencing was the initial resistance against it. I did just say … I guess I mentioned … that it changes. But that isn't really at the moment of the beep. That was just more from doing it a couple … 20 times. I learned! [laughs embarrassedly]
>
> A And then the soup pouring into the spoon. Is that part of your experience at the moment of the beep? Or…
>
> E: Yeah.
>
> A: … the shape of it, or whatever?
>
> E: Yeah. The shape, the way that it looked.
>
> A: And how is that in …?
>
> E: That was more, I mean, we've focused on the resistance thing, but the purpose of it [smiles abashedly] was so that I could see what it would look like. Um, watching like the surface tension build up in the edge. At the moment of the beep it was … the spoon wasn't completely through [smiles sheepishly] the soup yet, but there was still a little bit spilling over from the back end, and there was the residual from the last [laughs embarrassedly] … from the last attempt that was still there. Just watching the way that the liquid moved [laughs resignedly].

This is in some ways a typical relatively early (second sampling day) encounter with sensory awareness by a DES subject. We observe nine characteristics of the way this experience presents itself to Ephraim.

First, note that the sensory features are a primary focus of Ephraim's experience: he is aimed at, drawn to, interested in the resistance of the spoon against the soup and the shape of the pool of soup in the spoon.

Second, Ephraim's interest is in the sensory experience itself, not in the instrumental aim that employs the sensation. That is, Ephraim is interested in the resistance of the spoon against the soup for its own sake; he is not merely eating soup and making the sensory observations that that task requires. The eating-soup task is secondary or nonexistent in his experience at the moment of this beep.

Third, note the power of the sensory interest. Ephraim is not merely *idly* feeling the resistance and seeing the soup patterns — he is drawn directly to the sensory interests, they grab him to the exclusion of other aspects of his environment. There is music playing, but he does not hear it; there are doubtless other people and objects in his environment, but they don't exist in his experience at the moment of the beep.

Fourth, note the precision and confidence with which Ephraim describes his experience: he perceives the resistance in the scoopy part of the spoon, not in his hand; he's interested in the shape the soup makes and the paths it takes, not (for example) its color. This is not merely a dim sensation at the edges of his experience; the sensation is not a building block for some subsequent perception; the sensory is at the center of his experience. Ephraim has no doubt about his being focused on this sensory experience at the moment of the beep, no question about whether there is a fully differentiated sensation at the center of his experience.

Fifth, note that Ephraim is quite embarrassed or sheepish about reporting sensory awareness. This embarrassment/sheepishness is quite typical of subjects who frequently report sensory awareness, especially early in their sampling. Our aim is to describe the manner of appearing of sensory awareness; here we observe that descriptions of sensory awareness are frequently accompanied (at least at the outset) with embarrassment or sheepishness. It is not our aim to explain this embarrassment, although we will permit ourselves this speculation: Sensory awareness is a direct access to what looks good, what feels good, what attracts Ephraim, what repels him, in a very elemental, basic, sensual way. Sensual interests are intensely personal, by their very nature exceedingly private. To reveal one's basic sensuality is to stand naked before the observer, and sheepishness is a natural response. Some would say that Ephraim's sheepishness may come from having been 'caught' in a childish act (playing with his food), but we think the sheepishness is more elemental, arising from the experience, not the act: the sheepishness (in Ephraim and others) comes from the recognition and admission that the sensations themselves are *fun/attractive/alluring*, regardless of whether they are acted upon. We emphasize that this is speculation; it is in accord with our frequent casual observations but requires further study.

Sixth, all five of the samples on this sampling day contained sensory awarenesses. However, none of the samples from the first sampling day contained sensory awareness. It is not uncommon for sensory awareness to be overlooked or avoided on the first sampling day. Whether this is the result of a presupposition that attending to some sensory detail is too trivial to count as a feature of experience, or is a corollary to the embarrassment described above, or is the result of the punishment of talk about sensory awareness (see the Weihnachten Carousel below), or stems from some other factor remains to be explored. It does illustrate why an iterative approach to studying experience is necessary (Hurlburt, this issue).

Seventh, we note that the embarrassment/sheepishness is a sign that Ephraim is trying to report faithfully his actual experience. It is evidence that he is not making up his experience — why would he make up something that causes distress?

Eighth, there is one aspect that makes this cited example somewhat unusual: Ephraim here is *actively creating* the situation that makes his particular sensory awareness possible: he is actively, repeatedly pressing his spoon slowly into the soup just so he can see the flow and the shape of the soup into the spoon. Most sensory awarenesses, including all the sensory awarenesses in Ephraim's other samples, are not the result of direct creation of the situation, but rather merely involve the specific noticing of the already existing (inner or outer) environment. Ephraim's other samples on this sampling day have this incidental, not actively sought, observational quality: At sample 1, Ephraim was drawn to a shininess on a particular part of a traffic policeman's vest. He had stepped outside to have a cigarette, and the shininess simply attracted him. At sample 2: Ephraim is reading the booklet from a new CD, and while he's reading he happens to be attracted to the shadow that falls diagonally across the page. At sample 3, Ephraim was waiting for a computer game to load; at the moment of the beep he was particularly observing the '8' in '68% Done,' noting that the progress bar split the '8' perfectly in half. At sample 4, Ephraim was feeling the sharp edge of the Excedrin package as he opened it. In none of those examples was he manipulating the environment to observe some sensory aspect; on the contrary, it is as if the sensory aspect draws his attention unbidden.

Ninth, had this sensory observational experience not been interrupted by the beep, leading the subject to focus on it, it would likely have been forgotten, like a dream (or like a short-term memory not consolidated into long-term memory), almost immediately. If a friend were to ask him, in a few minutes, 'How was the soup?' Ephraim will almost certainly not recall the resistance or the flow patterns — even though that was actually what occupied most of his experience while eating the soup — and will instead respond that it tasted good.

Sensory Awareness: The Phenomenon

As we have seen in the examples, sensory awareness is the focused, thematic experience of a particular sensory aspect of the external or internal environment without particular regard for the instrumental aim or perceptually complete-objectness of that environment. To discriminate sensory awareness from non-sensory-awareness experience, here are some additional examples with brief commentary:

Example 6:
> Fatima was playing a computer game. At the beep she was focused on an orange gear that was rotating on the screen, meshing with another gear that lifted the elevator up to the next level. She was paying more attention to the color and shape of the gear than to its function as the mover of the elevator.

Fatima is paying attention to a sensory, non-goal-oriented, non-instrumental aspect of the environment. The color and shape of the gear occupy Fatima's attention, not the instrumental aspect of the gear. Therefore this is a straightforward sensory awareness.

Example 7:
> Georg was looking at the microwave clock to see what time it was. The clock read '4:28,' but at the moment of the beep he was focused on the pointy shapes of the line segments that made up the numbers. The appearance of these line segments, rather than the actual time, occupied his awareness.

Georg is not, at the moment of the beep, occupied with the clock as a time-telling instrument; he is occupied with the sensory aspects of the digits. Because he is focused on the sensory, not the instrumental value of his perception, this is a straightforward sensory awareness.

Example 8:
> Harold wondered what time it was and looked at the digital clock, which read 8:42. Harold was interested in the time-of-day represented by the 8:42 display, not its color or shape.

Harold looks at the clock for its instrumental value — to determine the time of day. This is *not* a sensory awareness. Examples 7 and 8 illustrate that sensory awareness is a feature of *experience*, *not* a characteristic of a sensory process. Georg's and Harold's sensory processes are doubtless quite similar: the pointy line segments impact their retinas the same way, and so on. But experientially (for reasons that we do not seek to explain), Georg apprehends the pointiness of the line segments whereas Harold apprehends the time represented by the line segments.

Example 9:
> Irma is waiting to cross the street. She is looking at the Walk / Don't Walk sign, which is displaying a red hand, so she doesn't cross.

There is not enough information here to know whether the red of the hand is apprehended only as a stop signal (in which case the red has instrumental, not sensory-awareness significance), or whether Irma is also interested in the red for its sensory qualities — that it is the same red as her lipstick, for example. Further questioning would be necessary.

The next examples illustrate that sensory awareness can be an aspect of inner seeing (aka seeing an image). The rules for determining whether to call an experience a sensory awareness apply equally to inner as to external seeing.

Example 10:
> Juan was talking with his wife Jill about Jill's mother, who is ill. At the moment of the beep Juan was innerly seeing Jill's mother in the hospital bed. Juan was particularly aware of the shininess of the oxygen tube in the mother's nose — the shininess seemed to stand out against the otherwise muted inner seeing.

This illustrates that sensory awareness can occur in an inner seeing. Had Juan been attending to the life-supportness (the instrumentality) of the imaginary oxygen tubes, this would be considered an inner seeing only; but because he is primarily drawn to the shininess, to a sensory aspect, DES would call it a sensory awareness as well as an inner seeing.

Example 11:
> Kevin was talking with his wife Kelly about Kelly's mother, who is ill. At the moment of the beep Kevin was innerly seeing Kelly's mother, seeing her as he had seen her the day before in the hospital. Kevin could describe the visual details of this seeing: she was wearing a blue hospital gown; there were oxygen tubes in her nose; he clearly saw the red sore on her cheek. Kevin understands

this seeing to be something like an illustration of the conversation he and Kelly were having.

This inner seeing has many sensory qualities (blue of the gown, red of the sore, etc.), but these qualities are not seen for the blueness or the redness themselves. The blueness and the redness are facts of the inner seeing, characteristics of the object being innerly seen, but they are not centrally or particularly in attention. This is *not* a sensory awareness.

Example 12:
> Linda was discussing the power steering of her car with her friend Lily. At the moment of the beep Linda was innerly seeing a schematic representation of a power steering system. She saw fluid-filled tubes and pistons; the different parts were in different pastel colors, as though represented in a textbook. Although she doesn't actually know how power steering works, she was imagining how it might work.

The question here is whether the pastel colorness of the inner seeing counts as sensory awareness, and the answer is that we don't know without further questioning. If these colors were merely incidental facts of the inner seeing, then they would not count as sensory awareness. For example, in Hurlburt and Schwitzgebel (2007), Melanie describes an inner seeing that accompanied a book she was reading. She saw a Greek woman on a road talking with a soldier. She reported that the image was quite detailed: the road went diagonally from close left to far right; there were green shrubs and lighter gray-green olive trees, and so on. In that image, the green and the gray-green were understood to be characteristics of the shrubs/trees, not particularly of interest in and for themselves, and therefore they are *not* sensory awareness. The same logic would apply to the pastel tubes and pistons. If Linda was imagining a schematic drawing of power steering, wherein the pressurized fluid happened to be pink and the low-pressure fluid happened to be green, then, like Melanie's shrubs/trees, this would not be sensory awareness. But if Linda was interested in the pinkness or the greenness; if she created these colors not because they represented a typical schematic drawing but because she was drawn to the pinkness and/or the greenness, then this would have been sensory awareness.

It is therefore not always entirely unambiguous whether a particular sample should be considered an instance of sensory awareness. Let's say schematic drawings are usually in primary colors, and Linda, who happens to be an engineer, knows that. Despite that, she creates an inner seeing of a schematic in pastels. But at the moment of the beep, she is interested in the pressures and is not paying attention to the pastelness of the pressure representations. Determining whether this image deserves to be called a sensory awareness would be a tough call.

The good news is that whereas some judgments are tough calls about individual samples, the characteristics of individual *people* are not usually that problematic. For example, Ephraim, in our examples, has a high frequency of sensory awareness *no matter how you make the tough calls*. Whether that high frequency is 75% or 85% might depend on the details of the tough calls, but it's a high frequency either way.

Example 13:
>Miguel is angry; that anger manifests itself in part by Miguel's sensing the hair on the back of his neck bristle.

DES considers the bodily aspect of a feeling to be *not* sensory awareness. This experience would be called the feeling of anger, not the sensory awareness of hair standing on end. This may seem an arbitrary distinction; should we call this both a feeling and a sensory awareness? DES seeks to apprehend experience. If the organizing principle of the experience seems to be the emotion, and the hair bristling is understood to be an aspect of the emotional experience, then the hair bristling is not considered to be a sensory awareness — there is not focus on the bristling for its own sake. The bodily aspect of an emotion is not called a sensory awareness by DES unless that bodily aspect is a focus of awareness apart from the emotional experience or any other perceptual/meaning aspect of awareness.[1]

Example 14:
>Steven was pacing around his condo engaged in a mental argument. At the beep he was innerly saying the word 'whatever' to himself in his own voice, as if directed at the person he was mentally arguing with. He was also

---

[1] Science is an evolving process, and we acknowledge that it may, at some future point, be desirable to reverse course on this decision. DES reveals that some people experience emotion with clearly available bodily aspects, whereas others experience emotion without any bodily aspects. Those experiences are phenomenologically quite different, but DES and the emotion literature refers to both as 'feelings.' We think that an adequate discussion of the phenomenology of feelings is yet to be performed, and when that happens, it may be clearer what to do about the common ground between sensory awareness and feelings.

aware of a sense of frustration and an accompanying sensation of heat and outward-radiating pressure behind his ears and eyes. Simultaneously, he was also aware of a 'frenetic' restless energy in his arms and legs which made him feel like he had to be moving.

It is possible to have a sensory awareness at the same time as a feeling. Here, the frenetic energy is itself a focus of experience along with (but not part of) the frustration. DES would consider this both a feeling and a sensory awareness.

Individual Differences in the Frequency of Sensory Awareness

Sensory awareness is a frequently observed phenomenon, occurring in roughly a quarter of all everyday experience samples. However, there are large individual differences in the observed frequency of sensory awareness. Heavey and Hurlburt (2008) stratified large introductory psychology classes on a measure of psychological distress (the SCL-90-R; Derogatis, 1994) and randomly selected 30 individuals. This stratified sample therefore was quite representative of the entering students in a large U.S. state university. They then applied the DES technique to each. Sensory awareness occurred in 22% of all sampled experiences. However, within subjects the observed frequency of sensory awareness ranged from 0% to 100%. The median frequency of sensory awareness across subjects was 16%, but 30% of subjects (9 of 30) had no sensory awareness at all. So while sensory awareness may be very common, it is by no means omnipresent.

Heavey and Hurlburt (2008) reported that the correlation between the subjects' frequency of sensory awareness and their psychological distress (SCL-90-R) scores was .04. This is only one study with only one measure of distress, but there is no reason to conclude that sensory awareness is unequivocally a beneficial or a detrimental characteristic of experience.

Jones-Forrester (2006, 2008) sampled the inner experience in women with bulimia nervosa, and discovered frequent sensory awareness, averaging about 40% across 18 subjects. For some of these women, the predominance of sensory awareness was striking. For example, Stella (Jones-Forrester, 2006) had sensory awareness in 35 of her 40 samples (88%). Here are some typical samples:

Sample 3.4 (the fourth sample on the third sampling day):
Stella was at work pulling a box off the shelf. She was

focused on the dry, dustiness of the box surface and waviness of the surface caused by the corrugations beneath it.

Sample 6.3:
Stella was playing with the tips of her hair and was aware of the grainy texture of the tips against her fingers.

Sample 7.4:
Stella was changing clothes in the bathroom and was aware of the aqua color of the floor tiles and also was aware of the sensation of cold pressure from the floor on the balls of her feet. (This is two simultaneous sensory awarenesses.)

In 7 of her 35 sensory awareness samples (20%) Stella seemed to be using sensory awareness actively to avoid potentially distressing stimuli. For example:

Sample 7.5:
Stella was at work eating her lunch. She was focused on the heaviness in her eyebrows as she intentionally furrowed them in an explicit, currently successful attempt to avoid the worry and upset that was currently just outside her awareness.

Sample 3.6:
Stella was on the phone with her father, who was screaming at her. Instead of hearing what her father was screaming, she was noticing the distortion of the sound as the speaker was being overdriven by the screams. She was also noticing the vibrating sensation in her skin next to her ear caused by the phone.

Sample 5.6:
Stella was stuck in traffic. She was actively trying to channel her frustration into a sense of calm by looking at the fuzzy blue outline of the sky framed by the spokes of her steering wheel.

Sample 7.1:
Stella was at work in conversation with her new boss. He had physically moved too close to her in a way that Stella found threatening. In response, Stella had leaned back. At the moment of the beep, Stella was feeling the

stretching sensations in her back as she arched away from him. Thus, at the moment of the beep Stella was *not* aware of feeling threatened by her boss' advance; in fact, she was not aware of her boss at all. She was focused on the relatively inconsequential arching sensations of her back.

Discriminating Sensory Awareness

When we describe sensory awareness to colleagues unfamiliar with the topic, they frequently jump to incorrect conclusions about the nature of the phenomenon. Here is what sensory awareness is *not*.

Sensory awareness is not merely some sensory aspect of a perception. If you are driving and you stop for a stop sign, the redness of the sign was doubtless an aspect of the perception that led you to stop. But that is *not* a sensory awareness as DES defines it *unless, as a central feature of your experience, you were drawn to or absorbed in or particularly noticing the redness.*

Sensory awareness is not part of the subject matter generally called 'sensation and perception.' Sensory awareness has little or nothing to do with the topics generally called 'sensation,' topics such as sensory threshold, receptor cells, adaptation, brain projection areas, and so on. Doubtless, sensory awareness depends on processes such as those, but sensory awareness is *the result of* those processes, not merely one more process among many others.

Sensory awareness is not a process, perceptual or otherwise, that occurs or is presumed to occur. Sensory awareness is a phenomenon in its own right, the figure of experience, something directly observed.

Some would distinguish between (a) first-order conscious perception (e.g., Andrew's seeing the shiny-blue patch) and (b) second-order conscious reflection or introspection (Andrew's reflecting upon the fact that he is looking at something blue). The concept of sensory awareness is orthogonal to that distinction. Sensory awareness is a directly apprehended phenomenon. Whether sensory awareness (or any other introspectable event) requires both a first-order perception and a second-order reflection is not known to us; we do not seek to explain how sensory awareness works, only that it exists as a phenomenon. We can say with confidence that we have inquired with substantial care on hundreds of occasions and only very rarely will a subject acknowledge that there is any hint of an awareness of a second-order process. We do not intend this to rule out the existence or necessity of a second-order process; we do intend to say that if there is a second-order process, it escapes the notice of subjects at the moment of the beep, including those subjects who are relatively skilled at knowing the difference between a first-order and a second-order process.

Sensory awareness is, however, the target of at least some forms of mindfulness training. For example, Segal, Williams, and Teasdale (2002) describe one of the techniques they use to teach people to be more mindful:

> If there is a window in the room, we ask people to look outside, paying attention to the sights as best they can, letting go of the categories they normally use to make sense of what they are looking at; rather than viewing elements of the scene as trees or cars, or whatever, we ask them simply to see them as patterns of color and shapes and movement. (p. 160)

This type of mindfulness training attempts to enhance the ability of individuals to focus on sensations without regard to their meaning, symbolism, or other informational significance and thereby to increase the relative frequency of the phenomenon of sensory awareness in the individual's ongoing experience.

We have found training DES investigators that sensory awareness is the most difficult of the main five characteristics for investigators to grasp. Unsymbolized thinking is difficult because many would-be investigators presuppositionally deny its existence (Hurlburt & Akhter, 2008). But sensory awareness is *more* difficult because many would-be investigators presuppositionally, but incorrectly, believe they *already know* what sensory awareness is, and therefore don't feel the need to try to master it. As a step toward ameliorating this difficulty, Hurlburt and Bensaheb have developed a multimedia training program comprising examples of moments of sensory awareness and moments of experience that in some way resemble sensory awareness but are not instances of sensory awareness. Bensaheb (2009) demonstrated that this training program increases the ability of naïve individuals to discriminate moments of sensory awareness from moments which are not sensory awareness. This increase is larger than that due to reading a written description of the nature of sensory awareness such as the one you are reading. This multimedia training program can be obtained at http://www.nevada.edu/~russ/des-imp-request.html.

Impediments to the Recognition of Sensory Awareness

We claim that sensory awareness is a robust phenomenon, identifiable by anyone who might look carefully at experience moment by moment, occurring in roughly a quarter of sampled moments. However, there is little or no discussion of the phenomenon in the literature. It is our aim to describe the phenomenon, not to explain the social psychology of its absence, but ten observations may be useful.

First, it may seem that there is nothing to understand, nothing unknown, about the phenomenon of sensory awareness. A common presupposition is that everybody has sensory awareness most of the time; *of course* we pay attention to sensory details — how else could we navigate our way through the world. That presupposition reflects a serious misunderstanding of sensory awareness as we define it. It is *not* true that everybody has sensory awareness most of the time: as best we can ascertain, roughly a third of people experience sensory awareness only rarely if at all. Navigating through the world around us does *not* require this thematic sensory awareness: I can easily stop at a stop sign without paying particular attention to the particular shade of its redness, listen to a lecture without paying particular attention to the timbre of the speaker's voice, and so on. A sensory awareness is *not* merely a building block out of which a perception is constructed. Sensory awareness is a center of interest, not a substructure, subpart, or ingredient of some other perceptual center of interest.

Second, as we observed above, sensory awareness is sometimes not reported by DES subjects on their first sampling day, even by those subjects who experience sensory awareness frequently. The iterative nature of DES (Hurlburt, this issue; Hurlburt & Akhter, 2006) can solve this potential under-reporting. But the non-reporting of sensory awareness on the first sampling day can be a problem for methods that rely on one-shot data gathering and for multiple-occasion methods that train subjects only on one occasion.

Third, and related to the second point, some people who have frequent sensory awareness do not know that they have sensory awareness at all. It is not until they examine the details of their experiences moment by moment that they recognize a frequent characteristic of their own experience.

Fourth, many people (including many students of consciousness) assume that everyone's experience is just like their own. We have tried to show that experience may differ dramatically from one person to the next (Heavey & Hurlburt, 2008; Hurlburt & Akhter, 2006, 2008; Hurlburt & Heavey, 2006; Hurlburt & Schwitzgebel, 2007), but the prejudice that everyone's experience is just like their own may lead people who do not have frequent sensory awareness (including many students of consciousness) to fail to recognize the occurrence of sensory awareness in others.

Fifth, it is difficult, if not impossible, to explore sensory awareness using armchair introspection. Hurlburt and Heavey (2004; cf. Hurlburt & Schwitzgebel, 2007) have argued against the use of armchair introspection in general. Armchair introspection is particularly problematic in apprehending sensory awareness because the hallmark of sensory awareness is that the sensory aspect grabs you, draws you, attracts you, as if unbidden. This unbiddenness is difficult for armchair introspection to simulate because armchair introspectors have already made themselves purposefully ready to observe.

Sixth, as we saw above, reporting a sensory awareness, at least at first, is often accompanied by a sense of embarrassment. That embarrassment is likely to cause a substantial (perhaps complete) under-reporting of sensory awareness except in those situations where subjects trust that the truth and the whole truth about experience is sincerely desired.

Seventh, as we saw above, sensory awarenesses, despite their at-the-moment vividness, are, like dreams, almost immediately forgotten. Although we are not aware of such a survey, this forgetting would likely lead to a substantial (perhaps complete) under-reporting of sensory awareness by all retrospective methods including questionnaires and interviews.

Eighth, the vocabulary that untrained people use to describe sensory awareness is substantially imprecise. In particular, people (including students of consciousness) frequently use the word 'feeling' in three quite distinct ways (cf. Hurlburt & Akhter, 2008): (1) to describe bodily sensory awarenesses (e.g., 'I was feeling a tickle in my throat'); (2) to describe emotional experience (e.g., 'I was feeling anxious'); and (3) to describe an inward impression or state of mind (e.g., 'I was feeling that I should take Elm Street instead of Pine Street because there would be less traffic'). That imprecision in the language makes it difficult at the outset to get a clear view of sensory awareness. It is difficult to reduce such imprecision unless an iterative method is employed (Hurlburt, 2009, this issue).

Ninth, as in the recognition of any phenomenon of inner experience, observers must bracket their presuppositions about what is observed; bracketing presuppositions is not easy (Hurlburt & Akhter, 2006; Hurlburt & Heavey, 2006; Hurlburt & Schwitzgebel, 2007).

Tenth, sensory awareness may be systematically punished. We give one example. The family is playing an informal game at the dinner table. It's the Christmas season, and the centerpiece is a candle-lit Weihnachten Carousel (aka windmill carousel or pyramid carousel): the updraft from the candles turns a balsa wood windmill which rotates carousels on the three levels of the pyramid. On these carousels is a Nativity scene: Mary, Joseph, the crèche, the wise men, the angels, the animals, and so on, all brightly painted and gaily rotating within the wooden framework. The game is a version of *I Spy*. 8-year-old Peter is 'it'; he has 'spied' an item on the carousel, and the rest of the family takes turns asking yes/no questions to try to guess which item Peter has selected: Is it moving? No. Is it made of wood? Yes. Is it white or partly white? Yes. The children love this game, which they have made up and elaborated over the years. Eventually the family gives up and requires Peter to tell what he has spied; he says it is the balls that sit on the fence posts around the base of carousel. 'Peter! There isn't any white on those balls! They're totally red!' And they are: the balls are, objectively, uniformly red painted, not a speck of white paint on them. The family has a light-hearted conversation about how much easier it would have been had Peter given the *correct* answer to his brother's 'Is it white or partly white?' question. Peter doesn't enter into this conversation.

However, a more careful look at the red balls reveals that each has the reflection of the two adjacent candle flames on it, two tiny spots of experienced white on the objectively uniformly red-painted balls. The spots are tiny, and they don't count as 'white' for anyone except Peter, who may be more sensorially aware than anyone else in the family. But they are indeed, looked at closely, experientially white. Peter has been punished (mildly, to be sure) for his sensory sensitivity, and he doesn't have the confidence to defend himself.

We speculate that inner experiences (sensory awareness, inner speech, inner seeing, etc.) are skills that may be acquired across development. Peter has learned a small lesson: that sensory awareness doesn't count; that talking about your sensory awarenesses will get you punished. We speculate that a long series of that kind of event — in the family, in the classroom, eventually in the workplace — may cause Peter's sensory awareness skill either to atrophy or to go underground: he will not talk about it, even to himself; he will be embarrassed if he is somehow cornered into talking about it (as was Ephraim); he will deny that he has it; he will not really identify the fact that he has it in his self-narratives.

We do not wish to claim that we know how sensory awareness does or does not develop. However, we think that this example may help the reader overcome the presuppositional stance against accepting the importance of sensory awareness and the individual differences of its occurrence.

Speculations about Sensory Awareness

Our experience of observing sensory awareness across many subjects leads us to believe its desirability can be thought of as something of a 'razor's edge.' On the one hand, sensory awareness seems a highly desirable characteristic of experience: it is a direct apprehension of the sensory features of the world around and within. As we discussed above, sensory awareness is the target of many forms of mindfulness training, which train individuals to focus on raw sensations. Mindfulness training has been shown to improve mental health (Segal, Williams, & Teasdale, 2002). This view has been confirmed by Hurlburt's unpublished sampling of the experience of adept meditators, whose inner experience was in fact dominated by sensory awareness.

On the other hand, we have sampled with a number of subjects whose inner experience was dominated by sensory awareness who did not enjoy good mental health. Stella, discussed above, is one example of a person for whom sensory awareness often appeared to serve as an escape or distraction from the meaningful demands/requirements of her situation. In Stella and others like her, the immersion in the sensory aspects of experience seemed to lessen the ability to cope effectively with the real world demands they faced. For example, Jones-Forrester (2006, 2008) demonstrated that sensory awareness was a frequent characteristic of women with bulimia nervosa.

Thus we are not in a position to say when sensory awareness is useful or a sign of health and when it is destructive or a symptom of pathology. Neither are we in a position to comment on the directionality of any relationship between sensory awareness and health (as we saw, its correlation with psychological distress is approximately zero). Our goal here has been to describe a frequent phenomenon of inner experience that deserves more attention so that questions such as whether or when sensory awareness is desirable can someday be answered. Some readers may find it frustrating that we provide few connections between sensory awareness and anything else. But that is the way, we think, of basic science. In 1957, Arthur Schawlow explored the coherent light rays that could be produced by stimulating rubies (a process later called a laser). He didn't immediately say, 'Aha! Grocery store checkout tool!' or 'Aha! Two hours of video in the palm of your hand!' Those came only at the end of a long series of observations, constructions, false starts, and refinements. For sensory awareness in Western science, it's 1957.

References

Bensaheb, A. (2009), 'Descriptive experience sampling interactive multimedia training tool' (Doctoral dissertation, University of Nevada, Las Vegas).
Derogatis, L.R. (1994), *The SCL-90-R: Scoring, Administration, and Procedures*, 3rd edition (Minneapolis, MN: National Computer Systems).
Heavey, C.L. & Hurlburt, R.T. (2008),' The phenomena of inner experience', *Consciousness and Cognition*, **17**, pp. 798–810.
Hurlburt, R.T. (1990), *Sampling Normal and Schizophrenic Inner Experience* (New York: Plenum).
Hurlburt, R.T. (1993), *Sampling Inner Experience In Disturbed Affect* (New York: Plenum).
Hurlburt, R.T. (1997), 'Randomly sampling thinking in the natural environment', *Journal of Consulting and Clinical Psychology*, **65**, pp. 941–49.
Hurlburt, R.T. (2009, this issue), 'Iteratively apprehending pristine experience'.
Hurlburt, R.T. & Akhter, S.A. (2006), 'The Descriptive Experience Sampling method', *Phenomenology and the Cognitive Sciences*, **5**, 271–301.
Hurlburt, R.T. & Akhter, S.A. (2008), 'Unsymbolized thinking', *Consciousness and Cognition*, **17**, pp. 1364–74.
Hurlburt, R.T. & Heavey, C.L. (2001), 'Telling what we know: Describing inner experience', *Trends in Cognitive Sciences*, **5**, pp. 400–403.
Hurlburt, R.T & Heavey, C.L. (2002), 'Interobserver reliability of Descriptive Experience Sampling', *Cognitive Therapy and Research*, **26**, pp. 135–42.
Hurlburt, R.T. & Heavey, C.L. (2004), 'To beep or not to beep: Obtaining accurate reports about awareness', *Journal of Consciousness Studies*, **11**(7–8), pp. 113–28.
Hurlburt, R.T. & Heavey, C.L. (2006), *Exploring Inner Experience: The Descriptive Experience Sampling Method* (Amsterdam: John Benjamins).
Hurlburt, R.T. & Schwitzgebel, E. (2007), *Describing Inner Experience?* (Cambridge, MA: MIT Press).
Jones-Forrester, S. (2006), 'Inner experience in bulimia' (Master's thesis, University of Nevada, Las Vegas).
Jones-Forrester, S. (2009), 'Inner experience in bulimia nervosa' (Doctoral dissertation, University of Nevada, Las Vegas).
Segal, Z.V., Williams, J.M.G. & Teasdale, J.D. (2002), *Mindfulness-based Cognitive Therapy For Depression* (New York: Guilford).

Claire Petitmengin, Michel Bitbol,
Jean-Michel Nissou, Bernard Pachoud,
Hélène Curallucci, Michel Cermolacce,
and Jean Vion-Dury

Listening from Within

Abstract: This article is devoted to the description of the experience associated with listening to a sound. In the first part, we describe the method we used to gather descriptions of auditory experience and to analyse these descriptions. This work of explicitation and analysis has enabled us to identify a threefold generic structure of this experience, depending on whether the attention of the subject is directed towards (1) the event which is at the source of the sound, (2) the sound in itself, considered independently from its source, (3) the felt sound. In the second part of the article, we describe this structure. The third part is devoted to a discussion of these results and the paths they open up in various fields of theoretical and applied research.

Keywords

Auditory experience, lived experience, pre-reflective, sound, structure of experience.

Introduction

What is it like to listen to a sound? The auditory experience has been studied relatively little. Whereas other traditions[1] give prime importance to hearing and sound, in our Western culture, sight is considered as the noblest of the senses. As Aristotle wrote, 'Seeing, most of all the senses, makes us know and brings to light many differences between things' (Metaphysics, A, 980a). Most of our understanding of knowledge is based on the visual model. Philosophical studies on hearing are rare, compared with the very large number of studies about sight and colours in particular. When sound is studied, it is studied from a physical or psycho-acoustic viewpoint, but rarely from a philosophical viewpoint (Casati & Dokic, 1994), and even more rarely as lived experience (Ihde, 1976/2007).

In the study presented in this article, we look at the experience associated with listening to a sound. Our aim is not — in what would be the resurgence of sensorial atomism — to try to isolate the sense of hearing from the other sensory modes, but to describe what we live, in the whole of our experience, when a sound occurs. In our view a description of this kind, by drawing our attention to dimensions of perception which are difficult to detect when we focus on visual experience, could enrich our understanding of cognitive processes.

In the first part, we describe the method we used to gather descriptions of auditory experience and to analyse these descriptions. This work of explicitation and analysis has enabled us to identify a three-fold generic structure of this experience, depending on whether the attention of the subject is directed towards (1) the event which is at the source of the sound, (2) the sound in itself, considered independently from its source, (3) the felt sound. In the second part of the article, we describe this structure. The third part is devoted to a discussion of these results and the paths they open up in various fields of theoretical and applied research.

I. Itinerary and Explicitation Method of the Lived Experience of Listening

1. Itinerary

We have constituted a multi-disciplinary research group consisting of philosophers, psychiatrists, a doctor specialising in neurophysiology, a doctor / therapist specialising in coma emergence, and a psycho-

---

[1] As in that of Veda in which listening to sounds (nada) is considered to be a privileged way of gaining access to supreme knowledge.

therapist. What brings us together is the conviction, for both philosophical and empirical reasons, that it is essential as a matter of urgency to introduce the 1st person viewpoint into cognitive sciences and neurosciences, as well as in the clinical field. Our work was carried out in three phases, following a preparatory phase during which we practised lived experience explicitation techniques, more exactly the explication interview, with the help of three of our members who were already skilled in these techniques (JMN, CP, BP). On completion of this preparatory phase, we then decided to concentrate on the explicitation of a particular type of experience, the experience of listening to sounds and music. We first chose the experience associated with listening to 'bizarre sounds'. In connection with his research in sound semiotics[2] (Aramaki *et al.*, 2009), one of our colleagues uses synthetic sounds which imitate for example the timbre of metal, glass or wood as it is hit. Changing one or more parameters makes it possible to obtain sounds with a timbre which is hard to identify, for example at some point between wood and metal, or metal and glass, sounds that we call 'bizarre'. Then we continued the project by listening to natural sounds, and then music. The three phases are as follows.

Phase 1

During this phase we spent two days listening to bizarre sounds and then making these experiences explicit. The procedure was as follows: (1) The group listens to a sound (lasting about 2 seconds). (2) Immediately after listening comes self-explicitation, i.e. each person describes in writing the experience he or she has just lived while listening to the sound (explicitation instruction: 'What happened as you listened to the sound'). (3) Cross-explicitation interviews, in groups of three persons playing in turn the role of interviewer, interviewee and observer. We thus listened to three sounds, and this was followed by self-explicitation and explicitation in sub-groups. The first sound was a transformed metallic sound, the second a glass/metal sound, and the third sounded like a rustling. This initial phase was followed by: (4) work in sub-groups to analyse the descriptions, in order to identify possible common experiential categories, and then (5) work in a large group to compare the categories detected by each sub-group, in order to point to the existence of any possible generic categories.

The main result of this initial phase was the detection of a generic process of attempting *to identify the source of the sound*: each of us,

---

[2] The semiotics of sound consists of identifying the acoustic clues which enable us to recognise a sound, and the cerebral processes associated with this categorisation.

for each sound, immediately tried to recognise the source of these bizarre (unheard-of) sounds. This process consisted in particular of identifying the means by which the sound had been produced, the action which could have generated the sound. We then asked ourselves whether the detection of this source identification process had not been made possible by a sort of slowing down or 'distention' of this process, which is usually very rapid and pre-reflective, a distention resulting from the ambiguity of the sounds listened to. Two other salient categories were identified: the specific *attentional disposition* enabling this recognition process, which itself is immediately enabled by a *process of generating this attentional disposition*.

Phase 2

Other types of sounds were used as material for the second phase: sounds from nature (in a garden and in a forest), the sound of a Tibetan bowl, short pieces of classical music (Brahms, Bach, Gregorian chant). On each occasion the protocol was identical to the previous one: (1) Listening in a group, (2) Immediately afterwards, self-explicitation, (3) Cross-explicitation interviews, (4) Analysis of descriptions and pointing up of existence of descriptive categories, and then (5) Comparison of categories detected.

This second phase, while confirming the existence of the process of identifying the source of the sound, enabled us to reveal two other dimensions of listening, two other ways of listening to a sound. The attention of the subject may in fact turn to the characteristics of the sound as a sound, independently of its source. It may also turn to the bodily felt sound, independently of the sound's source and characteristics. These three modes of listening correspond to three different attentional dispositions, each of which seems to have a different impact on the *structure of the lived space*. As the temporal structure of the auditory experience (in the form of the protention–retention process) has been described in detail by Husserl (1893-1917/1964), we decided to concentrate our efforts on the explicitation of this 'spatial' structure.

Phase 3

In a third phase, we considered this threefold structure as a hypothesis to be confirmed or falsified by the explication of other auditory experiences. For example, we tried to refine our descriptions of the attentional disposition specific to each listening mode. To do so, we fine tuned the explicitation questions which could trigger a reflective consciousness of each of these dispositions. One way of triggering this consciousness is to draw the subject's attention to the moment at which and the way in which he moves from one disposition to the other, in order to amplify the perception of the contrast between the two dispositions. This third phase — during which we listened to other natural sounds (such as that of a wood fire), and a short extract from a piece for 'Glass Harmonica' by Mozart — enabled us to refine the description of the structure of the listening experiences which we had identified during the two first phases.

2. Auditory experience explicitation method

To gather auditory experience descriptions, we used the explicitation interview method.[3] As we do not have the space here to describe it in detail, we will set out its main principles.

The goal of an explicitation interview is to bring a person to become aware of the pre-reflective part of his experience and to describe it with precision. The pre-reflective part of experience is that which is usually hidden by the absorption of attention in the object or content of the experience, and as a result is not spontaneously described by the subject.

The first key to the interview consists of explicitating an experience which is precisely situated in space and time, and bringing the subject back to this singular experience when he moves away from it — as is very often the case — towards the expression of generalities corresponding not to what he is experiencing but to what he knows or thinks he knows about his lived experience (and thus interpreting it rather than describing it).

In most cases, there is a temporal gap between the initial experience and its description. The second key to the interview is thus to help the subject to recall the experience, whether it is in the past or only just over, i.e. to return to it in all its sensorial and emotional dimensions, to the point at which the past situation becomes more present for him, at the time of the interview, than the interview situation itself.

The third key to the interview consists of helping the subject to redirect his attention from the content of his experience towards its

---

[3] The four main references in English are: Depraz *et al.*, 2003; Petitmengin, 2006; Vermersch, this issue; Maurel, this issue. Interested readers will find in these articles numerous other references in French.

diachronic and synchronic structure,[4] thanks to questions which are 'empty of content', which 'point to' the structure of the experience without bringing in any content. This questioning mode, which focuses on 'how' and excludes 'why' is based not only on linguistic indexes but also on non-verbal clues such as gestures which accompany (or replace) words in a pre-reflective way. The structure of an interview is an iterative structure which consists of bringing the subject to evoke again his experience several times, while guiding his attention towards a diachronic or synchronic mesh which is finer each time.

Once the descriptions have been brought together, analysis and comparison work is necessary to identify the structure of the experiences described, that is 'a network of relationships between descriptive categories, independent of the experiential content' (Delattre, 1971) and to detect any generic structures which are gradually extracted from the initial descriptions thanks to a succession of abstraction operations.[5] For example in the work we are concerned with, the bringing together of several descriptions such as 'I recognised the chirp of a blackbird', 'It is the sound of the wind in the trees' and 'It's Lucie I can hear' enabled us to detect an experiential structure which we have called 'identification of the source of the sound'. The recognition of a link between several descriptions of the type 'My attention is directed towards the fire over there' and 'I let the sound come to me' also enabled us furthermore to identify a synchronic experiential structure which we have termed 'attentional disposition'.

3. Self-adjustment of practices

Throughout our study, we have been at pains to be attentive to our practice, to acquire a reflective consciousness of it and to constantly move to and from between theory and practice, instead of remaining in the natural attitude, which consists of being absorbed in the object of the activity, i.e. here the production of results, particularly the production of generic descriptions of the structure of the auditory experience. As the format of this article does not allow a thorough analysis of this practice, which would require an article in itself, we will only mention the aspects to which we have been particularly attentive.

---

[4] The diachronic structure of experience corresponds to the stages of its unfolding in time. The synchronic structure of experience corresponds to its configuration at a given instant (sensorial registers used, type of attention mobilised, etc.)

[5] For more details on these operations of abstraction see (Petitmengin-Peugeot, 1999) and (Petitmengin, 2001).

In the gathering of descriptions, this reflective reconsideration of our practice, as interviewer and as interviewee, has been carried out by the means of 'interviews about the interview'.

— How does the interviewer understand the description, and thus the experience, of the interviewee? To try and answer this delicate question, we set up the following 'experiential protocol': an initial interview in which the interviewer elicits the evocation of an experience; a second interview in which the interviewer of the first interview makes explicit with the help of a third person his experience during this first interview.

— How does the interviewee evaluate the authenticity of his description? We have obtained some indications of an answer to this question by systematically gathering at the end of each interview a self-assessment by the interviewee, thanks to the following three questions: Does your description seem in your view to match up with the experience that you lived? (...) How do you know? (...) What did you do to answer my questions? These questions have enabled us to gather a description of precise evaluation criteria, for example, surprise because of the novelty of what is described:

> I have even been surprised to find things that I was not really thinking about, for example, these double pulsation movements (...). Yes therefore, I couldn't invent that. (Jean, Bach)[6]

For the same person, but another aspect of experience, the criterion is on the contrary a feeling of familiarity with what is described:

> All this is not at all new for me. I have always felt that. What I did this evening is to reveal the fine grain of what I have always lived. It is the musical experience I have *all the time*. I knew all that but I have got a finer consciousness of the music. It is as though things were taking on an extra dimension. (Jean, Bach)

This investigation has shown that throughout the work of explicitation, the subjects have precise internal criteria which give them information for example about the appositeness of a world, the effect of putting the experience into words, or the intensity of their contact with the experience. These criteria enable them to implement internal micro-regulations for example to adjust, continue or stop verbalisation, or to reactivate contact with the experience when contact is lost.

> I let myself become completely fascinated... I have the impression that my very repetition of words (for example, when I repeat 'filaments,

---

[6] Most of the interview excerpts have been slightly reorganised to facilitate the reading of this article: elimination of hesitations, redundancies, non-informative parts. A few excerpts are taken from interviews carried out with persons from outside the research group.

filaments'), finally almost makes me believe in the filaments, and I no longer give more than half my attention to what really happened. But as soon as I completely return to experience, I realise that 'filament' is not exactly the right word. I also realise that these filaments are sharp-ended filaments, filaments which make you scratch, and which are indeed associated with the impression of scratching given by the sound. (...) As soon as you asked me that: 'Does the experience match up with the description?', you immediately put me in the situation in which I absolutely had to return to experience, and stop describing it. This was a good way to return to the evocation, more intensely than before. (Michel, Brahms)

— We were also attentive to the impact of the modes of experience on its unfolding: for example, how the more or less 'constrained' nature of the experience — evoked experience or experience which is elicited in order to be made explicit (like listening to bizarre sounds) — influences the unfolding of this experience.

In the analysis of the descriptions, we were attentive to the following aspects:

— The process of emergence of descriptive categories and a shared vocabulary to describe the auditory experience: how did the abstract categories ('Source of the sound', 'Attentional disposition') emerge? How did we identify them from the descriptions gathered? In this phase of analysis, what did we do to 'understand' other people's descriptions? To what extent, in order to understand the description of another, did we have to access our own experience and through what process? How (and to what extent) did we arrive at an intersubjective agreement on these categories?

— The impact of the category on the experience, and the process of mutual refinement between descriptive categories and reflective consciousness of the experience: is the abstract category a vector of refinement or on the contrary of impoverishment or rigidification of experience? On numerous occasions, the emergence of a category describing an aspect of experience has enabled us to 'stabilise' in a way the reflective consciousness of this aspect, whose effect has been to further refine the consciousness of this aspect and thus to provide further details about its diachronic and synchronic structure.[7] For example, the fact of stabilising through a descriptive category the reflective consciousness of an 'attentional disposition' has made it

---

[7] Note in this respect the remark made by James: 'The snow that had just fallen had a very strange aspect, different from the usual appearance of snow. I decided to call it 'micacé', and it seemed to me, as I chose this name, that this difference became more distinct and more fixed than it was before' (James, 1890/1983, p. 484).

possible to detect a 'process of generating this attentional disposition', and thus to refine the diachronic structure of this disposition. The act of stabilising the reflective consciousness of the 'bodily zone where the sound is felt' has enabled us to refine the synchronic structure of this dimension of experience by differentiating between 'height of feeling' and 'depth of feeling'. What is interesting in the last example is that the 'depth of feeling' category has — in contrast to the previous one — emerged from the analysis of the interviews even before we had reflective consciousness of it: it is the category which, by drawing our attention to this dimension, enabled a reflective consciousness of this experience. In other words, the categorial refinement may precede and generate the experiential refinement.

It should be pointed out that one of us is a musician, and that two of us have regularly practised *samatha* and *vipassana* meditation for fifteen years.

II. Results: The Threefold Structure of Auditory Experience

The use of these interview and analysis techniques have enabled us to gather a description of ordinarily pre-reflective dimensions of the auditory experience, and to derive from these descriptions the following threefold structure.

1. 'Source of the sound'

1.1 Identification of the source of the sound

A sound is produced. If I am asked to describe my experience of the sound, what I ordinarily immediately describe is the physical event which is at the source of the sound: 'Someone has broken a glass in the kitchen', 'It is the sound of the wind in the trees', 'It is Peter who is sawing wood in the garden'. As Don Ihde writes: 'Sounds are "first" experienced as sounds of *things*' (2007, p. 60). The sound provides me with information about the characteristics of the objects which have produced it: their direction, their distance, their speed, the matter of which they are made, their density, their solidity or hollowness, and the consistency of their surface. But what is the experience associated with this act of identification? How do I know that it is the sound of the wind in the trees? What do I do to recognise this sound? This type of question — asked in self-explicitation and in explicitation interviews — has enabled us to begin to describe the ordinarily pre-reflective process corresponding to the act of identifying a sound.

— What these questions reveal first of all is the *result of the identification process* in the form of inner speech and images representing the source event. The subject pronounces the name of the source in an inner voice and/or sees an image or a visual scene representing the source.

> Very quickly, I imagine that it is air, wind. It is a powerful rush of air. I have the impression that it is something sweeping past. I saw a rush of air which was growing in force, from left to right. (Hélène, sound 57)

It may be an image which is precise in its size, location and colours:

> I see a frog in the form of an image about 20 cm square, although the image does not really have any sides. It is situated about 1 m 50 from me and about 20° above the horizon. The frog is brown and is cut out, that is it does not form part of the decor. (Jean-Michel, sound Adrien 37).

It may be a detailed scene — in which the subject finds himself in a specific 'perceptual position' (Andreas & Andreas, this issue):

> 'There is an image of monks... They have their hoods, they are contemplative, they are chanting. They are in the choir of a basilica or of a cathedral, it's a small group, they are at the back, I'm a long way from them. I am in the basilica but I am at a side door, relative to the choir, the side door on the right.' (Hélène, Gregorian chant)

...or an 'atmospheric' scene:

> Silence, forest interior, deep calm of the night... an atmosphere of vegetation. I 'recognised' the song-trill-chirp of a bird. Not 'this is a bird', but a complete atmosphere of peace, of attentive listening, of an evening in the unthreatening solitude of an unlimited forest. (Michel, sound Adrien 37)

The source of the sound can also be identified without words or images appearing. This experience, which has been described to us on several occasions, has been termed by Hurlburt (2009) *unsymbolized thinking*:

> This sound evokes the sound of a cow mooing. I didn't say to myself 'it's a cow', I did not see a cow, but I thought of it. But I don't know how I thought of it. I didn't say to myself, I haven't seen it. But it was nevertheless very present, the moo of a cow or of an animal... a bovine. (Claire, sound Y23)

— The *process* which culminates in the identification of the source is hard to apprehend because it is usually extremely rapid and pre-reflective. But we have gathered some clues about it. First of all, it sometimes takes place by successive approximations:

> I had the image of a flute. And immediately afterwards, of a creaking door hinge. Part of a door like that with the hinge... which opens. (Jean-Michel, sound Y17)

> I have the mental image of a helicopter and then very rapidly the mental image of a microlight plane. (Jean-Michel, forest).

In the following excerpt, the subject also describes an internal criterion which gives him information about the fact that the first 'candidate' object is not appropriate:

> I see a train, I have a feeling in my chest that it is not appropriate. So I see myself again with Claire in the forest at a moment when we heard this noise and we identified it together as the sound of wind in the trees. (Jean-Michel, forest).

In this last excerpt, the identification process is based on the *evocation of a memory*. Listening to 'bizarre sounds' has enabled us to detect another strategy consisting of *imagining the action of producing the sound*, in a constructed or remembered scene in which the subject can occupy several 'perceptual positions'. Here is the example of a constructed scene in which the subject is in 1st person perceptual position:

> I can very clearly see the fingers move. In fact I cannot see the fingers, I *feel myself* playing the notes. I am at the harpsichord. It is not even the vision but the feeling of the gesture. (Jean, Bach).

In the following example, the subject is in 2nd person perceptual position, i.e. he imagines himself in the place of Mozart:

> I can imagine myself perfectly in the process of touching this... this crystal and being him, and feeling the moment when pressure is just sufficient for the sound to appear. (Jean, Mozart).

Here the scene is seen in the 3rd person perceptual position:

> I see the keys of the piano and a hand which is playing.... it is the pianist's right hand. But I can only see the hand and a very small part of the piano, the keyboard, with the blacks and the whites clearly delineated, and the hand. (Hélène, Brahms)

1.2 Attentional disposition

The source identification process is associated with a special kind of attentional disposition: this is directional attention, focused on the source of the sound. The subject is only interested in the characteristics of the sound as a way of identifying the source, whose image rapidly blots out the auditory experience itself.

> My attention is directed towards the fire over there. The sight of fire blots out the rest of the experience. I forget the sound. It is as though the crackle becomes a quality of the fire, like its colour. (Claire, fire)

1.3 Structure of the experiential space[8]

In this process, the subject in a way is extended towards the source.

> I am in contact with the trees which are I don't know how many metres high, but I am over there, almost literally ... because it is over there that the sound is. It isn't in my ears, it isn't inside my body, it is over there, up there in fact. (Dorothée, forest)

> At a certain moment I identify the sound as the sound of wind in the trees. It is the forest. I quickly have an image of the whole forest undulating in the wind. I am over there, near the trees, at the top of the trees. I am going in this direction, I head over there, a certain distance away. (Claire, forest)

> Instantaneously my lived space is extended, changing itself to go and touch the source of the sound in geographic space. (Jean-Michel, forest)

The imagination of the source extends lived space far beyond the space which is visually perceived. The sound itself and the sound medium become as though they were transparent. The subject 'leaves himself' in a sense, to extend himself towards the source, and the body is in a way 'forgotten'.

To sum up, the process of identifying the source of the sound can be characterised as follows: (1) its result — the source — which appears in a verbal, visual or non-symbolic form; (2) an identification process which consists either of evoking a memory, or imagining the action of producing the sound (in a scene in which the subject can take various perceptual positions); (3) an attentional disposition which is focused on the source; (4) an extension of the experiential space in the direction of the source, with the sound and the body seeming to become transparent.

---

[8] What we are attempting to describe here is the way in which hearing a sound modulates the space experienced, while putting into parentheses what we know or think we know about geometrical space and bodily experience — notably the concepts of bodily scheme and the distinction between 'inward' space and 'outward' space. In other words, it is a matter of moving from 'the thought of the body or the body in idea', to 'the experience of the body or the body in reality' (Merleau-Ponty, 1945, p. 231).

2. 'Object sound', 'heard sound'

We have gathered the description of a second listening mode, consisting of listening to the sound independently of its source. The sound is not considered as a clue, a sign, a means giving me information about something else, but it is perceived immediately for itself. We take an interest in the characteristics of the sound independently of the event and objects which produced it, and of the meaning it may have. If it is a voice, we take an interest in the voice as a voice, independently of the meaning of the words. The qualities of sound as such are traditionally listed as volume, pitch, timbre[9] and persistence.

2.1 Characteristics of the sound

In the following excerpts, the subjects are trying to describe their experience of the sound as a sound:

> This sound is very difficult to characterise because it is a very special sound, there are high notes, there are low notes, there are many tones in this sound. It is a sound in which there are several sounds. (Jean-Michel, Tibetan bowl)

> A very pure sound, with these piano notes which are very clear, which come in to me through the right ear, with an impression of clam, because the notes are clearly distinct, and with a pretty and very sweet harmony. (Hélène, Brahms)

> When I hear the glass harmonica, I am surprised by its slight, fragile character, like a little garland, so fine that it could break with the slightest breath of air. And this little garland emerging from the magma of the other notes, subtle, I turn my attention towards it. (Jean, Mozart)

— When the sound is listened to as a sound, the *auditory qualities* seem to be closely associated with *qualities of a quasi-visual order*: the sound may have a certain luminosity, a certain colour, a certain form, and it may occupy a certain part of the visual space and move inside this space.

> Quasi-vision of the musical undulation. (Michel, Brahms)

> There is something visual, but without colours, it is more like transparencies which are more or less ... dense. (Claire, Brahms)

> I imagine a texture of glass, it is... a little transparent, bluish, slightly bluish, like crystal. It has colours yes, bluish white. (Jean, Mozart)

> I really see something like a kind of triangle which is growing from left to right, I see it. (Jean, Mozart)

---

[9] Timbre, which is very difficult to characterise, is what differentiates the sound of a piano from that of a clarinet, for example.

> Its chant appears to me like bowls which are enmeshed into each other, in growing sizes, parallel to the intensity of the sound. They are brown in colour, and start out from the lower left hand corner of my image. (Hélène, sound SA37)

> I see something as I hear the sound, I see something... angular. I cannot really say that I see it, but there is something visual and angular. I had an impression also, now it comes to me, also at the same time of... oh, of... it was accompanied by a kind of quite violent luminosity. Like a... beam of light. Like the sound, a beam. Like the sound which rises like that, with a kind of openness, it was also a beam of light, you see. A little angular, you see, like that [gestures]. The sound did not occupy all the space, it was as though it was closed up in an angle, in the space over there, you see.' (Claire, sound Y23)

These quasi-visual auditory qualities also sometimes seem to be associated with *qualities of a quasi-tactile order*:

> In fact it is difficult, this sound... it is intriguing.... Because it is at once breathy, rough, shrill... And when I say shrill, that means piercing... like small needles. (Jean, Mozart)

> The sound unfolds little filaments, which are rather like a scratching. Here again it is a little visual, that is from time to time I see small filaments of scratching which infiltrate to the left, to the right [gestures]. I see it very clearly... slightly low on the right. Small silver and white filamentous growths. (Michel, sound Y23)

> As soon as the sound starts I have the impression of something sharp, aggressive, grating. (Claire, sound Y23)

We may note a very clear difference between these auditory feelings, which are quasi-visual and quasi-tactile, and some very precise images whose content may be symbolic (scores, texts), elicited by listening to the sound as a sound, and particularly to music:

> The music appears, the melodic structure appears, with the rhythm, but there is neither a key nor lines. What appears very clearly white, pearl white, silvery white, are the notes... which unfold, which advance like that. They appear to my left. I see three or four notes and the vertical and the horizontal, three four notes and I see the two voices or the three voices depending on the case. I see the score. I see the essentials of the harmonic relations between the notes. (Jean, Bach)

— What *process* does enable the *identification of the qualities of a sound*, for example the differentiation of the timbre of two instruments or the appreciation of the volume of a sound? Although this process is particularly pre-reflective, we have gathered some fragmentary descriptions. For example, in the following excerpt, it is a change in the perceptual position which enables a classical pianist to evaluate the quality of the sound she produces during a concert:

> I become two in a way, in order to be present in the auditorium, as a spectator. I see myself play, I hear from a distance the sound which fills the auditorium, I can have a demanding ear, control the sound, and make people hear what I wish to hear. (Charlotte, piano concert)

2.2 Attentional disposition

The mode of attention required to listen to the sound as a sound is less directional, more open, more diffuse than the mode which is focused on the source.[10]

> My attention is directed towards the space between the fire and me. (Claire, fire)

> I hear the sound, not over there [at the location of its source], but I hear it in space, in a more diffuse way. The sound fills the space in a far vaster way. (Claire, forest)

This mode of attention however remains deliberate. It requires a tension, a slight effort.

> I stretch out towards these sounds in space, I make a slight effort to identify them. (Claire, fire)

> I go and look for the nature of the sound. I push my attention. It is a relative... effort. (Jean, fire)

The zone of the body mobilised is the region of the ears.

> It's as though I was going to meet the music... I don't know if you can say attention, my hearing... I listen out with my ear, that's it, I listen out with my ear. (Hélène, Brahms)

> Listen out with the right ear. Small movements of muscles inside the right ear, from the interior of the body to the exterior. Sensation of a rush of blood in this zone. (Jean-Michel, fire)

> To characterise the sounds, it seems to me I have to concentrate on my ears, in a movement which starts in my neck, moves up into the nape of the neck and then moves behind and in front up to the top of my skull. Like an internal periscope, like an internal horn of a snail which rises. I concentrate on opening my ears, as though the auditory canal became larger. (Jean, fire)

---

[10] Don Ihde describes the transition from a directional listening mode to a less focused listening mode as follows: 'The sparrow's song in the garden presents itself *from* the garden. But if I put myself in the 'musical attitude' and listen to the sound as if it were music, I may usually find that its ordinary and strong sense of directionality, while not disappearing, recedes to such a degree that I can concentrate on its surrounding presence.' (Don Ihde, 2007, p. 77)

— This listening mode enables the discernment of nuances which remain unnoticed when the attention is absorbed by the source of the sound.

> I hear nuances, different 'layers' of sound, irregular cracks which are more or less loud, and more continuous hissings, to which I was not paying attention. (Claire, fire)

2.3 Structure of the experiential space

This listening mode seems to cause a sort of 'densification' of the space situated between the ear and the source. The medium, which is as though it were transparent in the previous listening mode, takes on a certain density, a certain thickness.

> It is densified a little towards the sound. (Jean-Michel, Mozart)

> A rhythmical densification of the space. (Claire, Adrien 37)

The source of the sound, which in the previous listening mode masks the sound, fades away, it is as though it had been forgotten.

> I'm no longer interested in the fire. I don't even know that it is a fire. (Claire, fire)

But the sound remains 'external', on the surface, listened to only with the ears and not with the whole body.

> After reaching the top [of the hill] I try to concentrate on the sounds. But all these sounds remain in a way on the surface. They stay in my ears and in my skull, as though they are external to me. They never go down into my centre. This is absolutely not equivalent with music. It does not grab me like music. (Jean, forest)

> There is part of the music which does not penetrate, which I cannot succeed in feeling. It remains on the surface, outside me, an exterior sound which I listen to only with my ears. (Claire, Mozart)

To sum up, listening to sound as sound is characterised by: (1) identification of the qualities of the sound, auditory qualities closely associated to quasi-visual and quasi-tactile qualities; (2) an attentional disposition which is less directional than the disposition directed toward the source and yet deliberate, which mobilises the region of the ears, and enables the discernment of nuances which are not perceived when the attention is absorbed by the source of the sound; (3) a densification of the space between the ear and the source, and the occultation of the source of the sound.

3. Felt sound

A third listening mode consists of taking an interest in felt sound, 'what it does to me' when the sound is listened to. I divert my attention from the source of the sound ('what is this sound'), and from the sound as a sound ('what this sound is like'), to direct it towards the felt sound ('what the experience of this sound is like'). To use a visual analogy, I am no longer interested in the blue vase, nor in the blue of the vase, but I am interested in the felt blue, what it does to me to look at this blue.

3.1 Bodily felt sound

The sound 'resonates' in our body. This resonance is sometimes very easily perceptible, like that of the bass in a rock concert or a nightclub, or that of a pneumatic drill. But a certain amount of practice makes it possible to become aware of more subtle resonances, such as that of the voice (whether someone else's voice or my own voice), of music, of the sounds of nature, or of any other sound. Talking of 'bodily felt' sound is however an initial approximation. To describe the experience of felt sound, particular vigilance is required in order not to allow the description of the known bodily schema surreptitiously cover the description of the lived body.

Felt sound is characterised by the *zone of the body mobilised* and by the *sensorial qualities* of this felt sound.

— The resonance of the sound may be experienced as global, penetrating the whole body:

> The sound penetrates into us like the air we breathe. (Jean, garden)
>
> The music fills me. (Michel, Brahms)
>
> I feel the sound in me, I listen to it inside myself. (Claire, fire)

This resonance may also be felt at different levels of the body:

> The notes fill my head, and then it moves towards my plexus. It's a kind of undulation which fills my head from top to bottom and from right to left and then from left to right, and which gradually moves downwards. (Hélène, Brahms)
>
> I feel sense of slight tightening which begins at the top of the stomach and spreads upwards towards the centre of the chest before disappearing instantly. (Jean-Michel, Y17)

This resonance can be felt more or less deeply in the body:

Each time there is a sound, I am transfixed. In fact sometimes it goes through me, sometimes I am transfixed, and sometimes I am just lightly touched, on the surface.' (Jean-Michel, Mozart)

It can be experienced as correlated to the intensity of the sound:

The intensity of the bodily feeling is correlated to the intensity of the volume of the various sounds. (Jean-Michel, fire)

A sharpened attention enables the detection of a correlation between the pitch or the intensity of the sound, and the zone of the body which enters into resonance:

Each crackle of the fire passes pleasantly through my body. The deep sounds go through the stomach. The high sounds go through the chest. (Jean-Michel, fire)

The sounds go through my body: the high notes, the chest and the head, and the low notes, the stomach. (Jean-Michel, forest)

This sound, I feel it at the level of the heart, and I have the impression that it is opening up my heart, that it is opening something up, a space in the middle of my chest. (...) When the vibration becomes very very weak, I feel it at the summit and in the centre of my skull, inside. (Claire, Tibetan bowl)

— Sensorial qualities of felt sound. Most of the descriptions we have gathered of felt sound call on several sensorial registers: not only the auditory, but also the visual (transparent) and the tactile (smooth, fresh, sharp, prickly).

A happy, round, transparent freshness. I feel myself refreshed by the sound. (Claire, Adrien 37)

Welcoming, not warm because it was not in terms of temperature. Cosy. With a quilt, feathers, wool and all that, cotton... There is a thickness, a roundness. (Dorothée, Tibetan bowl)

It is a round rhythm, a round sound whose rhythm is smooth and round. (Claire, Brahms)

More precisely, we have noted that the submodalities most frequently used to describe felt sounds are movement, intensity and rhythm, i.e. 'transmodal' characteristics, which are not specific to any of the senses, but can be transposed from one sense to another (unlike for example temperature and texture which are specific to touch, or colour which is specific to sight).[11]

---

[11] Plato (*Théétète* 185a-186a) and Aristotle (*De l'âme*, II, 6, 418 a12 et 418 a18-20) had already noted these characteristics, which they termed 'common sensibles'.

> Straight away, I feel the pulsation of the music, and I feel it in my body. I feel inside myself something which is... sort of jumping... with the rhythm of the notes in my upper body, in my thorax, at the level of my heart and my solar plexus, something which is agitated like a dance. Inside myself it is as though there were... a rhythmicality which was completely in tune with the music and which meant that in my innermost being, muscles... or things contract, exactly as though I was dancing this music inwardly. (Jean, Bach)

The felt sound is a rhythm, a pulsation. It is what in music is not encoded by notes, but by dynamic notations such as 'crescendo', 'staccato', 'piano', 'forte'...

> In this famous solar plexus there are things that happen, which are pulsations which are those of the music, movements... of which I do not know the nature, pulsations which are those of the music and in fact there are two levels of rhythm. The intellectual rhythm is the succession of the notes themselves, quavers, semiquavers, etc., which I see in the score. And then at the same moment, there is this profound rhythm, which is the pulsation, which is not written in the music. There is this extraordinarily profound pulsation, which is absolutely not intellectual, that is not in the notes. I feel profoundly the pulsation in my innermost being as something which rises and falls, which contracts, like a sort of big heart that beats, but which is not going at the frequency of my heart but at the frequency of the specific pulsation of the music. A whole rhythmicality inside me which is in tune with the music. (Jean, Bach)

These inward movements, which are infinitely more subtle than emotions, and are described here as something of a 'pulsation', are easier to perceive in the experience of music. But fine attention also enables becoming aware of them in the feeling elicited by a voice:

> This song wraps itself around me and penetrates me, it is as though it were massaging me inside. (Claire, chant)

> I feel the vibrations of my patient's voice on my face, like a sort of weak electric current, a slight prickling. When the volume of her voice increases, my sensations increase in intensity. When the tone and the rhythm of the words change, my sensations are also modified. [Later in the session] her voice vibrates differently, I feel these vibrations and their variations in my chest, my stomach. (Jean-Michel, therapy session)

...or by a sound in nature:

> This poplar over there, it is as though radiated from it something, a shiver, a diffuse light, a very slight, very fine sound, which comes to me and touches me indescribably. (Claire, forest)

In this listening mode, the sound seems to lose its identity as a sound.

I feel this shiver in me. It loses its 'sound' identity. (Claire, forest)

3.2 Attentional disposition

— Special attentional disposition is necessary to become aware of the felt sound. This attention is unfocused, peripheral, and also passive and receptive:

> When I put myself in this disposition and that 'there, I am ready to listen', I feel like saying that my experiential space is my body and the whole room. (Jean-Michel, Mozart)

> There is openness, welcoming. You don't go looking, you wait for it to come. (Jean, fire)

> I let the sound come to me. (Claire, forest)

This attentional mode is easier to describe by contrast with the previous mode:

> Firstly, it's as though I was going to meet the music... I don't know if you can say attention, my hearing... I listen out with my ear, that's it, I listen out with my ear. And then the music penetrates me, penetrates into my head, that's it. It's as though at the start, I was going to meet the music, and that afterwards we met and it was the music which was penetrating me. (...) The passivity comes afterwards, once the encounter has taken place and the music is penetrating me. At that moment, I no longer need to... I am penetrated. (Hélène, Brahms)

In this listening mode, the bodily zone mobilised seems to be the front, and more particularly, the upper part of the body:[12]

> At the outset I am in a listening posture, my centre is open and ready to receive the sounds. (Jean, fire)

> And at that moment, I realise that what is mobilised in me, what is listening, is not only the ears, but a zone which is much vaster. And immediately, it's quite well delineated, it comes from there, in the middle of my chest, up to the head and even a little bit beyond the head, on the sides. It is as though my head was a little... bigger and I was listening with a sort of triangle, like that. (Claire, moped)

For the vibration to be fully felt, it seems important that this part of the body should be exposed to it, with no screen coming in between:

> The sound almost imposed... that I should put my back against something, not to relax or something like that but rather to open myself up... and it was really physical, it had nothing to do with a mental position. It

---

[12] The importance of the frontal zone of the body in this listening mode has been pointed out in particular by Don Ihde: 'The other, when speaking in sonorous speech, presents himself (...) as a 'presence' who is most strongly present when standing face to face.' (2007, p. 79)

had... become uncomfortable to feel this vibration in the stomach with the stomach compressed like that because I was bent over... So... to leave space for the vibration to spread out, or something like that. (Dorothée, Tibetan bowl)

I prepared myself, it was important for me to prepare myself physically... by adopting a listening position which for me is very physical, that is that I really need the sound to reach me... that there should be no screen between the sound and me. I was almost embarrassed to be seated because in fact there was the table which takes up space, which comes up to there, so all the lower part of the body does not receive... that is, it forms a screen. It's a little bit as though I needed my whole body to listen... to be really attentive to what it does to me to hear a sound. (Claire, Brahms)

— This attentional disposition is sometimes consciously prepared by a *process of generating this disposition*:

It is as though I was opening something up, which could be closed at certain moments, but that I open up to the maximum by making myself a little bit vulnerable, a slightly fragile zone that I am going to open up. (...) Before listening, I breathed deeply several times, I took breaths that were slightly bigger than usual... precisely in order to open up this zone and put myself in this position. (Claire, Brahms)

I am standing up, I absolutely needed to stand up to face the music, with both ears identically active, in an almost prayer-like attitude. My body has disappeared. All that remains is the centre, a yawning, open cavity, which awaits the sound, somewhat impatiently. I oscillate slightly around myself, as though to listen better. (Jean, Mozart)

Whereas in the previous excerpt the consciousness of the body is hidden, in the following excerpts it is on the contrary intensified by a systematic process of making contact with bodily feelings, validated by a very precise internal criterion (deep breathing).

I put myself into my body, I go down into my body. My whole body is mobilised. Breathing plays a role. I breathe in deeply which helps me both to enter into this state and indicates to me that I am (almost) in it. The breathing takes place on its own, at a very precise moment. (Claire)

I make contact with my sensations. It begins at the summit of the skull, and it ends with the soles of my feet. It is accompanied by an eye movement [eye movement in a downward direction]. In fact, I go to look for the feeling from the top of my head with my eyes, and I move down very very fast, with my eyes too. (...) And it is also accompanied by a movement of relaxation. That is to say when I do that I have a wave... an awareness of feelings which is accompanied by a wave of muscular relaxation. And while remaining in contact with my interior, with these feelings, I open up. I open up my ears, I open up my eyes. And I am in contact with what I see and what I hear too, and then at this point I wait, I wait. (...) This relaxation is validated by a deeper breath, which informs me about the fact that 'OK that's it'. At the end of this breath which comes like a sigh of relief. (Jean-Michel, fire)

3.3 Experiential space

— Sound vibration has an impact on the structure of the experiential space, it *transforms the texture of this space*. This transformation may be experienced as a relaxation, an opening, a softening:

I become relaxed [when music haunts me]. That is to say, I let myself be carried, I relax, in muscular terms, I relax. (Hélène, Gregorian chant)

This sound (...) I feel it opening my heart, opening something up, a space in the middle of my chest – that it is 'distending' it, 'tearing' it would be a little too strong. (Claire, Tibetan bowl)

I feel the first notes in my chest. It is as though something was softening in my chest and in my throat. (Claire, Mozart)

... or as a disruption: a tearing, a constriction. Felt sound may be unbearable[13] :

There are two sounds: a continuous gust and explosions. The explosions have a very strong impact. At the outset I am in a listening posture, my centre is open and ready to receive the sounds. The explosions attack me, they destabilise me rapidly, as if I had been struck a blow. (Jean, fire)

It is as though the sound went through the whole of the triangle [the body zone mobilised to listen], and it is like lightning, it scrapes and tears the triangle, from left to right, from end to end. *It is not even a sound, it is a disruption.* (Claire, moped)

Experiential space may retain a trace of this disruption:

Afterwards, the triangle is instantly formed again... But I have the impression that in this triangle, a small scar remains. (Claire, moped)

— This transformation of the texture of experiential space seems to be the result of a *process* of rhythmic attunement with the sound vibration:

It was really a... synchronisation of the rhythm with the vibration of the bowl, something like that. It was a vibration, it was an undulation which came from the bowl to me, and once it was in me, it was more a rhythm of... like a beat perhaps... but very very very small. And this

---

[13] 'This presence [of sound] is also a penetrating, invading presence. (...) This penetrability may be shattering, ultimately painful. The sudden scream at the moment of highest tension in the Hitchcock movie upsets my composure, and it is rightly described as piercing.' (Don Ihde, 2007, p. 81)

synchronisation was really interesting because the bowl vibrated increasingly slowly, less and less intensely, and thus, knowing that it was synchronised, that... it is as though my bodily functions had slowed down at the same time, that really gave this feeling... of going more gently from the interior. (Dorothée, Tibetan bowl)

It is as though the music entered inside me, got hold of me somewhere inside myself and forced me to follow, led me to follow on the rhythmical level. (...) I really feel an attunement between the sound and myself. (Jean, Bach)

—This synchronisation between inward space and outward space weakens, and makes less rigid, the distinction between the two:[14]

It is as though the exterior became denser and the interior more vibrant, less dense, and gradually the texture becomes identical. (Claire, Tibetan bowl)

This vibration abolishes the limits of my body. There is no interior and exterior, there is only this vibration. (Claire, Tibetan bowl)

The sound, it abolishes the limit between me and the outside. (...) There is no more skin, or a skin which is much more permeable. (Claire, forest)

The synchronisation of the two spaces may have the effect of removing the personal 'envelope':

There are pieces, moments when truly I am no longer there... (...) There is a coalescence at a given moment between what I am and the music. (Jean, Bach)

To sum up, felt sound is characterised by: (1) an attentional disposition which is unfocused, receptive, prepared by a process of generating this disposition which mobilises breathing in particular; (2) the bodily resonance of the sound, itself described by its level, its depth and its intensity, and its transmodal character; (3) a transformation of the texture of the lived space, associated with a synchronisation between interior space and exterior space, which makes the frontier between the two spaces more permeable.

---

[14] This synchronisation can be very gradual. Sometimes it can be immediate, which has the effect of instantly 'cutting through' the distinction between inward space and outward space. It is this experience which is remarkably described in the following lines by Rilke: 'He evoked the memory of the hour, in this other southern garden (Capri), where there was, outside and inside him, and putting one in tune with the other, a bird call which, in a way, did not break at the frontier of the body and reunited both sides in a single uninterrupted space where only remained, mysteriously protected, a single place of the purest, of the most profound awareness.' (Rilke, 1966)

Evocations

In the analysis of the interviews, we have noted many evocations generated by the sound, which themselves are associated with particular emotions or feelings. For example:

> Music elicits something old-fashioned which I connect with my grandparents, with the atmosphere I experienced in their home. A living room appears, it is the living room of my grandparents. With colours that are a little dull, faded. The living room is there, and the music makes me feel a sensation which I had when I was a child entering this living room. (Michel, Brahms)

The evocation may even appear before the source of the sound has been recognised:

> Something comes in through the skylight. Immediately, before even recognising it as the cooing of a dove, a particular atmosphere comes back to me of an abundance of plants and calm, with a hint of an earlier time. I recognise this earlier time as an earlier time which is not very distant, that of the time when I bought this house, ten years ago, when I discovered spring in the country. I realise that my body has just taken on a different texture, with a greater density in my back, with a particular sensation in my chest. (Claire, dove)

In these experiences, the evocation immediately elicits a bodily feeling which surreptitiously hides the felt sound – as one of us pointed out:

> It is the evocation which induces a bodily feeling. The evocations take me away from the experience of the sound. (Bernard, fire)

This is why we have noted these evocations, but have decided for the moment to leave them aside.

Interpersonal variations

For some of us, or at certain moments, the source of the sound, heard sound and felt sound are difficult to dissociate or stabilise:

> The source of the sound was it really first, or rather not first, it was… there were not two moments, not 'hey a sound, what is it' or 'hey a fire, that comes with a sound like this and like that', it was really all one I think. The sound itself, stripped of its source, that was difficult for me because for me it was really intrinsic to the sound to have a source: 'it's a tree', 'it's a car', as opposed to 'something produced a sound'. And so I have not necessarily succeeded in separating them, and I have tried to concentrate on my bodily feeling, on what I can feel when I listen to these sounds… which is even more difficult than the rest. (…) I don't think have succeeded… in listening to the sound as a sound. The sound

of the crunching of sand under the foot, it was not the sound that interested me in itself, it was the sound as contact with the foot.' (Dorothée, forest)

It is particularly difficult to abstract one's attention from identifying the source of the sound:

> When there is a rumbling, a crack, I immediately have a question about the origin of the noise. Why this noise. I cannot manage to abstract my attention from the question of the origin. (Bernard, fire)

For others, the distinction between the three modes and their stabilisation is easier.

> I carried out the experiment of listening by straining my ears to the outside, a little as though to seize sound outside, there, towards the loudspeakers. And it is very different from putting myself how I put myself at the outset, that is to say in this highly receptive position in which I open up to let something come, to let come something which does in fact come... into my heart, here in the middle. (...) I forget this zone (the heart) and what was happening there, to carry myself in a more intentional way towards something which is happening outside. And there, I hear *a sound*. I don't feel anymore, I don't see anymore, I hear a sound. I feel it much more outside. At that moment, I have the impression that the 'round rhythm' aspect, to sum up what I was feeling then, is transformed into a sound, into a simple sound if you like. In space. An auditory rhythm... gentle and pleasant... but it is something on the outside. Whereas in the first part of the experiment, it is happening inside me, and it is as if the music... was caressing me, yes in a sense was caressing me. (Claire, Brahms)

> In 1 the sound is over there. In 2 the sound is in the air, in the middle. I am no longer interested in the fire. I don't even know it is fire. In 3 I no longer know that it is a sound. I forget the sound, I forget the fire. (Claire, fire)

Some of us have developed a second-degree consciousness, i.e. a consciousness of the changes resulting from an increased consciousness of their sound experience.[15] For example, Jean-Michel realises that the attention given to the intrinsic properties of the sound strengthen the felt sound.

> When I try to distinguish between the different sounds, low/high, rhythm, my bodily sensations become more intense. That is when I focus on the characteristics of the sound, my bodily sensations intensify

---

[15] Shusterman (2007, p. 81) precisely identifies this sur-reflective level of bodily consciousness or 'soma-aesthetics'. At this level, we are not only conscious of being short of breath, or even of the way in which we breathe (for example, quickly and superficially by the throat), but we are conscious of the way in which our consciousness of breathing influences our actual respiration.

and become more precise. That is to say that I can locate the impact of a particular sound on my body. (Jean-Michel, fire)

Recapitulative table[16]

	Perceived result	Multi-modality	Attentional disposition	Experiential space
Source of sound	Object and/or procedure which could have been used to produce sound	Visualisation of the source	Focused on the source	Extension towards the source, transparent body
Object sound	Auditory qualities of the sound	Auditory qualities sometimes associated with, or translated by, quasi-visual or quasi-tactile traits	Non-directional but voluntary, centred on the region of the ears	Densification of space between source and ears. Obliteration of the source
Felt sound	Bodily resonance of sound	Transmodal feelings with visual, tactile, olfactory, kinaesthetic, somaesthetic resonances	Unfocused, receptive, prepared by a process involving the whole body	Synchronisation between inner space and outer space

III. Discussion

Our work of description and analysis thus leads to the hypothesis of a threefold structure of the auditory experience. The striking coherence of this structure with that revealed by the genetic realization method (*Aktualgenese*) — devised by Werner and his successors in order to obtain a description of the early phases of a perception — lends them both an element of mutual confirmation: 'When you play a series of notes on the piano, it is possible to show in the apprehension several stages in which a sound is heard more inwardly or outwardly. The

---

[16] This table sums up the descriptive categories of listening identified here, except for processes of evocation of scenes triggered by heard sounds (which is currently being analysed in more detail).

most frequent mode of apprehension is that in which the listener hears the sound as completely outward, as though coming from a determined sound source, as though linked to a certain object (for example an instrument). Such a sound may be called objective sound (*Gegenstandson*). On the other hand, there is often another variety of state of consciousness; the sound is not placed in the object, but it fills the auditorium; it is no longer an objective sound, but a spatial sound (*Raumton*). But there is still another way of experiencing a sound impression; the sound may be felt by the body of the listener; it is like a vase which resonates when it receives the sound. 'I am, says a subject, filled with this sound material, as though I had become a violin or a bell on which one might play." (Werner, 1934, p. 199).

However, this structure does not provide us with any information about the nature of the relationship between these three dimensions. Is it a static relationship of composition, with the auditory experience being constituted at each moment by the three dimensions? Is it a relationship of specialisation between three listening modes which are different and exclusive? Or is it a dynamic relationship, with each 'dimension' or 'mode' corresponding to a phase of a microgenetic process? A possible path towards answering these questions seems to lie in the distinction between several temporalities, which we hypothesise on the basis of our results: the double temporality of *becoming aware* of the experience on the one hand, and the temporality of the *unfolding* of the experience on the other hand.

Let us begin by looking at the first one, which is in fact a double temporality, that of the process of obliteration and of the reverse process of becoming aware of the auditory experience. The descriptions we have gathered have led us to make the hypothesis that the three dimensions we have detected — the identification of the source of the sound, heard sound and felt sound — correspond to aspects of experience which are increasingly pre-reflective, and which are hidden by one another. Ordinarily, when a sound is produced, attention is only directed to the heard sound to the extent to which it enables the identification of the source of the sound, an image of which quickly hides the heard sound. A sound is produced, and in a fraction of a second, I recognise this phenomenon as the song of a blackbird which comes in through my office window, without taking any further interest to the particularities of the birdsong.[17] The sound itself is as though it were transparent, I only have a pre-reflective consciousness of it, rather like

---

[17] 'The hunter intent on bagging his game misses the musical sonority of the birdsong, not because it isn't there, but it is the direction and location of his prey which motivates him.

a blind person who explores an object with the tip of his walking stick, but has only pre-reflective consciousness of the contact of the stick in the palm of his hand, to refer to a well-known example.

Directing one's attention to the characteristics of the sound consists in no longer considering the sound as a means of obtaining information about something else, as the sign of something, and taking an interest instead in the characteristics of the sound as a sound. For example, I listen to the blackbird's song as a sound, forgetting even that it is the song of a blackbird. Like the blind person who directs his attention from the object explored to the tactile characteristics of the stick in the palm of his hand. This redirection of attention towards the qualities of the sound enables me to acquire a reflective consciousness of them, and to discern nuances which are usually obliterated by the absorption of attention into the source. The French musicologist Schaeffer calls this listening mode 'acousmatic';[18] it is focused on the intrinsic qualities of the sound as a purely auditory object or 'sound object'.[19] This listening mode, which consists of parenthesizing or suspending the spatio-temporal causes of the sound to 'reduce' it to what one hears, Schaeffer also calls 'reduced listening'[20] (1966, p. 270). So, he writes, 'often surprised, often uncertain, we discover that much of what we thought we were hearing, was in reality only seen, and explained by the context' (1966, p. 93).

The absorption of the attention in listening to sound as sound occults an even more immediate experience: that of felt sound. But special circumstances enable the attention to be directed towards this feeling to acquire a reflective consciousness of it. For example, several of us carried out the experience of physically feeling the arrival of an aircraft or a boat several minutes before the sound was audible.[21]

So, too, with most daily concerns, directionality is that which stands out and is sufficient for ordinary affairs.' (Don Ihde, 1985, p. 79)

[18] The term comes from the Ancient Greek akousmatikoi, the name given to the disciples of Pythagoras who listened to their master through a curtain. The physical body of Pythagoras was hidden from them, and only the sound of his voice reached them. Shaeffer defines the term acousmatic as 'referring to a sound that one hears without seeing the cause of it' (1966, p. 91).

[19] In a recent article, Schmicking, following a suggestion of Husserl, proposes that the sound, considered independently of its spatio-temporal causes, should be called 'tonal phantom' (2008).

[20] Schaeffer has made of this listening mode the basis of his Musical Research Programme, whose aim was to discover the essential structures of sound, and to construct a taxonomy of sounds capable of organising not only the sounds of instrumental music, but all the sounds of the universe.

[21] This phenomenon has been related by Don Ihde: 'In Vermont while lying in bed at night my son often asked what the strange vibration of the earth was, until we noted that this

A certain attentional disposition makes it possible to become reflectively conscious of feelings which are even more subtle, such as that elicited by the voice of someone else, the song of a blackbird or even the rustling of foliage. Instead of going in search of the sound, 'listening out' towards it to characterise it, this disposition consists of making oneself receptive to it, of letting the sound come to you, of letting yourself be 'touched' by the sound. Like the blind man who could turn his attention away from the tactile characteristics of the stick ('smooth', 'cold') to internal sensations felt in the palm of the hand, who instead of touching the stick would allow himself to be touched by the stick.[22]

Pulsation, beat, caress, shiver... the dimension of the experience which is then discovered is made up of imperceptible dynamic modifications of intensity, orientation, amplitude, texture and rhythm, of a transmodal nature. 'These elusive qualities are better captured by dynamic, kinetic terms, such as 'surging', fading away', 'fleeting', 'explosive', 'crescendo', 'decrescendo', 'bursting', 'drawn out', and so on' (Stern, 1985, p. 54). This dimension, which Stern calls 'vitality dynamics', although 'hidden in full view' - he says – seems to be the very texture of our experience. The auditory experience and in particular music enable the drawing of our attention to these subtle transmodal bodily rhythms, which in fact are constantly with us.[23]

During the turning of attention away from the source towards the heard sound, and then from the heard sound to the felt sound, the effort made to seize and characterise an object is relaxed to make way for an attitude of receptivity and welcome. The process of becoming aware of increasingly deeply pre-reflective dimensions of auditory experience seems to be associated with a gradual loss of intentionality. This loss of intentionality is accompanied by a gradual synchronisation between the space perceived as 'interior' and the space perceived as 'exterior', a synchronisation which makes the distinction between the two spaces more permeable, and can go as far as to dis-

---

vibration modulated into the clearly heard approach of a high-flying jet airplane some minutes after the first 'felt' detection of its approach. Later we all recognized the transition of 'felt' to 'heard' sound that the jet displayed.' (2007, p. 44)

[22] To take the celebrated example of Merleau-Ponty of the hand which may be touching or touched (for example *Phénoménologie de la perception*, pp. 108-109, *Le visible et l'invisible*, pp. 164-165).

[23] This dimension has also been identified by Werner who called it 'physiognomic' (for example, in Werner, 1956).

solve it completely.[24] In other words, the more attention is detached from its absorption in outward objects to enter into contact with the inner experience, the more reduced is the distinction between 'interior' and 'exterior'. When listening becomes fully reflective, it is not listening 'from within' any more.[25]

In this hypothesis, the three dimensions of the auditory experience would be the phases of a gradual process of obliteration — the source of the sound masks the heard sound which masks the felt sound, together with a reverse process of becoming aware or gradual 'reduction' of the source to the heard sound, and then of heard sound to felt sound.

Let us now turn to the temporality of the *unfolding* of the experience. When a sound is produced, are the various dimensions of the sound — felt sound, heard sound and source of sound — given from the outset? Could they not be considered on the contrary as the successive moments of a process? In this hypothesis, which is suggested to us by the descriptions we have gathered, felt sound would be an early phase of a very rapid and pre-reflective microgenesis, of which only the latest phase — the recognition of the source of the sound — usually appears to reflective consciousness. This early phase is characterised by a less clear, or non-existent, differentiation between sensorial modes, between inward space and outward space, between knowing subject and known object. This phase is very rapidly followed by a differentiation process, which leads to the separation of an 'object' pole — the source of the sound — from a 'subject' pole. This separation is therefore not 'given', but created and maintained moment by moment by a pre-reflective micro-activity, constituted by tiny gestures of identification, recognition, categorisation and appreciation ... of which we have gathered an outline of description. In this perspective (adopted in Petitmengin, 2007), the process of becoming aware previously described would correspond to a process of gaining reflective consciousness not of elements which are given beforehand, but of

---

[24] 'The music is even so penetrating that my whole body reverberates, and I may find myself absorbed to such a degree that the usual distinction between the senses of inner and outer is virtually obliterated.' (Don Ihde, 2007, p. 76)

[25] We nevertheless use this expression in the title of this article to refer, not to a distinction of a spatial order between and outward world and an inward world separated by the limit of skin, but to a particular perceptual mode. In this we follow E. Behnke : 'The term 'from within', as used here, refers more to a manner of givenness than to a class of givens. (...) 'From within', then, can serve to indicate, not something spatially 'inside' something else, nor even a class of sensations belonging to a single privileged 'object' (e.g., my own lived body), but rather a 'style', 'attitude' or 'approach' that may be manifested in various modes of experience.' (Behnke, 1984, pp. 60-61)

the successive phases of this microgenesis, with each new stage in the reduction corresponding to the recognition of a more primitive phase.

In this context, several of us have sometimes caught a glimpse, particularly at the moment of waking, or when the sound surprised them, or on hearing an unfamiliar sound, of an instant of indifferentiation which is even more primitive: something happens, and for an instant, you don't know who you are, where you are, you don't even know that it is a *sound*. It is just an instant of consciousness which is neither inward nor outward, but which is nevertheless very vivid and clear, and is immediately followed by the unformulated question: 'What's going on? What is it?'

Another question raised by this structure is that of its transposability. Can this threefold structure be transposed from one sense to another? Could it not be a generic structure of perceptive experience? The following interview excerpts suggest for example its transposability from the sense of hearing to that of seeing (and perhaps to the sense of smell).

> I rediscover these 3 positions at the visual level: (1) I can look at the trees as trees; (2) I can look at the colours, the nuances of colours. (3) And then I can let the colour come to me, come and impregnate me and wash over me. I stop straining my eyes towards it. I let the colour come, it impregnates me like a perfume. When I remain for a long time in this disposition I have the impression that the limits of my body do not stop at my skin. Sound in this phenomenon, it abolishes the limit between me and the outside. And so does colour. (Claire, forest)

In the following excerpt, Jean realises that he cannot feel inside himself the sounds of the forest, but that on the other hand this experience takes place with colours.

> All these sounds remain in my ears without impact on my centre, as though external to me, not really interesting. And I become conscious that what music is, what en-chants me, what chants in me, what comes into my centre which the sounds of nature do not at the moment reach, is the spectacle of the forest. The harmonies are not sonorous, they are visual, coloured. The symphony here is almost silent, made of multiple greens, intense yellows, flamboyant ochres. (...) this musty odour, of forest mushrooms, combined with this admirable palette of colours. And it is towards this that my centre is open, it is with this that it is filled. (Jean, forest)

It is interesting to note that during his exploration of inner experience using the DES method, Hurlburt ('Sensory awareness', this issue) has noted many spontaneous descriptions of a phenomenon of focusing of the attention on the sound as a sound, which corresponds to the dimension of the experience we have termed 'heard sound' :

> Carol's friend Candy is telling Carol how to log into a computer web site. Carol is paying attention to the sweetly longish *a* sound in Candy's slight drawl; at that moment, Carol is not paying attention to what Candy is saying about the log-in procedure.

> Stella was on the phone with her father, who was screaming at her. Instead of hearing what her father was screaming, she was noticing the distortion of the sound as the speaker was being overdriven by the screams.

These excerpts illustrate the auditory version of an experience which Hurlburt has identified in all sensorial modes, an experience which 'involves the individual's being immersed in the experience of a particular sensory aspect of his or her external or internal environment without particular regard for the instrumental aim or perceptual objectness', and which he terms 'sensory awareness'.

This threefold structure of auditory experience is a hypothesis based on the descriptions we have gathered, which itself suggests further hypotheses. How can this set of hypotheses be tested, that is how can observations or experiments be devised which would enable them to become verifiable or falsifiable? The first possible path is to continue the work of description we have begun, for which this set of hypotheses and questions constitutes a fertile heuristic framework:[26] (1) by refining the description of the auditory experience in its various temporal unfoldings;[27] (2) by varying the experience and interview conditions: evoked experience freely chosen by the subject, experience immediately preceding a 'beep' as in the DES method, or experience carried out following a detailed protocol just before the interview; (3) by varying the type and level of expertise of the interviewees in the fields of music, meditation, etc.

The second possible path forward consists of creating a 'virtuous circle' of mutual enrichment and refinement of the 1st person analyses of the auditory experience and 3rd person studies of hearing. One way of doing this would be to use the experiential variables we have identified as neuro-physiological analysis criteria: for example, looking for the neuronal signature of the three attentional dispositions detected.

---

[26] 'The phenomena do not just 'speak out' themselves - they 'speak to' a question addressed to them.' (Ihde, 2007, p. 219)

[27] For example, the awareness of the dynamic of the auditory experience may be facilitated by devising 'experiential procedures' to disrupt or interrupt the process (such as listening to unfamiliar sounds). This type of procedure has similarities with the genetic realization method (*Aktualgenese*) devised by H. Werner (1956) and his successors to obtain a description of the early phases of a perception, which are usually hidden by its later phases.

Acknowledgements

This article was written under the auspices of the 'Réseau Philosophie et Neurosciences' (INCM-CNRS),and has been supported by grants from Cognisud. The authors wish to thank Don Ihde for his extremely helpful comments. They are also grateful to Peter Thomas for translating from French the initial version of this article, and to M. Aramaki, A Merer, R. Kronland-Martinet and Y. Solvi for supplying bizarre sounds.

Conclusion

What do we know about what it is like to hear a sound? Actually very little. Each stage of the reduction unveils an even more unnoticed dimension. The vastness of what a little sound may reveal is an inexhaustible wonder.

References

Andreas, C. & Andreas, T. (2009), 'Aligning perceptual positions; A new distinction in NLP', *Journal of Consciousness Studies*, this issue.

Aramaki, M., Vion-Dury, J., Schon, D., Marie, C., Besson, M. (2009), 'Une approche interdisciplinaire de la sémiotique des sons', in Dalmonte R. and Spampinato F. (eds), *Il nuovo in musica e in musicologia* (LIM, Lucques).

Behnke, E. (2002), 'World without opposite/Flesh of the World (A Carnal Introduction)', (http://www.lifwynnfoundation.org/worldwithoutopposite.html).

Casati, R. and Dokic, J. (1994), *La philosophie du son* (Editions Chambon).

Delattre, P. (1971), *Système, structure, function, evolution* (Paris: Maloine).

Depraz, N., Varela, F., Vermersch, P. (2003), *On Becoming Aware* (Benjamin).

Husserl, E. (1893–1917/1964), *Phenomenology of the Internal Time Consciousness* (Indiana University Press).

Hurlburt, R. and Akhter, S. (2008), 'Unsymbolized thinking', *Consciousness and Cognition*, 17 (4), pp. 1364–74.

Hurlburt, R., Heavey, C., Bensaheb, A. (2009), 'Sensory awareness' (this volume).

Ihde, D. (1976/2007), *Listening and Voice. Phenomenologies of Sound* (State University of New York Press) (First edition Ohio University Press)

James, W. (1890/1983), *Principles of Psychology* (Cambridge, MA: Harvard UP).

Merleau-Ponty, M. (1945), *Phénoménologie de la Perception*, (Paris: Gallimard).

Petitmengin, C. (2007), 'Towards the source of thoughts: The gestural and transmodal dimension of lived experience', *Journal of Consciousness Studies*, 14 (3), pp. 54–82.

Rilke, R.M. (1966), 'Erlebnis II', *Sämtliche Werke* VI (Insel-Verlag) (published in the *Insel-Almanach* 1919).

Schaeffer, P. (1966), *Traité des objets musicaux* (Paris: Seuil).

Schmicking, D. (Forthcoming), 'Sound as auditory sign of physical events and tonal phantom: A Husserlian analysis', in Dick C. and Banega H. (eds.), *Naturalization of Phenomenology* (Nordhausen: T. Bautz), to appear.

Shusterman, R. (2008), *Body Consciousness* (Cambridge: CUP).

Stern, D. (1985), *The Interpersonal World of the Infant* (New York: Basic Books).

Werner, H. (1934), 'L'unité des sens', *Journal de Psychologie Normale et Pathologique,* 31, 190–205.

Werner, H. (1956), 'Microgenesis and aphasia', *Journal of Abnormal Social Psychology*, 52, pp. 347–53.

Pierre Philippot & Zindel Segal

Mindfulness Based Psychological Interventions
Developing Emotional Awareness for Better Being

Abstract: *This paper presents and discusses the psychological interventions that are primarily based on the development of mindful awareness as a psychotherapeutic tool. Mindfulness based psychological interventions are defined and situated in their historical context, in the larger perspective of the evolution of psychotherapies in the Western world in the last two decades. A special focus is given to mindfulness based stress reduction (MBSR, Kabat-Zinn, 1982) and to mindfulness based cognitive therapy (MBCT, Segal, Williams & Teasdale, 2002). The structure and core elements of these interventions are presented. Then, we examine their effectiveness in improving psychological and physical well-being. In the next section, we speculate about the underlying psychological mechanisms that might account for the effects of mindfulness based interventions. Special attention is devoted to the cognitive processes underlying emotion regulation and self-awareness. Finally, we examine how a first person approach might contribute to the understanding of mindfulness based interventions.*

Keywords

Mindfulness, psychological interventions, psychotherapy, cognitive therapy, first person approach

The last two decades have seen the development of mindfulness based interventions (MBI) in health and clinical psychology. They have been originally proposed as an approach to better deal with stressful live situations (Kabat-Zinn, 1982) or as functional forms of emotion regulation strategies (Baer, 2003). In essence, MBI aims to develop the capacity to be aware of one's own present experience and to explore it with an open-minded attitude. Clearly, this constitutes direct clinical application of a first person approach to one's own emotional and affective life.

In the present contribution, we will present MBI in clinical psychology and relate them to the first person approach developed by Varela and Shear (1999). First, the notion of mindfulness, as understood in that specific context will be defined and located in its historical background. Next, we will present two short term MBI, Mindfulness Based Stress Reduction (MBSR, Kabat-Zinn, 1984; 1994) and Mindfulness Based Cognitive Therapy (MBCT, Segal *et al.*, 2002). Then, we will examine the effectiveness of these programs and speculate about the underlying factors that might be active in such interventions. Finally, we will discuss the reciprocal insights that MBI and first person approaches might offer to each other.

Mindfulness from a Clinical Psychology Perspective

Kabat-Zinn has defined mindfulness as a state of awareness resulting from 'paying attention in a particular way: on purpose, in the present moment, and nonjudgmentally' (Kabat-Zinn, 1994, p. 4) or as 'the awareness that emerges through paying attention on purpose, in the present moment, and nonjudgmentally to the unfolding of experience moment by moment' (Kabat-Zinn, 2003, p. 145). Every component of these definitions is necessary to understand the use of mindfulness in the domain of clinical interventions.

First, mindfulness does not refer to any specific content, but rather to a kind of consciousness resulting in a state of awareness that can be applied to any aspect of lived experience. It is thus a process, a way of relating to one's experience, whatever it is, without any attempt of generating a certain type of experience or of reaching a specific state. In this sense, mindfulness is fundamentally different from relaxation (Ost, 1987) or autogenic training (Schultz & Luthe, 1959), which seeks to reach a specific mental state and content.

Second, mindfulness emerges from the mental act of voluntarily orienting attention towards a specific target. Mindfulness is thus intentional and voluntary, and as such, it can be directly accessed. It does not refer to a state of consciousness that can only be accessed indirectly or unpredictably, like ecstasy, or that is dependent of a mediator, like hypnosis. The mere enactment of the intention of being mindful generates the state of mindfulness.

Third, attention is directed towards what is actually and presently experienced by the subject. Concretely, this means focusing all attention resources on a specific target (e.g., breathing or bodily sensation), and developing a reflexive awareness of any information arising from any sensory modality, as well as to the thoughts and mental images that spontaneously come to awareness. In mindfulness training, participants are first encouraged to focus on certain types of information, for instance, bodily sensations, or sensations generated by breathing. Further along in the training, the focus of attention might be directed towards a specific source of information (e.g., spontaneously occurring thoughts) while remaining aware of the other sources of information in the background (e.g., somesthetic sensations from posture, breathing sensations, etc.).

Fourth, a special note is given to the fact that these informational inputs, qualifying present experience, are changing from moment to moment. Thus, mindfulness is not only being aware of the present sensations, thoughts, and mental images, but also being aware of how they fluctuate in time and how the phenomenal world is always new and changing.

Finally, and perhaps most importantly, mindfulness is nonjudgmental. This does not mean that mindfulness practitioners must inhibit attitudes or judgments that are spontaneously and automatically generated by what comes to their mind. A painful sensation or thought will automatically trigger an aversive attitude and judgment, which are part of what the individual experiences at that time, and it would be non-mindful to attempt to change this experience. Rather, the mindful attitude is to take note of the automatically triggered attitudes and judgments, but not to 'follow them,' that is, to not allow them to automatically direct attention and trains of thought in a direction congruent with them. What is central in mindfulness is that the subject aims to govern his/her attention and to prevent it from being captured by affectively loaded sensations, thoughts, or mental images. Mindfulness practitioners seek to keep an open mind to any aspect of their experience and to explore it for what it is, be it painful or pleasant, attractive or repulsive. Thus, the nonjudgmental aspect does not primarily refer to a moral quality, but rather to a psychological capacity of voluntarily allocating attention to the present experience as it is, while preventing the capture of attention by automatic processes.

In sum, within the domain of MBI, mindfulness is defined as a psychological concept, involving psychological processes, mainly attention, perception, and consciousness. It is distinct from any spiritual, moral, or esthetic connotations. MBI can thus be defined as a psychological training program aiming at developing the capacity of being aware of one's on-going experience, including any automatic thoughts and processes that might otherwise remained unnoticed. This approach is akin to the basic stance of Varela and Shear (1999) when they state 'There are numerous instances where we perceive phenomena pre-reflexively without being consciously aware of them, but where a 'gesture' or method of examination will clarify or even bring these pre-reflexive phenomena to the fore. (...) Exploring the pre-reflexive represents a rich and largely unexplored source of information and data with dramatic consequences' (p. 3). In this perspective, MBI offer a structured training in developing conscious awareness of pre-reflexive phenomena.

The Historical Background of Mindfulness Based Psychological Interventions

The concept of mindfulness originates in the earliest Buddhist teachings (Gira, 1989) and it has been described as the heart of Buddhist meditation (Thera, 1962). This millenary tradition as been translated into a Western lay program by John Kabat-Zinn (1982) who sought to develop a short term group program to help people suffering from chronic health conditions to cope with resulting stress. Kabat-Zinn's program, MBSR, is almost exclusively based on mindfulness and consists of a progressive set of exercises and reflection upon these, aiming at developing a capacity to be mindful as defined in the previous section. MBSR has been applied to a large variety of patient populations, presenting with somatic or emotional health problems (Baer, 2003). It is now applied in hundreds of hospitals in North America and Europe.

MBSR has been adapted and manualized by Segal, Williams, and Teasdale (2002) who were designing an intervention for preventing depressive relapse. Their program, MBCT, is specifically targeting people who have suffered from recurrent depressive episodes in the past but who are presently remitted. It consists in an adaptation of the MBSR program with the addition of some psycho-educative and cognitive therapy components proper to depression. This program will be more extensively described in the next section.

MBSR and MBCT are considered as the two forms of psychological intervention that are predominantly based on mindfulness (Baer, 2003). However, other interventions include elements of mindfulness while not being predominantly based on it. One such intervention is the Dialectal Behavior Therapy (DBT), designed by Linehan (1993) as a treatment for borderline personality disorder. DBT's tenet is to promote a dynamic towards a central synthesis between acceptance and change. The basic idea is that for personal and emotional change to occur, people must first accept their own emotional experience and who they are, while actively working to change their behavior and environment to construct a life to which they aspire. Among the many skills taught in DBT is mindfulness, as a capacity to synthesize acceptance and change. Indeed, mindful observation of one's thoughts and feelings foster their acceptance while changing one's attitude towards them. Given its heavily disturbed target population, DBT is more progressive and longer in duration (around 50 weekly sessions) than MBSR or MBCT (8 weekly sessions).

Related ideas have been adopted by Marlatt (1994) in his program to prevent relapse in substance dependence. Marlatt (1994) focused on the notion of 'urge' for the substance as a prototypical example of non-acceptance of a present state of craving. As a cure, Marlatt proposed to develop the capacity to accept the discomfort of craving by adopting a mindful attitude of observing how the sensations, thoughts, and emotions related to the urge are changing from moment to moment. In this context, he has developed the notion of 'urge surfing.' Clients have to imagine that urges are ocean waves that grow gradually until they crest and subside. The client 'rides' the waves without giving in to the urges, thus learning that urges will pass.

Another form of intervention that includes elements of mindfulness is Acceptance and Commitment Therapy (ACT), developed by Hayes (1994). Together with non-judgment, acceptance is the most basic attitude necessary for the development of mindfulness (Kabat-Zinn, 1990). The notion of acceptance developed by ACT is identical to interventions that are primarily based on mindfulness. Clients are taught to develop an observing self that watches their bodily sensations, emotions, thoughts, and actions as distinct phenomena from who they really are. For instance, people are encouraged to consider that they have the thought that they are unworthy, rather than thinking 'I am unworthy.' In this perspective, they are encouraged to non-judgmentally observe their thoughts and emotions as they arise, without attempting to change or avoid them. However, unlike interventions primarily based on mindfulness, ACT does not propose meditation-type exercises. ACT also encompasses an important component related to 'commitment'. It consists of identifying personal values and goals of clients and in helping them to change the contingencies of their daily life in order to act more congruently according to these values and goals.

MBCT, DBT, Marlatt's relapse prevention program, and ACT all belong to what is conceived of as the 'third wave' of cognitive and behavioral therapies (CBT). These therapies share important premises. While classical CBT focuses on directly changing dysfunctional behaviors and cognitions and replacing them with more functional ones, the aim of the 'third wave' is to change the clients' attitude toward their behaviors and cognitions rather than specifically targeting behaviors and cognitions. For instance, rather than attempting to change an irrational cognition such as 'I am unworthy unless I act perfectly' into a more rational one, 'third wave' therapies attempt to change the attitude toward the cognition, considering it as just a thought (i.e., a product of the mind activity that does not necessarily reflect reality). The assumption here is that changes in dysfunctional behaviors and cognitions will result from this change in attitude.

Third wave psychotherapies also promote a different form of therapeutic relationship. While in classical CBT, therapists are experts who apply well established knowledge and procedures in a rather directive way, in 'third wave' interventions, therapists are coaches who encourage clients to explore their personal experiences and emotions. In MBI, therapists are encouraged to have a personal practice in mindfulness, applying to themselves the exercises they prescribe to their clients. Thus, socializing clients to this type of psychotherapy is not to convey well established knowledge, like in classical CBT, but rather to guide and explore personal experiences shared by the client and the therapist. This implies important differences in therapist training. Being trained in MBI is much more personally involving than being train to CBT.

To summarize, referring to the definition of psychotherapy proposed by Castonguay and Beutler (2005), MBI can be distinguished from classical CBT by the following facets: (a) While classical CBT focuses on symptom reduction, MBI focuses on developing self-awareness; (b) In classical CBT, the therapist has a more directive attitude than in MBI where his/her role is almost exclusively to facilitate exploration; (c) CBT stresses controlling and reducing the intensity of emotion, while MBI favors the of the attitude of allowing emotions. However, beyond these distinctions, it is important to note that there is no opposition between classical CBT and 'third wave' psychotherapies (Barlow *et al.*, 2004). As cognitive therapy came as an addition to behavior therapy, 'third wave' psychotherapies must be considered to complement classical CBT rather than replacing it (Teasdale, 2005).

Description of the MBCT Program

MBCT is an adaptation of Kabat-Zinn's (1982) MBSR program. The latter has been designed as a general program for dealing with stress in populations suffering from chronic conditions. MBSR has been described by Kabat-Zinn (1982; 1990), but it has not been published as a standardized treatment manual. MBCT however, has been specifically designed to prevent depressive relapse and has shown efficacy especially for individuals who have suffered from 3 or more depressive episodes (Teasdale *et al.*, 2000). MBCT has been published with a detailed session by session description (Segal *et al.*, 2002). In this section, we will briefly describe it, as an illustration of a structured MBI.

MBCT consists of eight weekly group sessions lasting two and a half hours. Each session is structured around the same caveat: it directly starts with a 15 to 40 minute mindfulness exercise in which participants practice their ability to focus their attention on their present experience non-judgmentally. The focus of attention varies according to the exercise: bodily or breathing sensations, auditory or visual perceptions, thoughts, and emotions. Following the exercise, participants are invited to discuss their experience of the exercise, and then to share their experience completing the homework exercises that had been assigned for the past week. The instructor then raises the specific topic of the session, rooting it in the comments and experiences just shared by the participants. One such topic, for instance, the concept of 'automatic pilot,' which is the propensity of our mind to function automatically and to govern our behavior without us being aware of it. Another topic is 'to stay present' to ongoing experience, while the natural tendency of the mind is to wander elsewhere. The session topic is embodied in a new mindfulness exercise that is practiced in session. Finally, homework is assigned (including 45 minutes of daily practice) and the session is closed with a short mindfulness exercise.

MBCT sessions are taught in a specific way. Analytical theorizing or abstract discourse is avoided. Rather, teaching always stems from the concrete personal experiences of participants and, if possible, from their direct experience with exercises practiced in session, or as homework during the previous week. Therefore, the importance of a regular and intense (45 minutes daily) practice during MBCT training is particularly stressed. In their comments and questions, participants are invited to stay as close as possible to their personally felt experiences and to refrain from abstract generalization. The instructor models this mental attitude. In other words, the mindful attitude of being aware of what is concretely experienced here and now, is practiced during the entire session.

Exercises practiced in session and for homework are diverse. They include the body scan, which consists of examining the body, part by part, in a relaxed, laying down position, while raising awareness of bodily sensations that may arise. Other exercises consist of various forms of sitting meditation in which participants focus their attention on a specific aspect of their present experience (e.g., bodily or breathing sensations, hearing or visual perceptions, thoughts, emotions, etc). Other exercises consist of accomplishing daily routine activities in a mindful way, for instance, brushing one's teeth while paying attention to any bodily sensation that may occur. From session to session, the exercises progress with the challenge they offer to participants. While the initial exercises use ample instructions and diverse sensory modalities or body parts as points of attentional focus, sessions gradually evolve by offering less instruction along with longer durations of attentional focus on body parts and sensations.

The MBCT program also encompasses psycho-educative and cognitive therapy components to specifically address depression. They consist of identifying symptoms of depressive relapse, the irrational thoughts characterizing depression, and the concrete strategies that could counteract the development of depression.

Efficacy of Mindfulness Based Interventions

It is beyond the scope of the present contribution to provide an exhaustive and systematic review of the effectiveness of MBI. The reader may refer to previously published systematic meta-analyses (e.g. Baer, 2004; Grossman, Niemann, Schmidt, & Walach, 2004). The general message of these reviews is that short term mindfulness interventions have an effect size of medium amplitude (average d around .60, i.e. that the means of MBI were on average 0.6 *Standard Deviation* higher than the means of the control groups) on psychological as well as somatic variables. This suggests that MBI are effective, over and above mere placebo effects. Yet, the amplitude of their impact is not as high as focused psychological interventions whose d are often above 1 (Ost, 2008). To date, we know of no RCT comparing MBI to a focused psychological intervention for a specific disorder.

However, it should be noted that the research on the effectiveness of mindfulness based interventions is confronted with several problems. First, with the exception of MBCT, designed for preventing depressive relapse, and DBT, designed to treat borderline personality disorder, most of the interventions studied were not designed for a specific disorder. This lack of a specific target implies more general, and hence, less sensitive outcome evaluation criteria, as specific effects might be diluted in general outcome measures. MBI might be at a disadvantage when comparing its efficacy with specific symptoms, while other interventions specially target these symptoms. In this sense, the effect magnitude of MBI designed for a specific condition (e.g. MBCT for depression) might be larger than 'general purpose' MBI.

An alternative strategy to validate MBI might rest in considering their impact on psychopathological processes rather than simply investigating the change they yield in terms of diagnostic criteria or in symptoms diminution. In other words, following a notion proposed by Barlow (2004), MBI should be validated in terms of processes rather than of symptomatology. Unfortunately, the processes by which MBI operate are still not well established. Baer (2004) has listed a number of potential processes (see next section) but this analysis is still speculative and the processes postulated are very general. Thus, even if research has established some efficacy for MBI, it has not yet provided a consensual model of the processes by which these effects might operate. As will be developed later, there are some indications that MBI may effect high order executive functions that are necessary for ending unhealthy rumination and other cognitive interlocks (Teasdale, Williams, & Segal, 1995). Still, the empirical validation of MBI would benefit from a sound theory accounting for the intervening factors and active ingredients.

Third, it should be noted that most MBI are very short term interventions (eight weekly group sessions for MBSR and MBCT). Their outcome should thus be appreciated in a 'dose-effect' perspective, keeping in mind that in a typical MBCT group of 15 participants, the total amount of therapist-hour per client is about 1.6. In this respect, MBI are very cost-efficient (Teasdale *et al.*, 2000).

In sum, the efficacy of MBI is partly established, although more research is still needed. In particular studies with random assignment to treatment conditions and credible control interventions are still scarce. The active factors accounting for MBI efficacy still need to be established. In contrast, it should be noted that the social dissemination of MBI clearly precedes its scientific validation. While indication criteria are largely unknown, and the efficacy is still under studied, there is a large enthusiasm for MBI in the public and in popular publications (e.g. Servan-Schreiber, 2007). Caution is thus recommended in the therapeutic application of MBI, especially as classic CBT intervention might be more effective than MBI in reducing symptoms in the case of acute disorders.

Underlying Factors Active in Mindfulness Based Interventions

As mentioned above, MBI primarily originated in a laic adaptation of a millenarian Buddhist tradition. They have not been directly derived from a psychological model that would specify *a priori* the processes by which MBI would operate. Nevertheless, different authors have speculated about the active processes in MBI.

The five mechanisms identified by Baer (2004)

Baer (2004) has proposed five mechanisms by which MBI might reduce symptoms. First, MBI entail exposure, especially exposure to emotional experience and painful sensations and thoughts. Clients are encouraged not to avoid painful aspects of experience, but rather to explore them and to develop a deeper awareness of them. In this process, people learn that the painful experiences do not have the catastrophic consequences that they are often *a priori* envisioning (Craske et al., 2008). In this sense, MBI work as a form of sensitive desensitization. Second, MBI promote cognitive changes by modifying the attitude towards thoughts and feelings. From a MBI perspective, thoughts have to be considered 'just as thoughts,' that is, as a creation of our mind, not as a reflection of truth or reality. Third, mindfulness training fosters self-management in several ways. The clients have to develop a strong personal discipline in order to fulfill the requirement of 45 minutes of daily mindfulness practice; they also have to learn to sustain uncomfortable states for extended periods of time (see the exposure point above). Fourth, although this is not an aim of MBI, in many cases, mindfulness practice often results in relaxation, which has been proven to be an effective approach for many psychological stressors (Carlson & Hoyler, 1993). Last, Bear (2004) mentions the acceptance component of mindfulness. Hays (2004) has defended the notion that acceptance, defined as 'experiencing events fully and without defence, as they are' (p. 30), is a major determinant of psychotherapeutic change. MBI greatly emphasise this aspect, encouraging participants to accept and explore (i.e., experience fully) all aspects of experience, including painful sensations, thoughts, and emotion.

The processes outlined by Baer (2004) have the advantage to refer to a well-established literature of processes known to be active in psychotherapeutic change (Castonguay & Beutler, 2005). However, this analysis also presents some limitations. First, most of the processes considered are common to many psychotherapeutic approaches. It is unclear whether MBI operate through the same processes as other forms of intervention, or whether they have some proper mechanisms of action. Second, the range of processes considered is large. Further, it is not specified whether some of these postulated processes bear more weight than others in accounting for the efficacy of MBI. Third, the five items listed by Baer (2004) represent broad psychological phenomena that are sustained by many different processes; these phenomena as such are too super-ordinate to be considered as processes. For instance, exposure is not a process but rather a procedure that is likely to mobilize many different processes (different types of conditioning, cognitive restructuring, change in self-efficacy, etc.), the involvement and relative importance of which are still objects of controversy (Craske *et al.*, 2008; McNally, 2007).

Mechanism of emotion regulation

In the perspective of overcoming some of these limitations, one way to further investigate how MBI operate is to approach them at a more molecular level: Which are the specific, concrete and operationalizable psychological processes that might account for the effectiveness of MBI? Our view is that MBI such as MBCT can be conceived of as prevention interventions aiming at developing psychological abilities that are central in emotion regulation and/or in preventing emotion dysregulation. These abilities address specific psychological processes that are involved in preventing or counteracting ruminations and other cognitive interlock phenomena that precipitate negative mood and promote emotional avoidance (Barlow *et al.*, 2004; Borkovec & Sharpless, 2004; Teasdale *et al.*, 1995). We propose that three types of such processes are particularly trained during MBI, each sustaining a specific ability. These abilities are attentional control, reflexive awareness, and the capacity to suspend automatic/immediate responses. They will be briefly reviewed in the following paragraphs.

Attentional control. MBI encompasses an extensive training of attentional abilities. In particular, every exercise that is part of the

MBI curriculum implies the training of (a) the ability to voluntarily focus attention on a specific object/sensation/thought, i.e. attentional engagement, (b) the ability to maintain attention on that object/sensation/thought, i.e., sustained attention, and (c) the ability to disengage attention from automatically activated content, i.e. attentional disengagement. These capacities are central to the cognitive regulation of emotion, especially as regards the capacity to disengage from automatic and recursive thoughts activated by emotion and to focus on situationally adaptive processing (for a full discussion of this point, see Philippot *et al.*, 2007).

Reflexive awareness. Another capacity that is systematically trained by MBI is reflexive awareness of personal experience. This is primarily accomplished through raising the awareness of body state and of automatically activated cognition and emotion during the mindfulness exercises, together with preventing the stream of consciousness to be carried away by automatic thoughts/judgements/perceptions. MBI also encourage participants to develop this type of awareness in their daily life and routines. Large individual differences exist in the ability to perceive bodily sensations (Pennebaker, 1982), as well as in emotional awareness (Lane, 2000). These individual differences bear important clinical consequences as poor emotional awareness has been related to negative health consequences, both at the somatic and mental levels (Taylor & Bagby, 2004; Ward *et al.*, 1988). It should be noted that several psychological models of emotional awareness locate its genesis in the conscious perception of bodily changes induced by emotion. For instance, Lane (2000; Lane *et al.*, 1990) has proposed that the most rudimentary level of emotional awareness rests in the perception of unspecified physiological arousal, and then evolves in the perception of specific body sensations, further followed by the perception of their integration in action tendencies. Higher levels of awareness include the perception of simple and then complex or blended emotional feelings. It is remarkable that MBI such as MBSR or MBCT are following a very similar path in raising awareness: During the first exercises, participants are encouraged to focus on their body sensations, first as separate entities, than as a whole body state. In later exercises, attention focus is extended to thoughts and emotional feelings.

Inhibition of prepotent response. Finally, MBI are also training the capacity to suspend automatic/immediate responses, in order to create a mental buffer in which to practice reflexive awareness. The notion is that automatic chains of stimulus-response are to be interrupted in order to allow for new, non automatized responses to take place

(Hays, 1994; Linehan, 1993). The notion that life challenges can be confronted via an automatic or an effortful route is a hallmark of psychology, especially in the domain of psychological and attitudinal change (e.g. Petty & Cacioppo, 1986). In the context of psychopathology, relationships have been established between impulsivity and the development of psychological disorders (Schachar & Logan, 1990). For instance, impulsivity is a characteristic of borderline personality disorder for which one of the most indicated treatment is DBT, a mindfulness based intervention developed by Linehan (1993). In MBI, the capacity to withhold automatic responses is developed by training the participants to observe and develop their awareness of the automatically activated action tendencies, without acting on them. This capacity thus directly entails the two previous ones: the capacity to focus attention (here on automatically activated action tendencies) and the capacity to raise awareness of the ongoing processes.

In a clinical context, the capacity to suspend automatic/immediate responses also implies the capacity to tolerate the emotional discomfort generated by not giving in to the urge to immediately respond. This is relevant for all types of MBI, but even more specially so in the case of the relapse prevention of Marlatt (1993). This capacity is akin to the notion of hardiness (Kobasa, 1979) or of resilience (Davidson, 2000). It refers the capacity of individuals to sustain stressful and negative experiences in a positive spirit, i.e. without loosing hope or developing negative affectivity. This capacity has been shown to be an important moderator of the impact of negative life events on subsequent health and psychopathological problems.

In sum, several psychological processes are intensively trained during MBI. For instance, in MBSR and MBCT, this training represents a minimum of 45 minutes a day during eight consecutive weeks. A significant psychological literature relates the three types of psychological processes to outcomes in terms of emotion regulation, as well as of somatic and psychological well-being. It is also noteworthy that the types of processes identified all refer to executive functions (Baddeley, 1996; Miyake et al., 2000). This suggests that MBI are specifically targeting executive processes that are involved in emotion regulation.

Evidence of the implication of emotion regulation processes in MBI

There are some recent research suggesting that indeed, MBI act on the above mentioned processes and that these might mediate the clinical outcome of the interventions. In a large clinical study, Bogels et al.

(2008) investigated mindfulness training as a new treatment for attention and impulsivity problems in adolescents with a variety of externalizing disorders. After MBI, participants self-reported substantial improvement on a diversity of variables including self-control, attention problems and mindful awareness. Importantly, they also performed better on a sustained attention test. Their parents corroborated these improvements. In addition, increased adolescent awareness after MBI predicted longer-term improvement.

Specifically addressing attentional focus, Jha *et al.* (2007) observed that mindfulness training modified subsystems of attention. In a control study, they examined three attentional subsystems: alerting, orienting, and conflict monitoring. They report that participants in an MBSR course improved the ability to endogenously orient attention as compared to a control group. Likewise, Valentine and Sweet (1999) observed that individuals trained in mindfulness meditation were displaying superior performance in sustained attention as measured by Wilkins' counting test, as compared to matched controls.

Regarding the capacity to disengage from automatic response patterns, some of our recent studies have started to explore whether the specific processes just outlined are active in MBCT intervention. For instance, Heeren and Philippot (2009) has shown that improvements in psychopathological symptoms following MBCT training were mediated by the reduction of unhealthy rumination, especially characterized by abstract and analytical thinking. Another study (Heeren, Van Broeck, & Philippot, 2009) has shown that MBCT training results in increased executive performance, especially in terms of semantic fluency, and that such executive improvement partly mediates MBCT effect on the improvement of healthy emotion processing capacities, such as the capacity of re-evoking emotional experiences at a high level of specificity (Williams *et al.*, 2000).

Obviously, this is just the beginning of the exploration of the processes sustaining MBI and a lot of work is ahead. Still, these preliminary investigations are promising and support the notion that MBI train some executive functions that might be specifically needed in the cognitive regulation of emotion.

Contribution of Mindfulness Based Interventions to a First Person Perspective

In this last section, three questions will be discussed. First, we will examine the extent to which MBI can be considered as a first person approach. Then, we will turn to a tenet of first person approach:

raising awareness of lived experience, and we will examine whether developing this capacities results in clinical benefits. Finally, we will speculate about how a first person approach might contribute to the understanding of MBI.

Mindfulness-based interventions as first person approaches

Can MBI be conceived of as a direct application of the first person perspective in the psychotherapeutic domain? According to Varela and Shear (1999), the first person approach is characterized (a) by an object, i.e. phenomenal experience, (b) by a set of procedures that allow the observation and study of that object, and (c) by means for the expression and validation of the observation and resulting knowledge within the community of researchers who have familiarity with the procedures.

Regarding the object, Varela and Shear (1999) define first person events as 'lived *experience* associated with cognitive and mental events' (p. 1). This is the exact definition of the object of mindfulness, and most exercises proposed in MBI are focusing attention on this lived experience with associated sensations, cognitions, and emotions. As explained in the section describing MBCT, reference to personal experience as directly lived by the participants as well as the instructors is strongly emphasised in MBI. Analytical and distantiating discourse, which is characteristic of a third person approach, is discouraged. The object of MBI and first person approaches thus appears to be very similar.

Regarding the set of procedures, Varela and Shear (1999) insist that a method for raising awareness (or for clarifying pre-reflexive phenomena) and training to that method are essential in first person approaches. A crucial point in first person approaches is 'to overcome the "just-take-a-look" attitude in regards to experience'. A sustained examination is necessary to 'produce phenomenal descriptions that are rich and subtly interconnected. ... The main question is: How do you actually do it?' (Varela & Shear, p. 2). MBI clearly consist in structured trainings which target the capacity to examine in a sustained manner phenomenological experience. They indeed produce rich and subtly interconnected knowledge about ones' self and emotions. Similarly, a basic attitude in first person methodology is to suspend ongoing mental processes and to redirect attention from content to mental processes. As describe above, this is again what is accomplished in any exercise which is part of the MBI curriculum. Both approaches are ultimately aiming at a meta-awareness: the awareness of the mental process rather than of the mere content. However, MBI and first person approaches differ somehow in what is attended to. While MBI focus on the experience itself, first person approaches emphasize the very process of description itself. Indeed, a central epistemological aspect of first person approach is to specify how one can become aware and describe his or her own mental processes (Petitmengin & Bitbol, this issue).

The last point, expression and validation of the knowledge, is relevant for the development of a scientific method, but it is not so for clinical applications. The first person approach as a scientific endeavour aims at creating, expressing, and disseminating knowledge in the scientific community. In contrast, the aim of MBI is ultimately to develop better being for individuals through the development of a mindful attitude and capacity. In this clinical context, a significant part of the knowledge that is created by individuals participating in MBI is considered as private and thus protected by ethical principles. Still within MBI groups, teaching mostly relies on participants'sharing of their experience. In this context, the medium of expression mostly consists in verbal accounts. Some (e.g. Kabat-Zinn, 1990) also use poetry to carry the meaning of complex notions, such as acceptance, to the intervention participants.

In sum, regarding object and procedures, MBI perfectly correspond to the definition of a first person approach. The third aspect, is only very partially met: Expression and description mostly consist of verbal accounts and validation is a scientific concern that is largely irrelevant for clinical applications. MBI can thus be considered as the application of the first person perspective in the psychotherapeutic domain.

However, this analysis opens new perspectives regarding the third criterion of Varela and Shear. Considering that MBI consist in an intensive training in observing one's own ongoing experience, one could propose to individuals participating in MBI to take part in experiments using a first person approach. Using an interview approach (e.g. Petitmengin, 2006) that would preserve the privacy and anonymity concerns raised above, MBI participants could be interrogated on a variety of issues, for instance the different modes of attention, the rising of emotion, the experience of observer versus field perspective, the 'gestures' that allow to fully explore experience, including its pre-reflexive components. As MBI train awareness to these phenomena, they might constitute a particularly interesting pool of subjects for such experiments. A further point of interest would be to consider longitudinal studies that would examine individual before and after MBI. This would allow to investigate how 'first person' knowledge evolves following an intensive mindfulness training, and thus, whether such training is effective in developing a set of procedure for observing phenomenal experience, i.e. the second characteristic of first person approaches as defined by Varela and Shear (1999). Another possibility is to recruit MBI instructors as participants in experiments using a first person approach. They indeed represent a population with extensive training in observing their present experience and in raising to awareness pre-reflexive processes.

Raising awareness as a therapeutic means

As developed above, first person approaches rest on the development of a specific type of awareness: the awareness of our mental processes, be it cognitions, emotions, or sensations. An important question is whether developing this type of awareness bears clinical consequences. This question has already been tackled in a previous section. Specifically, Bogels et al. (2008) have reported evidence that increased awareness following MBI predicts longer-term improvement in emotion regulation and psychological well-being in adolescents. Clearly, this question requires further empirical investigation.

Yet, useful information can be gathered in related forms of psychological intervention. For instance, Greenberg (2002) has designed a form of therapy aiming at developing emotional awareness: emotion focused therapy. Outcome studies on emotion focused therapy (e.g. Goldman *et al.*, 2005) have shown that the depth of experiencing and exploring emotion theme in the last half of therapy is a significant predictor of reduced symptom distress and increased self-esteem. Similarly, Holmes *et al.* (2008) have observed that adopting an actor perspective during emotional imagery (which implies visually experiencing the imagined situation through the eyes of the person experiencing it) results in a beneficial emotional outcome, while this is not the case if one adopt an observer perspective (i.e. distancing from experienced emotion).

To conclude, although scarce or indirect, existing empirical evidence suggests that raising experiential awareness might contribute significantly to improvement in psychological well-being. Enhancement of self-knowledge and emotion regulation capacities might mediate this effect. Indeed, raising experiential awareness is likely to result in a greater awareness of one's actual self, i.e. who one actually is. Recent research (e.g. Roelofs *et al.*, 2007), grounded on the Self-Regulatory Executive Function model of emotional disorders

(Wells & Matthews, 1994), has recently evidenced that discrepancies in self-perception were directly linked to symptoms of depression as well as indirectly via the cognitive process of rumination. Further, raising experiential awareness implies developing acceptance of one's experience, if only to just stay in the position of experiencing it. As developed in a previous section, acceptance is thought of as a major process in healthy emotion regulation (for a development of this claim, see Hayes, 1994). Still, more research is needed to investigate these largely speculative suggestions.

Direction for Future Research

Throughout this paper, we have repeatedly stressed that MBI require more research (a) to establish the extent of their efficacy and the conditions for which they are indicated and (b) to investigate the processes by which they operate. On this latter point, studies conducted in a first person perspective might offer a heuristic avenue for the understanding of MBI. As mentioned above, one difference between MBI and first person approaches is that the former focus directly on lived experience itself, while the latter consider the thought processes that enable the description of lived experience. Bridging these two perspectives, the focus of participants to MBI trainings could be directed to their ongoing thought processes as they attempt to develop their awareness of their lived experience.

As mentioned above, first person approaches have developed rigorous procedures to collect precise verbal descriptions of lived experience, for example, through interviews (Petitmengin, 2006), and to extract invariants from reports of multiple experiences from multiple individuals. These techniques would enable the MBI researcher to collect descriptions of a given type of mental process, and then to analyse and compare the collected descriptions in order to detect possible generic structures and variants of the process in question. Such an approach could be applied, for instance, to the executive processes operant in MBI.

For instance, traditional research at the third person is attempting to understand the higher order (executive) processes that come into play in emotion regulation and self-awareness. Presently, this research is importing concepts and measures that cognitive research has developed for the investigation of non-emotional problem-solving and processing. It might be that this conceptual framework is only partly adequate for the study of emotion regulation and self-awareness in clinically significant conditions. By a careful observation of the attentional processes and of their dynamics, a first person approach might usefully contribute in defining the exact processes that are mobilized during mindfulness training.

Very concretely, such an approach could tackle the following questions: Is it the capacity to focus and sustain ones' attention on a specific object that is central to the training, or is it the capacity for divided attention between a specific object (focal attention) and a broad state of alertness (open attention), or is it the capacity to move back and forth between these two types of attention? Using a first person approach, MBI participants could be interviewed regarding how they direct their attention to their ongoing experience and regarding the experiential consequences of different modes of attention (or attentional 'gestures'). These experiential consequences could concern emotional feeling (their nature and intensity), the types of cognitions (mental image and thoughts) that are automatically generated in a given attentional mode, etc. Another question that could be pursued pertains to the mental gestures that allow to establish a direct contact with one's experience and those that distantiate from it. Here again, the attentional mode might be of importance (see Genoud, this issue), but also the perspective adopted (field versus actor perspective). Participants could be interviewed about the steps that are necessary to come in touch mindfully with their experience. In a more fundamental perspective, MBI participants could be interviewed, using a first person methodology, on what, in their personal experience, makes mindful observation of their own experience therapeutic.

Conversely, as suggested earlier, MBI instructors as well as individuals who have been trained in MBI might constitute a particularly interesting subject pool for first person researchers. On the one hand, they have undergone an intensive training in mindful observation of their own ongoing experience. On the other hand, they constitute a wide and diversified array of individuals from the general population. Indeed, MBI are proposed to people of all ages and socio-economical conditions. Although most of these people are confronted with a difficult psychological or somatic condition, a significant proportion engage in MBI in self-development perspective.

To conclude, MBI and first person approaches are likely to cross-fertilize each other. MBI offer to first person approaches a structured training to develop and deepen the awareness of mental processes. Conversely, first person approaches provide an alternative (or rather complementary) rigorous scientific method to explore the processes by which MBI operate.

Acknowledgements

The writing of this paper has been facilitated by grants from the 'Fonds National de la Recherche Scientifique de Belgique' and 'Action de Recherche Concertée'. The authors appreciate the helpful comments of an anonymous reviewer on an earlier draft of this paper.

References

Baddeley, A. (1996), 'Exploring the central executive', *The Quaterly Journal of Experimental Psychology*, **49**, pp. 5–28.
Baer, R.A. (2003), 'Mindfulness training as a clinical intervention: A conceptual and empirical review', *Clinical Psychology: Science and Practice*, **10**, pp. 125–43.
Barlow, D.H. (2004), 'Psychological treatments', *American Psychologist*, **59**, pp. 869–78.
Barlow, D.H., Allen, L.B. & Choate, M.L. (2004), 'Towards a unified treatment for emotional disorders', *Behavior Therapy*, **35**, pp. 205–30.
Bogels, S., Hoogstad, B., van Dun, L., de Schutter, S. & Restifo, K. (2008), 'Mindfulness training for adolescents with externalizing disorders, and their parents', *Behavioural and Cognitive Psychotherapy*, **36**, pp. 1–17.
Borkovec, T.D. & Sharpless, B. (2004), 'Generalized anxiety disorder: Bringing cognitive behavioral therapy into the valued present', In S.C. Hayes, V.M. Follette, & M.M. Linehan (Eds.). *Mindfulness and acceptance: Expanding the cognitive behavioral tradition* (New York: Guildford).
Carlson, C.R. & Hoyler, R.H. (1993), 'Efficacy of abbreviated progressive muscle relaxation training: A quantitative review of behavioral medicine research', *Journal of Consulting and Clinical Psychology*, **61**, pp. 1059–67.
Castonguay, L.G., Beutler, L.E. (2005), *Principles of Therapeutic Change that Works* (New York: Oxford University Press).
Craske, M.G., Kircanski, K., Zelikowsky, M., Mystkowski, J., Chowdhury, N., Baker, A. (2008), 'Optimizing inhibitory learning during exposure therapy', *Behaviour Research and Therapy*, **46**, pp. 5–27.
Davidson, R.J. (2000), 'Affective style, psychopathology, and resilience: Brain mechanisms and plasticity', *American Psychologist*, **55**, pp. 1196–214.
Gira, D. (1989), *Comprendre le bouddhisme* [Understanding Buddhism] (Paris: Bayard).
Goldman, R.N., Greenberg, L.S. & Pos, A.E. (2005), 'Depth of emotional experience and outcome', *Psychotherapy Research*, **15**, pp. 248–60.
Greenberg, L.S. (2002), *Emotion-Focused Therapy: Coaching clients to work through their feelings* (Washington, DC: American Psychological Association Press).
Grossman, P., Niemann, L., Schmidt, S., Walach, H. (2004), 'Mindfulness-based stress reduction and health benefits: A meta-analysis', *Journal of Psychosomatic Research*, **57**, pp. 35–43.
Hayes, S.C. (1994), 'Content, context, and the types of psychological acceptance', In S.C. Hayes, N.S. Jacobson, V.M. Follette & M.J. Dougher (Eds.), *Acceptance and Change: Content and context in psychotherapy*, pp. 13–32 (Reno, NV: Context Press).
Heeren, A. & Philippot, P. (2009), *Changes in ruminative thoughts mediates impacts of mindfulness*. Manuscript submitted for publication.

Heeren, A., Van Broeck, N., Philippot, P. (2009), 'Effects of mindfulness training on executive processes and autobiographical memory specificity', *Behaviour Research and Therapy,* In press.

Holmes, E.A., Coughtrey, A.E. & Connor, A. (2008), 'Looking through or at rose-tinted glasses? Imagery perspective and positive mood' *Emotion,* **8**, pp. 875–79.

Jha, A.P., Krompinger, J., Baime, M.J. (2007), 'Mindfulness training modifies subsystems of attention', *Cognitive, Affective, and Behavioral Neuroscience,* **7**, pp. 109–19.

Kabat-Zinn, J. (1982), 'An outpatient program in behavioral medicine for chronic pain patients based on the practice of mindfulness meditation: Theoretical consideration and preliminary results', *General Hospital Psychiatry,* **4**, pp. 22–47.

Kabat-Zinn, J. (1990), *Full Catastrophe Living: Using the wisdom of your body and mind to face stress, pain and illness* (New York: Delacorte).

Kabat-Zinn, J. (1994), *Wherever You Go, There You Are: Mindfulness meditation in everyday life* (New York: Hyperion).

Kabat-Zinn (2003), 'Mindfulness-based interventions in context: Past, present and future', *Clinical Psychology: Science and Practice,* **10**, pp. 125–43.

Kobasa, S.C. (1979), 'Stressful life events, personality, and health: An inquiry into hardiness', *Journal of Personality and Social Psychology,* **37**, pp. 1–11.

Lane, R.D. (2000), 'Neural correlates of conscious emotional experience', In R.D. Lane and L. Nadel (Eds.) *Cognitive Neuroscience of Emotion,* pp. 345–70 (Oxford: Oxford University Press).

Lane, R.D., Quinlan, D.M., Schwartz, G.E., Walker, P.A. & Zeitlin, S.B. (1990), 'The Level of Awareness Scale: A cognitive-developmental measure of emotion', *Journal of Personality Assessment,* **55**, pp. 124–34.

Linehan, M.M. (1993), *Cognitive-Behavioral Treatment Of Borderline Personality Disorder* (New York: Guilford Press).

Marlatt, G.A. (1994), 'Addiction, mindfulness and acceptance', In S. C. Hayes, N. S. Jacobson, V.M. Follette, & M.J. Dougher (Eds.), *Acceptance and Change: Content and context in psychotherapy,* pp. 175–97 (Reno, NV: Context Press).

Miyake, A., Friedman, N.P., Emerson, M.J., Witzki, A.H., Howerter, A., Wager, T.D. (2000), 'The unity and diversity of executive functions and their contributions to complex "frontal lobe" tasks: A latent variable analysis', *Cognitive Psychology,* **41**, pp. 49–100.

McNally, R.J. (2007), 'Mechanism of exposure therapy', *Clinical Psychology Review,* In press.

Ost, L.G. (1987), 'Applied relaxation: Description of a coping technique and review of controlled studies', *Behaviour Research and Therapy,* **25**, pp. 397–409.

Ost, L.G. (2008), 'Efficacy of the third wave of behavioral therapies: A systematic review and meta-analysis', *Behaviour Research and Therapy,* **46**, pp. 296–321.

Pennebaker, J.W. (1982), *The Psychology of Physical Symptoms* (New York: Springer Verlag).

Petitmengin, C. (2006), 'Describing one's subjective experience in the second person: An interview method for the science of consciousness', *Phenomenology and Cognitive Sciences,* **5**, pp. 229–69.

Petitmengin, C. & Bitbol, M. (2009), 'The validity of first-person descriptions as authenticity and coherence', *Journal of Consciousness Studies,* this issue.

Petty, R.E. & Cacioppo, J.T. (1986), *Communication and Persuasion: Central and peripheral routes to attitude changes* (New York: Springer Verlag).

Philippot, P., Neumann, A. & Vrielynck, N. (2007), 'Emotion information processing and affect regulation:Specificity matters!', In M. Vandekerkhove *et al.* (Eds.). *Regulating Emotions: Social necessity and biological inheritance,* pp. 189–209 (London/New York: Blackwell Publisher).

Roelofs, J, Papageorgiou, C., Gerber, R.D., Huibers, M., Peeters, F. & Arntz, A. (2007), 'On the links between self-discrepancies, rumination, metacognitions, and symptoms of depression in undergraduates', *Behaviour Research and Therapy*, **45**, pp. 1295–305.

Schachar, R. & Logan, G.D. (1990), 'Impulsivity and inhibitory control in normal development and childhood psychopathology', *Developmental Psychology*, **6**, pp. 710–20.

Schultz, J.H. & Luthe, W. (1959), *Autogenic Training: A psychophysiologic approach in psychotherapy* (New York: Grune and Stratton).

Segal, Z.V., Williams, J.M.G. & Teasdale, J.D. (2002), *Mindfulness-Based Cognitive Therapy for Depression: A new approach to preventing relapse* (New York: Guilford Press).

Servan-Schreiber, D. (2007), *Anticancer* (Paris: Laffont).

Taylor, G.J. & Bagby, M.R. (2004), 'New trends in alexithymia research', *Psychotherapy and Psychosomatics*, **73**, pp. 68–77.

Teasdale, J.D., Segal, Z.V., Williams, J.M.G., Ridgeway, V., Lau, M. & Soulsby, J. (2000), 'Reducing risk of recurrence of major depression using Mindfulness-based Cognitive Therapy', *Journal of Consulting and Clinical Psychology*, **68**, pp. 615–23.

Teasdale, J.D. (2005), *Mindfulness-Based Cognitive Therapy and the Third Vague in CBT: Invited address*. In proceedings of the 34th annual Congress of the European Association for Behavioural and Cognitive Therapies, Manchester, United Kingdom.

Thera, N. (1962), *The Heart of Buddhist Meditation* (New York: Weiser).

Teasdale, J.D., Segal, Z.V. & Williams, J.M.G. (1995), 'How does cognitive therapy prevent depressive relapse and why should attentional control (mindfulness) training help?', *Behaviour Research and Therapy*, **33**, pp. 25–39.

Valentine, E.R. & Sweet P.L.G. (1999), 'Meditation and attention: A comparison of the effects of concentrative and mindfulness meditation on sustained attention', *Mental Health, Religion & Culture*, **2**, pp. 59–70.

Varela F.J. & Shear J. (1999), 'First-person methodologies: What, Why, How?', In F. Varela and J. Shear (Eds), *The View from Within: First-person approaches to the study of consciousness*, pp. 1–14 (Exeter: Imprint Academic).

Ward, S.E., Leventhal, H. & Love, R. (1988), 'Repression revisited: Tactics used in coping with a severe health threat', *Personality and Social Psychology Bulletin*, **14**, pp. 735–46.

Wells, A. & Matthews, G. (1994), *Attention and Emotion: A clinical perspective* (Hove: Lawrence Erlbaum).

Williams, J.M.G., Teasdale, J.D., Segal , Z.V.& Soulsby, J. (2000), 'Mindful meditation reduces overgeneral autobiographical memory in depressed patient', *Journal of Abnormal Psychology*, **109**, pp. 150–55.

Daniel N. Stern

Pre-Reflexive Experience and its Passage to Reflexive Experience
A Developmental View

Abstract: *Taking a developmental perspective, experience is divided into three domains: the pre-reflexive; and two reflexive domains, the non-verbal reflexive and the verbal reflexive. This splitting of the reflexive domain is done in part because infants spend the first two years of life with only the pre-reflexive and non-verbal reflexive modes during which so many basic interpersonal skills are learned. The structure of experience in these first two domains is very rich. In particular, the role of 'dynamic forms of vitality' as a global organizer of interpersonal experience is presented as playing a major role in the structuring of pre-reflexive experience. The process of the passage of experience between all three domains is also explored, with the following question in mind: what is special about the passage into the verbal reflexive domain? We suggest this process requires acts of 'soft assembly', as described by dynamic systems theory. The soft assembly process, however, is not unique to the verbal reflexive domain but is needed in all passages between domains to link different modes of experience.*

Key Words

developmental perspective, domains of experience, pre-reflexive experience, non-verbal reflexive experience, verbal relfexive experience, dynamic experience, 'forms of vitality', passage between domains of experience, soft assembly

Introduction

This article is concerned with three main domains of experience and the passage between them. They are: the pre-reflexive experiences which are immediately lived, involving 'first order' ('primary') consciousness; and two types of reflexive experience, 'non-verbal reflexive' experience; and 'verbal reflexive' experience.

The reasons for this redivision of phenomenal experience comes largely, but not exclusively, from the developmental perspective adopted.

Experience in these domains can become or already is in 'reflexive consciousness'. What distinguishes the three domains is not the type of consciousness that attaches to them, or they are attached to, but what is the nature of their phenomenal experiencing.

A brief preview of terms is useful to orient the reader.

'Pre-reflexive' experience will refer to phenomenal experience as it is happening – as it is directly lived. This is 'first order' or (primary consciousness). The experience remains as a trace or sketch. The trace exists before or without it is ever being transposed or refigured into one of the other domains of experience. It is in this sense that the trace is pre-reflexive. These traces can become reflexively conscious and when they do they have a particular form, namely, the experiencing of the dynamics of a happening (its movement, force, temporal profile, directionality, spatial excursion. We will call these dynamic experiences 'forms of vitality', see below).

'Non-verbal reflexive' experience refers to (pre-reflexive) experience that is refigured into some corporal, or sensori-motor or affective structure. But not into language. In other words there has been a bending back upon the original (pre-reflexive) trace and refiguring it. It is for this reason we call it reflexive. Reflexivity does not necessarily imply a revision into language. This level includes 'implicit knowledge', body concepts, and other similar non-verbal concepts.

'Verbal reflexive ' experience is what we mean by the experience of language, both comprehension and production. It consists mainly of non-verbal reflexive experience and pre-reflexive experience that has been refigured into language. It is of second order consciousness, constructed after the fact.

The reasons for positing 'pre-reflexive' experience and for splitting apart reflexive experience into non-verbal and verbal is largely developmental. The infant goes through an initial long period of roughly the first two years when he cannot verbalize but is capable of experiencing directly and of non-verbal reflexion upon that experience. Why has nature arranged it so? Perhaps because children need a repertoire of basic non-verbal reflexive experiences to build language upon. This notion is confluent with the ideas of the large extent to which language is based in non-verbal models (eg., Lakoff & Johnson's 'primary metaphors' 1980; 1999). The relatively sudden arrival of language on the scene at roughly two years may contribute to the overestimation of its specialness as a new and totally different lens on experience. This has had several consequences for studies of reflexive experience (and clinical psychology). There has been an underestimation of the complexity and richness of the structures of non-verbal reflexive experience, especially and not only in pre-verbal infancy. Finally, we tend to give a privileged place to language as the port of entry to 'first person experience'.

The Nature of Pre-reflexive Experience

What are the possible organizations of pre-reflexive experience? Whatever is experienced pre-reflexively must already be structured or organized to some extent. If not, all of its later refigurations as seen reflexively would have to emerge (from what?) in the process of its passage to verbal or other forms of reflexive expression. There must be a structure to pre-reflexive experience, or else there is nothing to build upon. And the structure must derive from what the infant can experience.

There are many descriptions of experiences that have the flavor of the pre-reflexive. Each with different but related organisations: 'felt sense' (Gendlin,1996); 'felt meaning' and 'intuitive experience' (Petitmengin, 2007; 1999); 'background feelings' (Damasio, 1999); 'forms of feeling' (Langer, 1953); 'vitality affects' (Stern, 1985); 'image/gesture' (McNeil, 2005). These vary in many ways such as complexity and scope, yet commonalities emerge.

One of the main features of these phenomenal events is that they are wholes. The gestalt, or 'emergent property' seems to be the most useful concept for dealing with holistic experience. The leap to a gestalt is mysterious, but that is what we have to work with, that is how the mind works. Still it is helpful to identify the various features that play a role in creating the whole. Granted that the global pre-reflexive experience is refigured in the sense that the whole experience emerges progressively during the direct living, i.e. during the present moment of the event. But it is not necessarily refigured later after the event is over and the present moment exited.

* * *

A methodological point is needed about including developmental material from pre-verbal infants to understand pre-reflexive experience. The disadvantages are several. The most obvious is the impossibility of a first person verbal account. (However, it is worth asking whether forms other than the verbal are less convincing and useable for inferring subjective phenomena). Another potential disadvantage is the comparability of subjective experience in pre-verbal infants relative to verbal adults. They may differ in the capacities available to structure pre-reflexive experience. Also they have never had the influence of language in their initial perceptual pre-structuring.

There are also advantages. The infant offers a purer 'preparation' having had no significant prior traffic with language (only sound and music). And the infant has a huge repertoire of mental capacities that have been identified over the past several decades. These are less dissimilar to adult capacities than one might have thought.

Finally, an imagined 'second person account' of an infant is conceivable but very unreliable. Still, I have tried that earlier but in a very rough and non-systematic manner (mostly for the benefit of parents) using a fictive baby (Stern, 1990). Such an exercise is the most common of activities. Parents try to glimpse their baby's subjective landscape innumerable times every day and often, every few seconds, when needed, in order to know what to do next. This is carried out via deduction and more to the point, via empathy. Empathy is a 'second person' path to accessing another's subjective state (Varela & Shear, 1999). Empathy provides essential information for intuitive parenting and for all intersubjectivity.

* * *

Returning to pre-reflexive (and pre-verbal) infants, what are the central forms of experience that could structure the pre-reflexive domain? There is one gestalt that plays a crucial pre-reflexive structuring role. This is 'the-phenomenal-experience-of-human-action'. It will interest us particularly as it has been little studied as a whole experience. This experience of human action arises regardless of whether the action is real, virtual, anticipated, or imagined, or whether it is visual, auditory, tactile or otherwise perceived, or whether it is performed by the self or seen in another. This experience is key in interpersonal and intersubjective interactions, especially of the intimate kind that involves family, friends, lovers, parents with infants, and psychotherapy.

Several phenomenal experiences available to pre-verbal infants can accompany the-experience-of-human-action. The most relevant for our purposes is that of 'dynamic forms of vitality' or 'vitality forms'. Dynamic forms of vitality are a member of the larger family of dynamic experiences. While dynamic experiences in general are not often considered in themselves, with important exceptions (eg., Langer, 1953; 1969-1972; Merleau-Ponty, 1962.), 'dynamic forms of vitality' (see below), is even less studied. The gestalt of 'dynamic forms of vitality' arises from five un-reflexive components or features: movement; force; temporal contour; space and directionality/ intentionality.

What is meant by dynamic forms as a holistic unit is exemplified by a statement attributed to Albert Einstein. He was once asked whether he thought in words or pictures. It is said he answered, 'Neither, I think in terms of forces and volumes moving in time and space'. As used by Einstein, force-movement-volume-time-space, is a basic unit — a whole — a dynamic image to describe the happenings of the universe.

Now, zoom in to describe the basic dynamic units, the gestalts of the very small events, lasting seconds, that make up the interpersonal, phenomenal moments of our lives: the force, speed, flow and felt meaning of a gesture; the timing and stress of a spoken phrase or even a word or laugh; the way one breaks into a smile or the time course of decomposing the smile; the manner of shifting position in a chair; the time course of lifting the eyebrows when interested and the duration of their lift; the shift, the flight of a gaze; the rush or tumble of thoughts; the unfurling of a sense; the cresting of an emotion. These are examples of the basic wholes of movement-force-time-directionality/intention that occupy our subjective experience of interactions in everyday life, and make up a large part of the infants' sensory world. The scale is small but that is where we live and it makes up the matrix of experiencing ourselves and others. The same is true for the time-based arts of music, dance, theatre, cinema, poetry.

This global dynamic experience of forms of vitality is the main candidate we propose for structuring the traces/sketches of pre-reflexive experience of interpersonal events..

The notion of vitality forms is applicable to human interactions, not to the inanimate world where natural laws apply. However there is a close relationship between these two worlds. In going from physics to phenomenology, natural laws (like gravity or entropy) are replaced by intentions and motives, and mathematics are replaced by subjective dynamic forms of vitality. The basic units are, nonetheless, similar.

This is not a trivial resemblance. I would speculate that developmentally the first version of motion-force-time-space and intention is acquired during infancy when human action (both by the self and by others) is encountered. The resultant sensori-motor gestalt becomes the pre-reflexive base from which our view of the inanimate world of physics evolves. Later observations of the workings of inanimate nature then use this early sensori-motor experience as a mode of perceiving and understanding the natural non-human world. It is interesting that Einstein says that he must first get an experience in his body, a sensory-motor feel, before he can write a formula.

Let us then examine the separate features making up the whole that is the dynamic form of vitality.

Movement

A gestalt is the result of detecting partially independent features and then combining them, in one step to make a whole. The whole experience of movement-force-temporal contour- directional space - intention, together, is the gestalt that makes up a dynamic form of vitality. Phenomenologically, the features that compose the gestalt all turn around movement. From the point of view of psychology, force, time, space, and intention are the daughters of movement. All taken together compose forms of vitality.

For instance, force is not felt alone but only when embodied in movement, real or imagined. Movement is not instantaneous, it has a time course, a temporal profile. Directional space is created by movement and its trajectory. Finally, intentions depend on the execution of a movement or on the planning of a possible movement. As seen by humans, intentions presuppose a possible or real movement.

Movement is our most primitive and fundamental experience. Many thinkers have long argued that movement comes first in evolution and in development. It has a primacy in experience throughout life. It is widely thought that during evolution, approach and withdrawal emerged from the general capacity to move. The different emotions then differentiated out from approach and withdrawal. Bodily concepts and then progressively, language evolved from this movement base (Panksepp, 1998). The philosopher Maxine Sheets-Johnstone has written a book entitled *The Primacy of Movement* which also proposes that movement comes first in both phylogeny and ontology (1999). This point is driven home with force when watching a fetus move, via echogram, even at 12 weeks gestation. At this stage of fetal development, generalized (whole body) and specific local movements (gestures/acts) occur frequently (Piontelli, 2007). It is startling at first view, to see the vigor, almost violence of movement at the very beginning of life.

Langer gave movement a foundational role in feeling (1953). Lakoff & Johnson (1980; 1999) and McNeil (2005) give it a fundamental role in thinking and language. Gallese and Lakoff (2005) suggest that images, concepts, and language itself, are born in the integrative activity of the sensory-motor cortex. Husserl considered movement to be the mother of cognition (1962; 1964). Similarly, Polanyi states that thoughts come out of bodily experiences, from the tacit knowledge embedded in the body (1962).

There is also mental movement. It is experienced as internal motion. When we think a thought or feel emotion or have sensations, the mental experience is not static. Subjectively, a thought can rush onto the mental stage and swell, or it can quietly just appear and then fade. So can an emotion. It has a beginning, middle and end. Physical movement seen in others is also felt in the self at the same time, via the mirror neuron system (Rizzolatti *et al.*, 1996; Gallese, 2001; Rizzolotti, Fogassi & Gallese, 2001). It can also be felt when imagined (Jeannerod & Frak, 1999). The feel of movement can come from music which is 'sound in motion' (Kurth, 1925/1991; Eitan & Granot, 2006), from a touch or pain or a changing taste (a swallow of wine). When we hear or read language, or let free the imagination we can experience virtual worlds of forces in motion. The experience of movement (physical or mental) traces a small journey. Mental movement while it is happening, traces a profile of its rising and falling strength as it is contoured in time.

Human physical movement is analogic, fluid, flexible, intention bound, shaped and constrained by our anatomy, our characteristic speed of movement, and by the human motives which direct it. Together these give it the distinctive signature of human movement. The dynamic forms of vitality that emerge are multisensory and apply across all domains of physical and mental life. The following list of adverbs illustrates this well.

Exploding, surging, accelerating, fading, drawn out, fleeting, forceful, powerful, feeble, cresting, pulsing, tentative, pulling, pushing, relaxing, floating, fluttering, effortful, easy, tense, gliding ... and many more.

While these words are common enough, this list is curious. Most of the words are adverbs or adjectives. The items on it are not emotions. They are not motivational states. They are not pure perceptions. They are not sensations in the strict sense as they have no modality. They are not direct cognitions in any usual sense. They are not acts as they have no goal state and no specific means. They fall in between all the cracks. They are dynamic forms of vitality. They do not belong to any particular content. They describe a separate kind of experience that structures the pre-reflexive and helps constitute what passes across the mental stage.

However, forms of vitality are rarely divorced from a content. More accurately, they carry a content along with them. They are not empty forms. They give a temporal and intensity contour to the contents, and with it a sense of an alive 'performance'. The content can be an emotion (i.e. shifts in emotion), a train of thoughts, physical or mental movements, a memory, a phantasy, a means-end action, a sequence of dance steps, a shot in a film. The vitality dynamic gives the content its form as a dynamic experience. The contents, by themselves, need not conform to any particular dynamic experience. Anger can appear on the scene explosively, or build progressively, or arrive sneakily, or coldly, and so on. So could happiness and its smile.

The content material provides the goal; the specific behavioral patterns to reach the goal; and the qualia. But only when the contents are yoked to arousal do they take on a dynamic form of vitality (Stern, 2004; 2010). This is what gives them the feel of flowing and aliveness — of being human.

While we often merge the dynamic vitality forms with the experience of its content to create a holistic event, they remain separable. Usually, it is the experience of the contents (the thought or emotion, etc.) that attracts our human interest, but not always. For instance when someone reaches for an object, the goal-directed reach is the content of the act, the What? was done. But suppose they reach violently, the How? of the act. We can focus on the reach-to-goal or the explosion of the act, or back and forth, or merge them.

The only time we could experience a pure dynamic form of vitality, devoid of content, would be in the earlier phases of life, or in the first milliseconds after a stimulus when the arousal system has already fired, but before the emotions and cognitions have had time to kick in. This too may have a phenomenal existence such as what accompanies a jolt of arousal, ' a something is starting to happen'.

The idea of content free dynamic forms of vitality as phenomenal experiences in infancy is quite plausible. In older people capable of reflexive experience one might only see content free vitality forms as the result of 'dissociation'. But the infant might first have to 'associate' vitality forms with content events.

In practice, dynamic forms of vitality are flexible gestalts that are assembled slightly differently each time they are used in the real world. Each 'feature' has a range of variability in type of movement, time course, force, direction and intention. So that in every particular instance a slightly new gestalt is composed for the immediate context and gives rise to a somewhat unique form of vitality.

Force

Objectively, the force of physical movements is measurable. Subjectively, force is inferred and felt. Movements are experienced as caused and guided by forces. The sense of force within movement arises from how the mind processes dynamic experience from any source, 'real' or imagined. Force is experienced as acting 'behind' or 'within' the event and at its inception. We read in the feeling-perception of force, energy, power to human movement. This is expectable given that we feel the effort and force behind our own movements. It is also due to the mirror neuron system which probably provides a parallel simulation of the experience of our own muscular effort.

This fundamental tendency to experience force within movement appears to be a 'mental primitive' (how the mind evolved to process certain events).

Intentionality

The motives that initiate and guide movement go by many names and related concepts. Psychology, in general, speaks of 'motives' and 'intentions' or volition; cognitive psychology and neurosciences of 'values' that attract; psychoanalysis of 'desires', 'wishes', and 'drives'; ethology of triggering activation or releasing fixed action patterns; and philosophers speak of 'will' or of the related concept of 'aboutness'.

Recent studies attest to the very early appearance of 'proto-intentionality'. In the second trimester of pregnancy, fetuses show a prospective control of movement, a sort of action planning en route so their movements have a 'soft landing' (Zoia *et al.*, 2007; Piontelli, 2008). Neonatal imitation depends on matching a goal state, (Meltzoff and Gopnik, 1993; Kugiumutzakis, 1999; Nagy, 2005). Imaging studies reveal that an 'intention detection center' 'lights up' in infants when they see an intentional movement. Infants will 'imitate' a complete action which they have seen only in uncompleted form without the goal realized. They infer the goal and enact it (Meltzoff, 1995) (see below). These indicate how movement and intentionality are inextricably tied together from very early in life.

There is the phenomenal experience of an intention in the process of unfurling and revealing itself. For instance, when someone raises their hand towards the side of their head, as it moves a viewer cannot know if it will arrive to touch the ear, scratch the head or adjust the glasses. Its path is simply watched to discover its finality – phenomenally it is an 'intention unfolding' experience.

Temporal Contour

Temporal contour is the time profile of a movement as it unrolls. It includes rhythm, tempo, duration, accent, and all the other temporal indices of how something is done. This is readily seen in the time-based arts where dynamic forms of vitality are a fundamental aspect of performance. Dynamic forms of a piece of music are written into the musical score. And beyond that, the difference between a technically adequate performance and a transporting interpretation lies in the unique forms of vitality a great artist can bring to the work and transmit to an audience. The power of dance and cinema lies beyond the story-line and resides in the dynamic experience of the story's enactment. The different forms of art could never collaborate, fuse or create new 'totalities' à la Wagner (Borchmeyer, 2003) without dynamic forms of vitality to act as their common language, their 'esperanto'. Neither categorical emotions nor abstract ideas can do that, and moods are too slow changing. Only forms of vitality can shift within an art form at the time scale of phrases (Stern, 2010).

Vitality

The sense of vitality, of aliveness, arises from the gestalt of movement, force, temporal contour and intentionality. This gestalt is the primary manifestation of being animate, and provides the primary sense of aliveness.

We move all the time, both physically and mentally. If our mind and body were not in constant processes of change when awake, we would not feel alive and vital. Our respirations rise and fall over a cycle repeating every three seconds or so. Our bodies are in almost constant motion: we move our mouth; twitch; touch our face; make small adjustments in head position and orientation; alter facial expression; shift the direction of gaze; adjust the muscular tone of body position.

These go on even when not visible from the outside. Gestures and larger acts unfold in time, They change fluidly once an act has started. We can be conscious of any of this or it can remain in peripheral awareness.

There are at least three events accompanying movement that turn it into a subjective dynamic form of vitality from early in life. First there is proprioception that gives movement a constantly changing representation in the mind. Secondly, prior to a movement, there is a discharge in the motor cortex lasting a hundred or so milliseconds before the movement even starts. These are rarely conscious in the ordinary sense. These discharges launch the movement. They are 'intentions' at the neural level. The relation between the psychological intention and the later executed movement corresponds to what is meant phenomenologically by 'will', or the experience of 'volition' — a powerful element in the sense of vitality. Of course there are also conscious intentions that are realized in action, providing the sense of intentionality and agency as usually meant in psychology. Prior to conscious intentional acts there are often very small, short 'intentional movements' that start at the very beginning of the intended act then stop abruptly with the act uncompleted. These are 'trials', lasting split seconds, of the whole act, (Kendon,1994). These partial acts remain out of consciousness, but they give the phenomenal sense of 'leaning forward', of 'wanting' even without consciousness of the specific goal desired.

And finally, our own mirror neuron systems fire not only with the movements of others, but with our own movements. This may provide a virtual experience in parallel with proprioceptive experience. This adds to the sense of our own vitality as an intending, moving center of activity. And so it is likely to be for infants.

The mirror neuron system permits us to virtually experience the intentions of others as read in their movements. Accordingly, their intentionality and vitality can be experienced by us in large part.

Seeing someone dead is immediately shocking because they do not move, nothing moves, even the almost subliminal vibrations of tonicity stop. We grasp this in a glance with focal and peripheral vision. Without motion we can not read or imagine mental activity, nor force, nor intentionality within. That is how we know there is no vital presence.

Similarly, when a mother goes 'still face' while facing her infant, i.e. not moving her face at all, not even slight expressions, babies, even neonates get upset within seconds (Nagy, 2008). Newborns already have working peripheral vision. Accordingly, stillness is registered no matter where their focal vision is on the face.

The ongoing changes of almost constant movement reignite and maintain our sense of being alive, of 'going on being' à la Winnicott (1971). And if movement did not have a dynamic flow, but was a sequence of discrete steps, we would be digital organisms, whatever that would be like.

Variations in the intensity (force and effort) of the movement, the shape of its temporal contour, and the urgency of its intention give the impression of vigor, zest, and 'life force'.

Dynamic forms of vitality are possibly the main form in which the pre-reflexive infant experiences self and others. It is likely the central axis around which other pre-reflexive and later reflexive organizations form. This highly global way of experiencing persists in all of us, and is crucial in artistic creation and collaboration.

We have in hand, then, a rich repertoire of lived pre-reflexive experiences, each with its own structure. These must somehow find their way into the reflexive domains.

Passage from one Pre-Reflexive System of Organization to another Pre-Reflexive System

Let us first look at the passage of experience staying within the pre-reflexive domain. This may shed light on the later problem of going from pre-reflexive systems to reflexive ones.

Even neonates show a switching from one pre-reflexive organization of experience to another. They can imitate a human model by protruding the tongue (Meltzoff, 1981). Even more surprising, during the first day of life, they can raise the first finger as if pointing up in imitation of a model. To do this they must form a visual representation or trace of the model's finger which is pointing up (or of the protruding tongue). Then, they must transform that into a physical act. This implies a cross-modal transfer from a visual experience to a proprioceptive-kinematic one. (Recall that the infant has no conscious knowledge that he has a face or tongue or fingers.) Many such passages between different modal organizations are known, between vision and touch, audition and vision, etc. This can be passed off as simple 'cross modality' but it involves switching the nature of the experience, in this case from visual to sensori-motor-proprioceptive. But is the switch noticed by the infant? If his major concern is the dynamic experience, in what way does it matter that the form of vitality is carried in the visual or sensori-motor modes. In any event, it would appear that initially the dynamic experience would take precedent over the experience of modality.

A fascinating aspect of this imitation is that sometimes an observer can see the effort of trial and error involved in this passage. For instance, some neonates can slowly get their first finger into the upright pointing position, when imitating. Others move both hands initially, then one, then open up the entire hand so all fingers are pointed straight up, then progressively fold back down all the fingers except the first which is left in the pointing position. It is as if one is watching the soft assembly of the act in slow motion (Nagy, 2008).

We shall see again and again how effortful and stumbling the process of passage between organizations can be, even when the passage is within the same pre-reflexive domain. This will also prove to be the case when passing from pre-reflexive experience to both non-verbal reflexive experience, and to verbal reflexive experience. We are so intrigued by language that we give the passage into language a very special status in almost all respects.

The passages between different pre-reflexive experiences are usually not thought to be accompanied by consciousness, except perhaps for the feelings of the dynamic vitality forms of effortfullness, of 'something starting to happen', of 'intention unfolding' and similar experiences mostly related to emergence and becoming.

One can pass directly from pre-reflexive experience into language. If a pre-reflexive experience does pass directly into language, what could its phenomenal experience be like, beyond an effortful or effortless emergence into language? If effortless, as is so often the case, it would be akin to Merleau-Ponty's 'upsurge of a fresh present' (1962), in the form of the sudden but natural presence of a word or phrase on the scene.

Passage from Pre-Reflexive Experience to Non-Verbal Reflexive Experience

Most often, pre-reflexive experience first passes into the non-verbal reflexive mode where it acquires more structure before going into a verbal reflexive mode. Since so much of pre-reflexive experience passes into language by way of the non-verbal reflexive experience, let us turn to these passages.

To pass from a pre-reflexive experience to the non-verbal reflexive mode, the trace/sketch is taken up by a reflexive process in the non-verbal domain. 'Affect attunement' as seen in the latter part of the first year in the pre-verbal infant provides an excellent example. It is dependent on the capacity for 'secondary intersubjectivity' as described by Trevarten & Hubley (1978) (The simultaneous sharing by two minds of the same mental landscape evoked by a referent.) The key observation is what mothers do when they want to show the baby they understand or share what the baby feels, and how babies respond to such efforts (Stern, 1985). Here is an example.

A ten-month-old girl was seated on the floor facing her mother. She was trying to get a piece of puzzle into its right place. After many failures she finally gets it. She then looks up into her mother's face with delight and 'opens up' her face (her mouth opens, her eyes widen, her eyebrows rise) and then closes her face back down, in a series of changes whose time contour can be described as a smooth arch, a crescendo, high point, decrescendo. At the same time her arms rise and fall at her sides. Mother responded by intoning, 'Yeah' with a time-line that rises and falls as the pitch climbs and then falls, and with it the volume crescendos and decrescendos: ' yeeAAAAaahh'. The mother's prosodic contour matches the child's facial-kinetic contour. They also have the exact same duration (Stern, 1985, p. 140.)

What else could the mother have done to let her daughter know that she understood and shared the baby's excitement and joy of that moment? The mother can't just say, 'Oh! I do know how that feels.' After all, the girl is only ten months old and would not understand. Alternatively, the mother could imitate what the girl did, i.e., open up her own face then close it down in a fairly faithful imitation of what the girl did. But there is a different problem with this. The girl could 'say to herself', 'OK, you know what I did, physically. But how can I be sure that you know what it felt like to do what I did? You could be a mirror, or a Martian. How do I know you even have a mind?' The mother resolves this by doing a selective imitation, an 'affect attunement'. She switches to a different modality (from seen action to heard sound) but she keeps the dynamic features faithfully, i.e. there was a matching of the form of vitality. With that, the act takes on the mother's personal signature. The girl then understands that her mother is not just imitating but that a similar experience is in the mother's own repertoire of experience and is sharable between the two. The match thus becomes a match of internal feeling states via overt behaviors. A transfer between systems of organization has occurred. It is striking that a specific non-visible feeling state is signaled by a specific, non-classical (non Darwinian) behavioral expression (eg. pride, shame, embarrassment, guilt). Some sense of mutual understanding has been established.

There is also 'under-attunement' and 'over-attunement' (Stern, 1985). For example, a child expresses delight in using a toy machine gun found in a friend's house and lets out a yelp of joy. If the mother is not delighted but does not want to squash his enthusiasm entirely, nor censor him in public, she can under-attune. So, if the child's yelp was quite intense and prolonged, she can let out a sound that is considerably lower in intensity and of slightly shorter duration. In other words, she 'purposely' mismatches and sends back to the child a dynamic form of vitality that says, 'I am not as enthusiastic about that machine gun as you are, in fact, I discourage it, but I do understand that you are enthusiastic'. Similarly, 'over-attunement' can encourage as much as 'under-attunement' can discourage.

In such affect attunements there are two possible ways in which a passage from pre-reflexive to non-verbal reflexive can be seen. When the mother said, 'Yeah' she was probably not reflexively conscious of her act. But in most 'over' and 'under attunements' the mother is reflexively conscious, not always of exactly what she did but of the intention to send a message to her child — an evaluation. Mothers comment on this conscious aspect readily. (Among adults, detailed exploration of first person accounts by a second person, can reveal the phenomenal presence of some of these non-verbal reflexive experiences. The 'Micro-Analytic Interview' by a 'second person' on the subject of an adult's first person accounts can do this. It is based on the behavioral micro-analysis applied to mothers and infants [Stern, 2004].)

From the infant's side in the 'Yeah' example, right after the mother says 'Yeah', her daughter looks at her, smiles, then turns to play – indicating that she is satisfied with that maternal response and she can now go on by herself. This seems to require that the immediately previous two events (the child's enthusiasm and the mother's response) are registered and compared. This is tantamount to a reflexive experience.

In this fashion the matching/mismatching of dynamic forms of vitality can shape what the infant does and how he feels about doing it. It is like sculpting his mind from the inside-out. It is a powerful tool in the parent's ongoing socialization of the infant into the family and wider culture. It has another advantage. It is well suited for negotiations. It is not a set of rules. It opens the door to the diplomatic dealings that characterize the compromises about what you can, and not do, and where the real limits are to be set in different contexts. These negotiations are essential for learning some degree of subtleness in the ordinary dealings with others as well as crucial judgments such as evaluating 'sincerity conditions'.

Delayed imitation later in infancy (when secondary intersubjectivity is present but not speech) provides another example: An infant sits across a table from an experimenter. A vase is on the table. The experimenter takes an object and passes his hand above and towards the mouth of the vase but lets the object fall from his hand too soon before he gets it above the mouth of the vase, so it falls to the table. In a second try he lets the object fall too late so it falls to the table but now on the far side of the mouth of the vase. The infant is then sent home. He comes back the next day and they sit across the table with the vase as before, only this time the infant is given the object. He immediately takes the object and makes it fall directly into the vase. (Recall he has never seen the act completed, i.e. the intention realized.) The infant, then, looks up to meet the experimenters eyes, as if to say, 'I got ya'.

In this example, several passages of experience from one organization to another have been accomplished. At minimum, the infant has experienced the act as performed by watching another (not quite) do it; experienced the act as performed by himself; and experienced his performance in the other's eyes.

Most implicit knowledge about 'what-it-is-like-to-be-with-a-specific-other' involves a refiguring and elaborating of pre-reflexive impressions into implicit knowledge of being with the other. In other words in passing from the pre-reflexive to the non-verbal reflexive

To summarize this subsection, even in infancy there are many passages from pre-reflexive to non-verbal reflexive experience while staying within the non-verbal domain. Language is clearly not essential for all passage into reflexivity.

We have yet to consider the more difficult passage from non-verbal reflexive experience into language.

Passage from Non-Verbal Reflexive Experience into Verbal Reflexive Experience (Language)

The passage from non-verbal reflexive to verbal reflexive experience presents new problems. It is generally thought that the structures of non-verbal reflexive experience are impoverished compared to linguistic experience, and that the passage from a simpler organization to a complex one is more difficult. First, it is not so clear that the non-verbal reflexive systems are more simple and impoverished. They are analogic which permits infinitely more graded information than digital systems such as language. As soon as a word replaces a non-verbal experience, much is gained and much is lost.

Secondly, we have seen that that experience can be treated reflexively in the non-verbal domain. Reflexivity, itself, is not the exclusive property of language. Accordingly, it is not likely to be the cause of the difficulty with this passage.

Third, does the intrinsic power and potential of the code belonging to an organization (eg. language) make the process of passage into it a larger leap? For instance, the Arabic number system is intrinsically more powerful with greater potential for extension and new combinations of thinking than the Roman number system. Does that make the passage, itself, from Roman to Arabic more difficult or of a different order? Yes, for some mental operations, no for others.

Finally, might it be that the passage from non-verbal reflexive to verbal reflexive involves an extended and more complex form of second order consciousness.

Before pursuing this issue further it is useful to look in detail at the act of passage between the non-verbal reflexive and the verbal reflexive. We find some of the same characteristics seen in shifting from the pre-reflexive to the non-verbal reflexive domains of experience. In particular one observes the effortful trial and error process of 'soft assembly'. ('Soft assembly' describes the process of putting together the elements of an unpracticed goal oriented action [or idea] so that it is functional, but where there is not only one way to do it. This is most easily seen in first-time actions or at least not highly practiced ones. Development, by its nature, provides multiple examples of this process [Thelen & Smith, 1994]).

Two examples of a passage from the non-verbal reflexive to the verbal reflexive domain of experience are illustrative

Kathrine Nelson (1989) put together a group of us to study the speech of a precocious girl, Emily, who engaged in dialogues and monologues before her second birthday. These were audiotaped and the group studied them for over a year of the girl's life.

Emily's monologues occurred after a 'good night' dialogue with her father, after he left her bedroom for her to go to sleep. She raised the pitch of her voice. These monologues serve many functions such as representing real life experiences, narrative recreation of the world, problem solving, text forming function, a speech genre, a reinforcement of previous dialogue, a construction of self in time. What strikes me at this reading is the effort and difficulty for Emily to get her experiences into language and even harder into a narrative form. She shows a trial and error path similar to that seen for the pre-verbal infants in going from one pre-reflexive organization to another, eg.

finger imitation. The following monologue illustrates this (Nelson, 1989. Episode 1.3 [24;1] p. 65).

Maybe the tow truck come back,

and then tow truck nother car(?) ...

maybe my tand by the tow truck with the (ho-) ...

maybe tow, the tow, tow, (woo-) h-,

go back and then yellow car come (back).

And then leave the blue car.

The it's broken.

Now the (big) tow-tow truck back with the blue car...

And then my tanta get Momor,

and, and maybe Tanta saw the tow truck,

and Mormor.

Maybe this broken my ...

And then we go back to Tanta.

And then we go back Tan- ...

Maybe Daddy come back here, we go back my ...

And then ...

the tow truck come back and tow nother car ...

and then come back tow different kind ... car

But then we,

This go to my house,

And we come back.

And then..different time ...

Somebody come and get ...

The little.

No one with, keep the (whether anyone) like the (with) and put (with)

And come in the house ...

And then the tow truck come back ...

For little car ...

But then ...

FROM PRE-REFLEXIVE TO REFLEXIVE EXPERIENCE 325

She is struggling for ways to make the passage of a lived experience into a verbal-narrative form. The question can always be asked is she having trouble with the putting already known and structured experience into words? After all, she is just now learning a larger vocabulary and has not yet fully mastered narrative form. Or does the problem lie in the lack of structure in her pre-reflexive experience?

This next episode comes from a frequent experience for her, going to the beach. It is a memory, expectation and a bit of world-making (Nelson, 1989. Episode 1.5 [28;0] p.67–68).

We are gonna ...

at the ocean.

Ocean is a little far away.

Baw, baw buh (etc.)

Far away..I think it's ...

Couple blocks ... away.

Maybe it's down, downtown,

And across the ocean,

And down the river,

And maybe it's in,

The hot dogs will be in a fridge,

And the fridge (would) be in the water over by a shore,

And then we would go in,

And get a hot dog and bring it out to the river,

And then sharks go in the river and bite me,

In the ocean,

We go into the ocean,

And ocean be over by ...

I think a couple of blocks away.

But we could be,

And so on

Is the difficulty of passage attributable to a relative lack of structure in the pre-reflexive or non-verbal reflexive experience or to the immaturity of her vocabulary and narrative-making (which we know becomes more fully adult-like only at 4 years), or is it in the act of passage itself, i.e., of coupling these two systems of experience.

Maybe this is a false question since each of these are influencing the others profoundly.

When we observe many forms of spontaneous, non scripted speech we are offered a picture not so different from what is seen in young children at the beginning of this developmental journey.

A closer look at spontaneous, unscripted speech among adults about human interactions is helpful. Most dialogues and trialogues within the family, in couples, among friends and in the talking psychotherapies are of this kind. Recall that speech production requires physical as well as mental movement. It involves voluntary movements of the vocal chords, tongue, mouth, lips, breathing, etc. Movement remains primary. Dynamic forms of vitality remain relevant. That is what makes it human and belonging to the experience-of-human-action.

In unscripted speech which has never been told before, or not been told often, or told each time in different ways depending on the audience, there is something in mind that wants expressing. Let us call this 'something in mind' an image, in the broadest sense of the term or sequence of images. The image can be an idea, a movement, a gesture, an emotion, a dynamic form of vitality, a background feeling, an event. These are initially pre-reflexive or non-verbal reflexive. Now comes the messy work of fashioning spontaneous speech. A task of soft assembly. There is an intention to link the image(s) to words. For almost each phrase, the intention enters into a dynamic dialogue with the speaker's repertoire of pieces of language to find the best fits. This is an 'intention unfolding process' — where intention and language get yoked. Emergent properties form. New linkages are created, tentatively accepted, revised, rejected, reintroduced in a different form and mixed with all the other creative products of an intention unfolding process.

This process, which usually takes split-seconds or seconds, is unpredictable, messy, widely distributed in the body and mind and usually involves conscious and unconscious bodily happenings. This non-linear process is perhaps what makes us most human. It would include how the word search gets performed, with what deliberation or rising excitement, with what burst of enthusiasm or calm when it 'catches' a word. It is a process that can rush forward, hesitate, stop, restart gently, etc. It can express itself in various dynamic forms of vitality. It is quintessentially a process of soft assembly — a continual improvisation to fit found reality.

It is these dynamic qualities that give the impression of an 'inhabited body' — an 'inhabited thought process', that is in action and alive, now. Without this, we would not experience a vital human being behind the words being said.

This verbal processing of implicit material makes it possible for a psychoanalyst and patient on the couch, not even seeing each other face-to-face, to know so much about each other, implicitly, and to share an intersubjective space, akin to a 'second person' knowledge of another.

Also, the process of talking involves another person, a partner in dialogue. The two find their way in a rapidly changing field. The person who is listening has their own shifting vitality dynamics. That is a crucial part of the field. In other words, there was never an exactly specified goal. There were tendencies in search of a finality. And on the way they found a series of evolving goals and intentions constantly updated.

The idea of goal directed movement being soft assembled on the spot to meet the immediate context, may help to ease these problems. The nuances of soft assemblage require that dynamic forms of vitality do the job of fine-tuning to the found context, i.e., the actual interpersonal situation the speaker (or thinker) is in.

One reason for these problems is that we tend to consider events when they are completed and seen retrospectively. From this vantage point it seems reasonable to imagine that a specific initial state somehow found the means to arrive at a predestined end state. However when an event is viewed while it is still ongoing and its assembly still unfinished neither the initiating state not the end state is so clear. We move from an inquiry about intentions — means — goal states to an inquiry about processes of creation — emerging — and becoming. But the reflexive process operates during the happening not just after. The work of the Boston Change Process Study Group (1998–2005) uses these ideas in describing micro-change and macro-change in the psychotherapeutic process. Gendlin has well explored this clinically in another fashion (1996).

Experienced therapists are peripherally aware of many of the above dynamic features of their patient's speech that influence their overall clinical impressions. However, because of the emphasis on word-meaning in talking therapies, the dynamic non-verbal features of speech are less often the central focus of attention.

Nonetheless, they can reveal what is hidden in the words or behind them, such as the degree of authenticity, of hesitation, conflict, difficulty and fear in telling, the amount of excitation or engagement, the distance of the narrative stance from the 'here and now', boredom, deadness, disavowal, the amount of defensive blockage in the passage from mind to speech, and much more. This kind of sensitivity requires sensibilization to dynamic forms of vitality so as to disembed them from the rest of the verbal flow.

Here is an example. If a patient says, 'I've told this story so often that it has become the reality of what happened ... I even sort of believe it... but it isn't what really happened.... What really happened was ...' (Then the patient tells what really happened). The therapist will naturally be interested in what 'really' happened and will explore why the distorted first version was needed. But if the therapist waits and first focuses on the dynamic forms of vitality and the experience of the telling, not its explicit verbal import, he or she can take a different path that might go further, faster, or elsewhere. The therapist could say (if it were true), 'You said that like it finally burst out of prison.' This might lead to the patient telling of the forces that created the revision in the first place.

Or if the patient spoke differently, the therapist might say, 'You said that like you were afraid to bump into the furniture in the dark.' This might evoke the patient's fears of being punished or hurt or humiliated by revealing the real story. In other words the experience of the defenses in the form of vitality dynamics can be evoked well before exploring the conflict leading to the defenses, as understood explicitly. This focus on the dynamics of telling will, in fact, facilitate the exploration of the conflicting content. If that is fruitful the patient will, himself, directly get to why the 'real version' was disguised. In addition the patient will get a first hand experience of how his defenses operate and what the therapeutic relationship can tolerate and contain. In short, the focus is on the dynamic form of how he expressed himself, not the explicit sense of the words.

This clinical approach is yet another, granted indirect, general way to creep up on first person phenomenal accounts.

Finally, in considering the passage into language, the distinction between what is brain and what is mind must be respected. The brain, as interconnecting neural networks, does not mark the passage from non-verbal reflexivity to verbal reflexivity as phenomenally special compared to a shift between other neural organizations, except in the sense that more or different neural networks may be involved.

It is interesting that brain studies show that the language centers are intimately connected to the centers for other brain functions. If one hears the words 'cry', or ' yell', or 'scream', the receptive language areas will, as expected, be activated but they will in turn simultaneously and unexpectedly, activate the sound production areas of the cortex, as if one had actually yelled, etc. Or if one hears the word 'run', 'jump', or 'skip', the appropriate motor centers will be activated along with the receptive language centers. Upon hearing the word one can have the conscious phenomenal experience of an image and a meaning, but remain unaware that their body has been acted upon and been primed to act, virtually. Neural circuitry and phenomenal reality need not line up.

The inexact, messy, trial and error process of soft assembly can be seen in passages between domains of experience be they between the pre-reflexive and non-verbal reflexive or between the non-verbal reflexive and the verbal reflexive The assembly process is most evident when the linkages are first forming but evidence of them persists even after the passage is well practiced. Soft assembly is key.

In summary, what gives the phenomenal specialness to language experience and to the passage into the verbal reflexive mode? The process of the passage into the verbal reflexive domain, in itself, may not be so special. It shares the same messy, trial and error process of soft assembly as do the passages between other domains of experience. The passage process is perhaps not the best candidate for specialness. Alternatively, is there an extension of second order consciousness in the verbal reflexive domain, an enlargement of scope and increase in complexity? Or does the specialness arise from aesthetic and functional considerations (but this is beyond our immediate scope). Nevertheless, one cannot forget that the value given to language is in part chosen by the culture including the scientific climate.

It may prove helpful to isolate out these interdependent but separable elements to advance the inquiry.

We have also tried to call attention to the key role for dynamic forms of vitality in the structuring of pre-reflexive experience and in its passage from one form of experience to another.

We have reached a point where the phenomenological questions have become the most urgent ones. The neurosciences are continuing their productivity and are finding that most of the brain is remarkably multisensory as well as interconnected among functional units, so much so that the functional anatomy of the brain as we have learned it may need to be drastically redrawn. This leaves so many of the more interesting problems of mind and experience outstanding, and up to phenomenology to lead the way.

References

Borchmeyer, D. (2003), *Drama and the World of Richard Wagner* (Princeton, NJ: Princeton University Press).

Boston Change Process Study Group (BCPSG)(2005), 'The "something more than interpretation" revisited: Sloppiness and co-creativity in the psychoanalytic encounter', *J. Am. Psychoanalytic Assoc.*, **53** (3), pp. 693–729.

Boston Change Process Study Group (BCPSG), Stern. D.N., Sander, L.W., Nahum, J.P., Harrison, A.M., Lyons-Ruth, K., Morgan, A.C., Bruschweiler-Stern, N. & Tronick, E.Z. (1998), 'Non-interpretive mechanisms in psychoanalytic therapy: The "something more" than interpretation', *International Journal of Psychoanalysis*, **79**, pp. 903–921.

Damasio, A. (1999), *The Feeling of What Happens* (New York: Harcourt Brace & Co.).

Eitan, Z. & Granot, R.Y, (2006), 'How music moves: Musical parameters and listener's images of motion', *Music Perception*, **23** (3), pp. 221–47.

Gallese, V. (2001), 'The "shared manifold" hypothesis: From mirror neurons to empathy', *J. of Consciousness Studies*, **8** (5–7), 33 – 50.

Gallese, V. & Lakoff, G. (2005), 'The brain's concepts: The role of the sensorymotor system in conceptual knowledge', *Cognitive Neuropsychology*, **21**, pp. 1–25.

Gendlin, E. (1996), *Focusing-Oriented Therapy* (New York: Guilford).

Husserl, E. (1962), *Ideas Pertaining to a Pure Phenomenology and to a Phenomenological Philosophy. First book: General Introduction to Pure Phenomenology*, trans. B. Gibson (New York: Collier. Original Work published in 1913).

Husserl, E. (1964), *The Phenomenology of Internal Time-Consciousness*, trans. J. S. Churchill (Bloomington, IN: Indianana University Press).

Jeannerod, M. & Frak, V. (1999), 'Mental imaging of of motor activity in humans', *Curr. Opin. Neurobiol.*, **9**, pp. 735–39.

Kendon, A. (1994), 'Do gestures communicate? A review', *Research on Language & Social Interaction*, **27**, pp. 175–200.

Kugiumutzakis, G. (1999), 'Genesis and development of early human mimesis to facial and vocal models', In J. Nadel & G. Butterworth (Eds.) *Imitation in Infancy*, pp. 36–59 (Cambridge: Cambridge University Press).

Kurth, E. (1925, 1931 orig./1991), *Selected Writings*, trans. and ed. R.A. Rothfarb (Cambridge: Cambridge University Press).

Lakoff, G. & Johnson, M. (1980), *Metaphors We Live By* (Chicago, IL: University of Chicago Press).

Lakoff, G. & Johnson, M.(1999), *Philosophy in the Flesh: The Embodied Mind and its Challenge to Western Thought* (New York: Basic Books).

Langer, S. (1969–1972), *Mind: An essay on human feeling, Vols. 1–3* (London: Johns Hopkins Press).

MCNeil, D. (2005), *Gesture and Thought* (Chicago, IL: University of Chicago Press).

Meltzoff, A.N. (1988), 'Infant imitation after a 1- week delay: Long-term memory for novel acts and multiple stimuli', *Developmental Psychology*, **24**, pp. 470–76.

Meltzoff, A.N. (1981), 'Imitation, intermodal coordination and representation in early infance', In G. Butterworth, (Ed.) *Infancy and Epistemology*, pp. 85–114 (Brighton: Harvester Press).

Meltzoff, A.N. & Gopnik, A. (1993), 'The role of imitation in understanding persons and developing theories of mind', In S. Baron-Cohen, H. Tager-Fusberg, & D. Cohen (Eds.), *Understanding Other Minds: Perspectives from autism*, pp. 335–66 (Oxford: Oxford University Press).

Merleau-Ponty, M. (1962), *Phenomenology of Perception* (London: Routledge).

Nagy, E. (2005), 'The first dialog: Conversation through imitation with newborn infants', *Behavioral Brain Sciences*, Supplementary Commentary.

Nagy, E. (2008), Personal communication, Dundee, October, 2008.
Nelson, K. (Ed. 1989/2006), *Narratives from the Crib* (Cambridge MA; Harvard University Press).
Panksepp, J. (1998), *Affective Neuroscience, The foundations of human and animal emotions* (Oxford: Oxford University Press).
Petitmengin, C. (1999), 'The intuitive experience', In F.J. Varela and J. Shear (ed.), *The View from Within: First-person approaches to the study of consciousness*, pp. 43–77 (Exeter: Imprint Academic).
Petitmengin, C. (2007), 'Towards the source of thoughts: The gestural and transmodal dimension of lived experience', *Journal of Consciousness Studies*, **14** (3), pp. 54–82.
Piontelli, A. (2007), 'On the onset of fetal behavior', In M. Mancia (Ed.) *Psychoanalysis and Neuroscience*, pp. 391–418 (Amsterdam: Springer Verlag).
Piontelli, A. (2008), Personal communication. Milan, November 2008.
Polanyi, M. (1962), 'Tacit knowing and its bearing on some problems of philosophy', *Reviews of Modern Physics*, **34**, p. 601.
Rizzolatti, G., Fadiga, L., Gallese, V. & Fogassi, L. (1996), 'Premotor cortex and the recignition of motor actions', *Cognitive Brain Research*, **3**, pp. 131–41.
Rizzolotti, G., Fogassi, L. & Gallese, V. (2001), 'Neurophysiological mechanisms underlying the ununderstanding and imitation of action', *Nature Neuroscience Reviews*, **22**, pp. 661–70.
Sheets-Johnstone, M. (1999), *The Primacy of Movement* (Amsterdam / Philadelphia: John Benjamins).
Stern, D.N. (1985), *The Interpersonal World of the Infant* (New York: Basic Books).
Stern, D.N. (1990), *Diary of a Baby* (New York: Basic Books).
Stern, D.N. (2004), *The Present Moment: In psychotherapy and everyday life* (New York: WW. Norton).
Stern, D.N. (2010), *Forms of Vitality: Dynamic experience in psychology, neuroscience and the arts* (Oxford University Press), In press.
Thelen, E. & Smith, L.B. (1994), *A Dynamic Systems Approach to the Development of Cognition and Action* (Cambridge MA: MIT Press).
Thevarthen, C. & Hubley, P. (1978), 'Secondary intersubjectivity: confidence, confiding and acts of meaning in the first year', In A. Lock (Ed.) *Action, Gesture and Symbol: The emergence of language* (London: Academic Press).
Varela, F.J. and Shear, J. (Ed. 1999), *The View from Within. First-person approaches to the study of consciousness* (Exeter: Imprint Academic).
Winnicott, D.W. (1971), *Play and Reality* (London: Tavistock/Routledge Publication).
Zoia. S., Blason, L., D'Ottavio, G., Bulgheroni, M., Pezzette, Scabar, A. & Castiello, U. (2007), 'Evidence of early development of action planning in the human foetus: a kinematic study', *Exp. Brain Res.*, **176**, pp. 217–26.

Eugene Gendlin

What First and Third Person Processes Really Are

Abstract: *'Implicit understanding' is much wider than what we can attend to at one time, and it is in some respects more precise. Examples are examined. What is implicit functions in certain characteristic ways. Some of these are defined. They explain how new concepts come to us in a bodily process that goes beyond previous logic but takes implicit account of it, without new logical steps.*

All concepts can be considered 'explications' of implicit body-environment interaction. 'Explication' provides an overall model within which the objectivity of logical concepts can be explained and preserved.

Section III concerns new kinds of operational research. Section IV shows how a theory of logically connected terms can always be formulated from something known implicitly. Section V shows how the explication model affects the theory of language.

Keywords

Body, body knowledge, implicit, consciousness, space, motion, theory construction, concept formation, proprioceptive, kinaesthetic, focusing.

I. Implicit Understanding

This article will present a different view of 'first person process', not what most of its proponents and objectors think it is. The new view will also enable us to understand the third person perspective differently.

First person process involves something I call 'implicit understanding' (IU). Among many roles, implicit understanding functions in the coming of new concepts. How new concepts come will show us a lot about first person process.

I begin with the question: How do we generate new concepts? How do they come? Scientists and philosophers don't say much about how their concepts came. We are told why the new concept is better, but hardly ever how it came. Someone might say, 'It came to me in the shower.'

The concepts of science change every few years and become more numerous and complex. It is well known that the new ones are not logically deducible from the old ones. But the existing concepts can only explain what follows logically from them. Novelty cannot be denied but it seems inexplicable. We have no logical account across the changing concepts of science.

To study the role played by *implicit understanding* in the coming of new concepts will not undermine the concepts we already have. Those concepts work *explicitly*, with logical implications. Logic is *their own* power for precise consequences. To use their power we must let them work as if they were alone, without us. Logical inference requires that we don't let anything upset the concepts. For example, while calculating our bank account we don't double one deposit because it came from a special source. All our technology depends on logical inference. Seven billion of us couldn't all live on the planet without it. To undermine logic and explicit concepts is not sensible.

Of course we know that we operate the concepts. How they work 'alone' is something we let them do. This isn't very puzzling. Whatever else concepts are, they are tools. For example, a screwdriver must be allowed to keep its own narrow head, and to engage the screw with it. We are holding it, of course, but the screwdriver's own pattern turns the screw. Obviously, more complex machines produce their own results. Concepts similarly have *their own* logical inferences, quite apart from what is implicitly involved in the coming and having of concepts.

We keep the system of existing concepts inviolate and separate. Then we can also have a second system in which we study how something implicit works in the coming of new concepts. We will be concerned throughout with the necessary separation, contrast, and relationship between the system of explicitly formed concepts and our second system about how something functions implicitly. Far from being in conflict, this article will show that if the two systems stay separate, they expand each other reciprocally.

Let me cite some examples of 'implicit understanding' (IU):

- From just a few words we can grasp a complex situation. Someone reports: 'Jim said no.' The single statement of a single fact brings a new understanding of the whole situation. The single occurrence is not just itself; it is also the change in our implicit understanding.

- In the opening scene of Ibsen's *Hedda Gabler* a man comes to deliver a telegram. From how she treats him we suddenly understand the kind of person she is.

- The coming of a new thought can also reorganize a situation. 'Oh, he's afraid of George!' we think, and immediately a great deal has changed. We would like to understand how such a new thought can come. Right here I am only pointing out the relationship between the occurring *one* and the implicit *many*.

- One sensation can also change our understanding of the whole situation, for example one smell: ('Oh!...'). Laid out in words it might be 'Oh! That's the sauce burning! I left it on the stove when I went to answer the phone, and I don't have more stuff to make the sauce again, and there isn't time to go to the store, and ...' Only the 'Oh!...' has actually occurred, but the '...' includes much more: who is invited for dinner, and why, and what sort of reactions they are likely to have, and many past events with them, and what could still be cooked, and much else. All of that is implicit and understood in one 'Oh!...' How can so much be implicit in one syllable?

What is implicitly understood is much more than we could separate out one by one. We saw that one event can change the implicit many. Now I add: the changed many will change the next event, what we actually say or do next. So the one–many relation is really a one–many–one relation. The one occurring event can change what functions implicitly, and that can change the next event — which again changes the many. It is a 'process': *implying–occurring–implying*.

The many are not thought separately. They change implicitly without ever having formed. Changing without ever forming is a hallmark of implicit functioning, as we will see.

We can always say some of the many, if we are asked. This is already being studied and can reveal a lot to the researcher about what was actually happening at any one moment. The 'describing' is itself a behaviour with many observable variances. Brief references to IU enable one to say more and more. There is hardly an end to what can be said just to 'describe' one moment. About an hour's worth is typical (see Petitmengin, 2009, this volume).

But usually we move on. The implicit understanding (IU) implies the next saying or doing, the occurring of which will change the implicit understanding so that it implies a further next saying or doing. We can study that process as well.

Usually we move on smoothly, but sometimes we cannot say what the IU implies. Then we have a problem; it might be practical or theoretical. It might be obvious ('How can I make a good dinner without a sauce?') or subtle ('This tastes a little funny. What does it need?'). A theoretical problem may also be obvious ('How do new concepts come?') or subtle ('I don't know what is wrong with this explanation, but something is.').

Let us observe what we do when we try to solve a problem. We use not only statements. *We think with something implicit as well.* We state a problem in words as far as we can. Many things feed into the problem. We can repeat some of what we know, but we are just stuck if we have nothing but statements and an empty blank. To think further, we must attend to something implicit. We refer to it in shorthand by calling it 'this' or 'this but also that ...'. We hold on to the spot where we sense the problem: the spot is 'this', but also 'that' and the dots. The '...' is where we can hope for new thoughts, where they could come.

A great gamut of things functions implicitly at such an *edge*: much common knowledge, our own special knowledge, everything we have read, heard, why we think it's important, and much else. We refer directly to 'all that'. It is an implicit understanding (IU). When there is a problem, we also 'understand' that we don't understand some of it, although it is all one situation. It is important and remarkable that we sense this 'edge' of our IU where further thoughts are implied.

If we look for the sensed quality of the edge, it can become something bodily-sensed and palpable, a 'this' or an 'it' that we 'have a hold of'. I call that a '*felt sense*'. Or, we can refer to the IU just in passing. But most of the time we don't refer to our IU at all. We go from event to event, from concept to concept, from what we can say to what we can say, or from one action to the next.

This is a range of very different kinds of talking and thinking. There are observable marks and many well-replicated studies of this range: palpable direct reference to IU, touching IU only in passing, no direct contact with IU. There are many correlations with the differences it makes (see Hendricks, 2009, this volume). Implicit functioning is quite open to research.

There is always IU, although there is no 'it' when we don't refer to it. What we do is always implicitly determined by IU. We understand implicitly what we are doing, and what is happening. If the ever-present IU disappeared, we would not understand our surroundings; suddenly we would not know what we are doing and how we came to this moment. The IU is always there, but direct reference changes it. Then the next events and the ensuing process come differently.

If we refer directly so that a palpable 'it' comes, and if we refer to it again and again for a minute or two, some new aspects may emerge, for example: 'Oh, it has something to do with how it relates to that other thing.' That small step is felt as a distinct advance, and can lead to a further step, for example: 'Oh, it's not so much that other thing, it's more this third thing.' The contents may contradict, but the change made by each step enables the coming of the next. Direct reference changes the implicit many, and then each step changes them further. So these hard-won new statements differ from the many which we can always easily say (for example, the many that were implicit in 'Oh!...').

The aspects we state from IU were not separate units before we separated them out. We could never separate them all, even if there were a finite 'all'. But there cannot be. In implicit understanding there is no all. The implicit many are not a finite number. They have no separate identity.

Let us examine 'separate identity':

What has identity is 'self-identical'

Once we separate something out, it has its own identity. It becomes self-identical. It is a unit. I say it functions 'as itself'. But it was not like that before being separated out. When the many are only implicit, they are not units located each in its own position in time.

The contrast is sharp: something self-identical has identity conditions and occurs in its own time location. It is a unit. But before we separate some of them out, they don't exist separately. Below we will see how they do function.

Existence includes the implicit

With so much happening implicitly, of course we cannot deny that the implicit exists. Existence includes not just single events and self-identical units, but also what functions implicitly.

It was long held that what exists must be self-identical. Since self-identicals have space and time locations, it was assumed that only what fills space and time can exist. I will argue that what exists is not only in the kind of space and time in which things are self-identical units. There are other kinds of space and time.[1] The model of self-identical units is not an all-encompassing way to understand everything.

To exclude the implicit from existence and from science has been a gigantic omission. Currently this is already being remedied.[2]

Implicit understanding is a crossing

The usual concepts bring the unit model. They make everything seem to consist of self-identical units. With the usual concepts we can only say how the implicit does *not* function. Then it seems that the implicit cannot be studied.

In my larger work I have formulated many characteristics of implicit functioning, more than I can take up in an article. Here I am only trying to show that we can have an explication system about concept-making and implicit functioning. But I must discuss two characteristics:

We saw that we understand many together. Each thing which we could separate is already affected by the others that are already affected by it. This is an odd pattern, more intricate than the usual kind of 'many'. It is also more intricate than the usual kind of 'one'. Let us allow this more intricate pattern to stand. I name it 'a crossing'. Rather than being side by side, each is a modification of the already-modified others. They are one understanding (IU) because of the crossing. Implicit understanding is a crossing. That is how they are able to

---

[1] Time can be viewed as within happening, and generated by it. Happening need not be within pre-given time locations. I will discuss this further below. For a full treatment see *A Process Model*, chap. I-B (Gendlin, 1981/1997).

[2] Gallagher (2006) establishes a term ('prenoetic') that refers to the implicit. He writes: 'The *prenoetic* function of the body schema . . . [is] *ordered according to* the intention of the actor rather than in terms of muscles or neuronal signals. . . (p. 38). 'When in the context of a game I jump to catch a ball, that action cannot be fully explained by the physiological activity of my body. The pragmatic concern of playing the game . . . even the rules of the game . . . may define how I jump. . .' (pp. 142–43). '[T]he schematic adjustments . . . do *not appear as explicit parts* of the perceptual meaning, although *implicitly* they help to structure such meaning. (p. 141) '[This] is not itself a perception of . . . an object; for if it were, it would require . . . a spatial frame of reference . . . [It is a] non-perspectival awareness' (pp. 137–38) [my emphasis].

With just one term that refers to implicit functioning ('prenoetic'), Gallagher has empowered something everyone has always known to become a source for new concepts.

imply *one* actual next event. Because they are a crossing, they can change all at once, and without forming separately.[3]

'Crossing' (or something that functions like crossing) is a necessary concept for understanding the implicit, as we will further see.

Now a second all-important characteristic of implicit functioning: the IU retains the single events (perceptions, cognitions) after they have occurred. They don't just disappear. Their effects are included in the IU from then on. Cognitions bring their logical implications along with them when they become implicit in the IU. When they become implicit they actually have more effects than when they were self-identical. Now their inferences cross with everything else we understand implicitly, and participate in a much larger result. In a crossing, if more inferences participate, *more* novelty can result, because the inference from each generates precise new effects in the many others.

We often observe this bodily novelty. Dreyfus (1992) points out that computers cannot recognize new language formations (for example, new metaphors). People come up with new phrases. People can understand them but they stymie the computers. Computers use only the already-existing forms.

Dreyfus cites research showing that chess masters make superior new moves without deliberating, even when playing against quite good players. Many other examples can be cited. For example, musical improvisation is often better and more intricate than what one can deliberately construct. Our bodies can implicitly employ our knowledge in new formations that don't consist only of already-existing forms.

With our characteristics of implicit functioning we can now understand how the body does this. The many old moves that the master knows function implicitly in the coming of a new move. Their implicit functioning includes the inferences from each possible move, as well as the logical consequences many steps ahead for both players. Thinking ahead to the consequences of each move takes the average chess player so much time to deliberate. For the master, implicit functioning is inference-inclusive. In the coming of the new move, the many moves and their inferences are 'taken account of' without ever occurring separately. Therefore the chess master doesn't deliberate.

---

[3] Philosophy's 'one' was always known to include the many, but those were its 'particular' instances. However, we now see a 'one' which includes a very different 'many' which function implicitly. Their implying of one next event is a future in the present. Implying is part of every occurring and has no separate time-position. This is a more intricate model of time (see *A Process Model*, chapter IV-B).

The coming of a new move is not logical, but it is certainly not *not-logical* either, since it takes account of the logical implications. It consists *neither* of the same moves *nor* is it something simply different.[4] Our familiar concepts can say this only as two denials. Let us take this more intricate pattern itself with us. I say that all the implications are 'carried forward' in the new occurring.

From the master's implicit understanding of the situation, the stupid moves don't come to mind for consideration. A few possible moves might come, but not the many possible ones. Similarly, Churchill said about Marlborough that a great military commander understands a complex situation immediately, while others understand it only after the battle.

At any stage of knowledge there are many stupid things that would never occur to any of us. We don't deliberate about sitting down on a wet bench, or about taking a picture into the sun. The ever-present IU is the bodily knowing. In much of life, especially our own fields, we may be confident of handling the next situation. We know that if there is a problem, the new moves will come.

But what if nothing comes? What if our bodily knowledge is enough so no stupid moves come, but nothing else comes either? Then we need direct reference to the IU. I say more about direct reference below.

Since the body implies the next move, the word 'body' changes its meaning

What functions implicitly is the body. We were taught that we understand things just with the brain, but brains only work through the whole body. In *A Process Model* (1981/1997) I have written at length about this. Organisms encounter the environment not only with brains and perception. *All living organisms concretely are environmental interactions* (an odd phrase). Their very stuff is environmental, and they imply their next moves in the environment long before some organisms develop perception and brains.

Since we understand and think with the body, the meaning of the word 'body' is changing. No longer does 'body' mean just the chemicals that are left when we die. The body is not only what is defined in physiology (or what used to be so defined). Now 'the body' means the living body that functions implicitly, and behaves with perception and IU.

---

[4] Implicit functioning goes beyond the ancient pair: 'the same and the different'.

The body's functioning seems much wider than IU. For example, toenail growth does not seem part of IU. But there is not one distinct line between the body's implicit functioning and implicit understanding.[5]

The word 'consciousness' is also changing

IU is an implicit consciousness. We live always in implicit consciousness. The word 'consciousness' has long been considered merely as the content of attention. But attention is very narrow. *Consciousness is vastly wider than attention.* We could never attend to each thing of which we are implicitly conscious.

Consciousness is not a separate 'reflection'. We humans can, of course, 'reflect' on behaviour and perception after they happen, but consciousness is not that kind of separate reflection. *Consciousness arises in behaviour formation and is present in all animals.*[6]

We are definitely not unconscious of our IU. If it suddenly disappeared we would be horribly disoriented. We would suddenly not know what we're doing or how we came here. So the word 'consciousness' greatly expands its meaning here.[7]

Our two systems are clear. We use our existing concepts with their explicit logic, and we also develop an explication system in which we study the process of implying–occurring–implying, how all concepts are explications from implicit functioning, and how it is possible to generate something new, including new concepts.

---

[5] Once we separate a process (and specify it with our instruments and concepts), it may seem not to be in IU. But *in the body* the processes are not simply separate. They occur separately in some ways during some phases, and are one interaffecting process in other ways during other phases. There is not one line. Psychosomatic medicine also shows that behaviour and thought involve one implicitly multiple body process.

[6] Behaviour-formation is felt; it is inherently conscious. Perception and the bodily feel of the perception is part of how behaviour forms. Behaviour elicits and consists of environmental carrying forward of the body process. Animals feel their doings. Rather than saying that we are 'conscious of' behaviour, we should say that the formation of behaviour is what generates consciousness.

[7] Other words also change: the IU is often called the 'background', so named from the visual experience of 'a figure and the background around it'. Even my term 'edge' invokes that notion. But 'background' has meant something undifferentiated, lacking in figures. The implicit understanding contains a great many 'figures'. The IU is very precise and governs what we say and do next. When we speak, the implicit is what we centrally mean (for example, we centrally mean the sauce burning and all that this involves; we don't centrally mean just 'Oh!'). Now the word 'background' changes to mean something precise, and central.

The words 'proprioceptive' or 'kinaesthetic' also change. 'Proprioceptive' has meant sensing one's muscles; 'kinaesthetic' meant sensing one's motion. The bodily way in which we can find our IU is similar to how we find our muscles and movements. Therefore both words have been confusingly used to name the IU, since there was no word for IU. It seems hard to believe that there has not been a word for it!

II. Deriving the 'External' World

I will now try to show that the distinction between external and internal is not a given. I will derive it. This will also show how third and first person originate.

First I will give some examples of direct reference and carrying forward. Then I will argue that bodily knowledge is environmental interaction, and that this is prior to the distinction between external and internal.

As we saw in the chess example, the IU is the reason why the many stupid thoughts don't come. So the IU functions in the 'nothing comes'. The fact that nothing comes is an achievement. But if nothing comes, we need direct reference to get a palpable sense of the problem. Once we have that sense, then small steps of carrying forward come from it, and eventually a large step. The palpable sense (the 'felt sense', a 'direct referent') comes a few seconds or a minute *after* we refer to it while it is still not there. This is an odd kind of referring, but it is easy when we become familiar with it.

There are occasions when everyone has a felt sense. For example, when someone did not understand what we said, we rephrase it. We do that by referring directly to what we meant ('Let me see, what was I trying to say?'). We separate 'it' from the words we have just used. From separating, alternative words come. Let us notice that they come from the separation. We will see this again as we proceed. The separation is the effect of referring directly to the implicit as such.

Another such occasion is when we have forgotten what we were about to say. That can happen, for example, when we wait while others are speaking. By the time they stop and turn to us, we may find that we have 'lost hold of' what we were going to say. The readiness to say it was a cluster of implicit statements that had never actually formed. We never had it in words. Now we search for 'it', to get it back ('What was I going to say?'). We refer directly to our bodily sense of it, so that it can return, and words can come from it.

Sometimes something palpable comes of its own accord. For example: suppose you have an oddly gnawing feeling. Then you realize it's something that you were supposed to do today — it's now Monday afternoon — what was it ...? You don't know, but what it was *is* there, in that gnawing body-tension. You think of many things you ought to have done today, perhaps very necessary things, but no. None of them are 'it'. *How do you know that they are not what you forgot?* The gnawing knows. It won't release. You burrow into this gnawing. Then suddenly — you remember: Yes, someone was waiting for you for lunch. Too late now! *This might make you quite tense. But what about the gnawing? That particular tension has eased.* Now the '...' no longer hangs there. Why not? Because the one next thing which the gnawing implied has now occurred (not the original lunch, of course, but this remembering, now). This occurring has carried your whole body forward. You can tell that this now is what you were going to do, and not those other necessary things.[8]

The same kind of carrying forward process can come with quite new things, not only with things we had and lost. When we have the sense of a problem, we can tell when seemingly right and relevant thoughts fail to carry it forward, whereas some little minor step does (for example: 'Oh, it's more like that other thing').

How is it possible for the body to 'know' what we cannot yet think? Why does the '...' hang there until we get it right, as if it knows what we don't know. *What is bodily knowledge?*

The concrete body is environmental interaction

The body, also behaviour, and then also cognition, *is* body-environment interaction. The whole body consists of environmental events. And every cell *is* an interaction with its local environment in the body and in the whole body's environment. The body is environmental interaction through and through.

Body process is a carrying forward by the environment, and it always implies further environmental events. So the body is concretely ongoing 'knowledge' of the environment, not first as representation but first as interaction. The meaning of the word 'knowledge' changes to include concretely ongoing (bodily-implicit) knowledge.

All organisms *are* environmental interactions, but animals *are and have a sense-of* the environment. The body process which *is* always environment interaction develops a field *of objects* (and behaviour possibilities with objects).[9]

The body implies behaviour space

Animal bodies perceive objects with which they have behaviour possibilities (what Gibson [1966] called 'affordances'). *The objects are spread out side by side, but the possible behaviours are not spread out side by side.* Rather, any one behaviour changes how a great many

---

[8] There may always be still further steps: You may suddenly realize you forgot that the person cancelled the appointment last week. Remembering is always a present process which we can study, not only the repetition of something recorded. I am pointing to the pattern I call 'carrying forward' which characterizes all process.

[9] See *A Process Model*, chapter VI, where the 'of objects' is derived.

other possibilities can be enacted. For example, if we throw an object to the other side of the room, we can no longer take it there and lay it down. If we are already taking it, we can stop and throw it, but it will be a shorter throw. If we turn and go to the telephone, we will be too far to throw it at all. Each possible behaviour is implicitly also the changes it would make in the other possibilities. This crossing of implicit (not occurring) sequences has the characteristics of implicit functioning which we saw above.

A crossed cluster of behaviour possibilities is implicitly part of every object and every single behaviour. *Behaviour possibilities constitute the 'space' we perceive, and into which we behave.* The perception of behaviour possibilities does not consist of separate colours, separate sounds and smells ('sense data'). The sense-modalities are not yet separated, as I will show.

Humans have behaviour space as all animals do, but humans can also do more: In a further and different development, the human body implies not only behaviour but also cognitions. Speaking and thinking is a kind of body–environment interaction.

Human bodies imply patterns *as patterns*

Humans have the capacity to perceive patterns not as things but *just as patterns*. For example, speech consists of just sound patterns. We can see visual patterns as just visual, apart from what we hear or touch. We can perceive a pictured cat and also perceive that it is only a visual pattern on a piece of cardboard. Dogs cannot do both; they will either push the cardboard around, or growl at the cat. The dog sees patterns but not as patterns, only as the thing with which it behaves.

Animal perception is only 'of' objects. The human perception *of* separable patterns *of* objects involves a doubled 'of', an essentially human development.[10]

What we can do with patterns (including speech) becomes part of the human behaviour context. But the body implies its objects in all five unseparated senses. The analysis in terms of separate organs must not make us miss the fact that objects are implied by the body in all its sense-modalities. We see the cat on the chair as a cat we could pet, not as a picture. The analysis only in terms of sense-data is mistaken.

---

[10] See *A Process Model*, chapter VII-A for the derivation of the doubled 'of' in human pattern responding.

Sense-intakes are incorporated into the five-sense objects which the body already implies.[11]

The priority of behaviour space

The bodily-implied space of behaviour possibilities is clearly always prior in animals and humans. Why do we tend to assume that the divided sense-modalities are prior? It is because of the explanation in terms of separate organs. Should we not accept the explanation? Of course we accept it. But we can find a way to consider it within a wider model, rather than assuming it as the only view. This wider model will also explain a lot that the analysis in terms of separate senses doesn't explain.

For example, considered in the wider system we see not just colours but the chairs and our friend's typed papers stacked on one of them. And not just the chairs and the papers, rather we see that we can't sit down in this chair unless we first remove the papers (which might disturb them, and where would we put them?) whereas we could sit down in the other chair if we first turn it to face into the room. We always perceive the situation into which our behaviour forms. The perception of a situation cannot possibly be constructed only out of colours and sounds.

If we assume that we see and hear only separate sensations, then the meaning of 'perception' becomes narrow. Environmental interaction seems to be just the organ-intake. The behaviour possibilities are considered 'interpretations' added to the organ-intakes. The essential interactive contribution by living organisms — the implying and carrying forward — seems merely subjective, merely added on, not perceived. We seem not to perceive the space of possibilities in which we act.

For example, consider an animal running away from a predator. If it has gotten far enough away, the current view holds that the predator behind it is not perceived. So we have to say that the predator is now being 'imagined', or 'remembered', something internal because not perceived by a sense organ. But I argue that isolating the organ-intake introduces a secondary (although valid) distinction. *The predator is*

---

[11] See *A Process Model*, where this has been carefully derived. Although we can prove that purely visual geometric triangles excite butterflies more than the irregular triangles of a sexual partner, the butterfly's body does not imply visual triangles, only another butterfly — in all five senses. Even if only visual perceptions are coming in at the moment, the body implies behaviour possibilities *with the thing*. Behaviours are bodily implied, and can form even if just one sense is now coming in. Then, if another sense becomes active, its input joins the ongoing behaviour formation. This further explains the 'intermodality' Gallagher (2006) has very rightly presented.

obviously still in the perceived space of behaviour possibilities. The animal would not, but could, turn and go toward the predator. It runs away from something in the perceived space in which its behaviour forms. While the animal runs, every tree whizzing by is perceived as distancing the predator. The trees and the running occur in the perceived space of behaviour possibilities which includes the predator.

Similarly, it is assumed that we don't perceive the space behind us when there is no organ-intake from the rear. But I argue that what is behind us is part of the *presently perceived* behaviour space in which we act. We perceive where we could now turn around. We would be quite startled if we suddenly perceived an absence back there, an abyss of nothingness. *The space behind us is always part of our perceived space, the space into which our behaviour forms.*

We need to understand more clearly why the concept of 'perception' has been narrowed so that the space of behaviour possibilities seems unperceived. What would be involved in claiming that perception of behaviour space is and always remains prior and more encompassing? Why does it seem to disappear? The analysis in terms of organs and parts denies behaviour space and replaces it with the ordinary space we are accustomed to assume. That 'space' doesn't contain behaviour possibilities; it is empty except where things fill it. *How does that empty space arise? The answer to this question will let us assign the proper role to both spaces.*

The space of behaviour possibilities is perceived in first person process. The third person perspective is analysis in empty space. If we can trace the empty space to its source, we will be able to determine the priority.

Moving patterns generate empty space

Humans can move just a pattern from one thing to another and another. We take a pattern from a thing that has it, and move it to cardboard, wood or steel. Human making is moving patterns. This is how we make our wonderful machines. We make new things by moving patterns. We are *homo faber.*

When a pattern is moved from one thing onto another, the pattern ignores all the characteristics of the thing that had the pattern, as well as all the characteristics of the thing onto which we moved it. It is the *same* pattern in both places, regardless of what else the things may be. When a pattern is moved, nothing changes but its location. *Moving patterns generate a space of locations (points). As far as the moving patterns are concerned, space is empty.* Things seem to be located in an emptiness around them.

The moving patterns create the concept of 'motion', not behaviour, not action, just motion. *Motion is only a change in locations, from one point to another point. Mere motion is first created when humans move patterns to make things.* Then mere motion comes to seem basic. But behaviour is prior to motion by billions of years. We make wonderful things by considering things in motion-space. The only way we can be misled is if we explain the body, behaviour, and perception in no other way than within the empty motion-space.

Motion-space separates itself, and separates everything else from itself

If behaviour is viewed as motion,[12] the motion separates itself from the rest of behaviour. What it cuts away from itself seems unobservable. The behaviour space disappears and is replaced by two new segments, one observable and one unobservable. Both are new products made by the way motion splits them. Now the environment seems to be something 'external'. The rest has to be considered 'internal'.

The implying of behaviour comes to seem not to be environmental interaction. Rather it seems to be merely something inside an externally-observed body. *We have derived the external and the internal.*

Motion-space splits body from 'mind'

The leftovers from the externalized body become 'the mind'. The 'mind' seems hidden, 'internal.' But we can derive this split from the empty space made by moving patterns.

We need not uncritically assume the external and the internal as two givens. They are both products from the human activity of making things. The activity of making *produces* external and internal spaces; making is not itself within external or internal space.

Of course we don't deny the externally-observed body, medicine, organic chemistry, and neurology. We need only to recognize that behaviour space is prior. *Behaviour space does not happen within 'external' motion-space. The analysis in 'external' motion-space develops within behaviour space.*

---

[12] There are current proposals for a 'sensorimotor coupling'. Current researchers are looking for a tie between perception and motion, not between perception and behaviour. But living things never just change location; there is always more involved and perceived in behaviour (O'Regan & Noë, 2001).

We design the machines and their parts in the empty motion-space of moving patterns, but we build the machines in behaviour space. And behaviour space is also where we test what we have built. There is no empirical testing of concepts. We only test operations. We operate machines which were designed in the concepts of motion-space. We turn the machines on and let them operate directly in environmental interaction. That is why the results can differ from what we logically inferred from the concepts alone.

In modern quantum physics, for more than a century, the empty space of motion-locations has not been the conceptual map. But empty location space continues to be assumed in all the other sciences.

There is much puzzlement over the fact that physics has a different conceptual map than the other sciences. But in an explication model the conflicting conceptual systems pose no problem. We don't assume that there has to be only one, since conceptual systems do not represent nature; they are explications within the body–environment interaction.

The objectivity of our concepts

Elsewhere I have shown that our concepts have a kind of objectivity which is still largely misunderstood. No loss of objectivity results from knowing that nature is an implicit intricacy, not a system of self-identical units that could be represented by one conceptual system.[13]

Our concepts are truly the patterns *of things*, because the things reveal their patterns on our patterns. Seen through our patterns, the things cast their profile — *their* patterns on ours. That is why our analyses are really about the things, even though on our patterns.

Two different patterns can both have that objectivity. Conflicting systems don't leave us in limbo. Different patterns bring different results, but always more data from the direct environmental interaction than could ever follow from the conceptual patterns alone.

Since it was not understood that operations are environmental interaction, it was for a long time the great puzzle of Western philosophy, why nature upholds our concepts. Malebranche said that thought and nature are like two wound-up clocks that show the same time (no interaction between them). The current assumption of 'correspondence' and 'representation' is not very different. This epistemology has been endlessly criticized, but there has been no alternative. Now we are developing an alternative model.

---

[13] This is discussed at more length in my 1997 paper 'The responsive order'.

People have long felt they had to assume that nature consists of the unit parts science has made — this year's version. Supposedly our representations approach ever closer to nature's one set of unit parts; we were just wrong last year. But we were not wrong. We would still obtain the result we predicted last year, if we performed the old operations with the old equipment. But this year we can build and do more, and predict the outcomes of more complex operations and concepts.[14]

The explication model explains why the computers we design really work, and the airplanes really fly. *The results of analysis are not 'only' constructions*. The Postmodernists were wrong to deny the objectivity of scientific concepts (especially when they wrote the denial on computers, and took airplanes to conventions to say it). Their real contribution was destroying the representational assumption. But since they saw no alternative, they glorified 'limbo'. We see exactly how logic builds the world further, and how logical consequences add to implicit understanding. We see why our two systems must be kept apart, and also how they relate.

It does not take away from the objectivity of concepts that they came from first-person process, from implying–occurring–implying. On the contrary, we can only explain their objectivity within the explication system we are developing. The unit concepts cannot supply the overall model of nature. We need not only unit concepts, but also what I call 'process concepts', some of them directly about implying–occurring–implying, many more about various kinds of organismic events. In the next section we will consider how process concepts enable new kinds of research.

The first person process is not a 'perspective'

First person process has been widely misunderstood as being inside an externally-observed body.[15] I have tried to show that first person process is bodily-implied environment interaction. Our conceptual systems are explications developed from within environmental interaction, and then tested in it.

In the usual view there is an unbridgeable gap between first and third person 'perspectives'. But only the third person is a *perspective*, a view (the 'view from nowhere', the observed without the observer).

---

[14] See Robert Crease's 'Interview with Feynman,' cited in his article 'Philosophy of science' (1997). See also his *The Play of Nature* (1993). Scientists play in the lab till they do something that has some regular result. 'If we do x we get y' creates an 'it'. Then attributes 'belong to it'.

[15] Along these lines, phenomenology is often misunderstood as if it were limited to the 'inside' of a person in a little corner of the encompassing externalized world.

The word 'perspective' assumes that the environment is something merely viewed, not interacted with and behaved in. First person process is not a perspective.

If first person process is understood *from first person process*, we can explicate how it is bodily, implicitly conscious, far exceeding the objects of attention (of viewing), always an implicit understanding, needing no added observer.

Everyone is a first person process. IU is used by everyone all the time, but certain procedures are necessary to refer to it directly and to use it systematically. They are discussed in the next Section. Then Section IV concerns working in a theoretical or research field when we sense a new concept which cannot be formulated in the current terms of that field.

III. Training and New Territories

Training

With training, people become able to go from no direct reference at all, to reference just in passing, to palpable direct reference. This range is measurable by characteristic modes of language. What people can tell us with training is not what was there before. Direct reference carries the IU forward. But now we can study this 'carrying forward' itself. At first most people don't report much of what happens. We don't need to trust what the reports are *about*. Talking is not only about something; talking is behaviour and can be studied.

In any kind of research, if we ask subjects to describe what happened when we administered a measure, we may be shocked. We may discover totally unsuspected variables. Then we can measure those directly. *Measurable indices can be found for any experience, however 'internal' it might seem. External and internal are not actually divided.*

Researchers also need to refer directly to their own IU. Administering a measure to oneself can quickly reveal what it really measures. This is needed to choose a measure. For example, if one hypothesizes that the variable one is studying is affected by anxiety, just choosing any measure of 'anxiety' isn't sufficient. Without taking the measure oneself, one cannot find out if it taps *the kind* of 'anxiety' that would have the effect one predicts. Very different variables are called 'anxiety'.

There is a tendency just to assume that a unit event corresponds to one's concept. But assuming it isn't enough. One needs independent indices of what the measure makes happen.

It is often assumed that operational variables must come only from 'external' observations. But by referring directly to IU, researchers can distinguish many variables which can *then* be operationally defined and quantified. Without direct reference these variables will never be found.

Direct reference can also save one from arbitrary measures that have little hope of success. For example, in one study ordinary dream reports were compared with reports from survivors of sexual abuse. No differences were found. The measure was the frequency of 100 common words. But someone familiar with abuse victims could recognize phrases such as 'they didn't believe me'. Measures often fail to correlate when they have no experiential relation to what one wants to measure. Meaningless syllables may not produce the kind of process that significant words would produce. Taking the measure yourself might reveal, for example, that deciding a 'preference' between a lovely and an ugly picture is not the same process as between two equally attractive ones.

Once identified, new variables will have observable indices. It is certainly not more 'objective' to remain lacking in distinctions and variables only because they must first be found by direct reference.

The skill of directly referring can be developed through training. There is now an international network of such training (www.focusing.org) which offers two practices 'Focusing' and 'TAE', each with precise steps. 'Focusing' teaches referring to the implicit. It has many uses in many fields. 'TAE' (Thinking at the Edge) is based on Focusing, and is a new way of thinking and concept formation.

The instructions for Focusing grew out of quantitative studies of tape-recorded psychotherapy. The studies used a scale of observable linguistic indices of the degree to which clients directly referred to something implicit during therapy. We predicted that clients would move up on the scale during the course of therapy, but they did not. If they began low, they failed in therapy even after years. (Currently we integrate Focusing into therapy so that starting low on direct reference no longer predicts failure.)

We first identified this variable from directly referring to our own IU. Then we were able to define and quantify its observable indices, and produce findings which contradicted our prediction.

Direct reference opens many different territories

Direct reference opens quite a large territory, in which many advances have already been made. They need to be collected, interrelated, and evaluated. We need a new Bacon to create a public science from these advances.[16]

I call it them a 'territory of territories'. People sometimes want to think of them all as one thing, but that would confuse different territories. Focusing and TAE (concept formation) constitute only one such territory. Another includes meditation, autogenic training, deep relaxation, and hypnosis. Still others are Feldenkrais, hands-on body work, and movement. I don't know enough to classify. Even within one field the specialties may utterly differ.

There are also very different ways of relating to IU. For example, in one kind of meditation we merely observe and welcome what 'comes up the stairs' without identifying with it. This opens a different territory than Focusing does. In Focusing we welcome without identifying, but we 'go down the stairs' to the murky edge where a new felt sense of 'all that' can come. We enter and go a few steps, or many. The relaxation is not nearly as deep as in meditation.

In Focusing the felt sense brings a larger and stronger kind of 'I'. 'I' am here; the felt sense of my whole situation is over there. In contrast, some kinds of meditation can bring an 'absence of self'. But meditation can also build resilience in the face of whatever comes. There are different territories, and there is no reason to lose any of them.

Body sensations are not all of one kind

What we refer to may at first seem just bodily, 'just' the physical discomfort, excitement, or nameless physical quality. But one soon senses when it is implicitly complex. A beginner might ask: 'Is this a felt sense or just indigestion?' Either is possible in the same bodily location, but implicitly they exist very differently.

Of course we want all physiological and neurological analysis of experiences. Every analytic advance also makes further advances in IU possible. But a given instrument may or may not define what happens.

We cannot cut the bodily sensations off from the IU if they carry it. We may describe them in the same words at first, but we must guard against dividing them according to the current units and categories. The intricacy of what happens does not fit under the units of the current conceptual model. If these factors are considered, the study of bodily variables in direct reference is very promising.

---

[16] Don Johnson and I called for the creation of such a science in our 2004 article.

IV. Training In Concept Formation

In theoretical and research situations it pays to keep track of what we sense but cannot yet conceptualize. Of course we want to do this, I argue. My usual example: If your lab equipment is acting funny today, would you ignore it because you don't know what the problem is?

One doesn't want to be the kind of scientist or philosopher who ignores unclear edges and says only what is already well known. To think something new, one must often enter a murky physical feeling which might not seem promising at first.

When a felt sense comes from something that we cannot formulate, we may be excited about it. Why is a palpable 'edge' sometimes so exciting? The coming of a felt sense is a bodily event in which a great many implicit statements that have not occurred have all just been carried forward. Of course that can be bodily exciting.

And, why is becoming able to explicate such an edge even more exciting? The explication creates a whole field in which we can do and make new things and create new analyses. That is so much more, and we still have the felt sense (now carried forward) as well.

TAE is designed for people who are tracking something they sense, but have been unable to say. This is usually because what they sense involves a new kind of conceptual pattern, a kind that cannot be subdivided into self-identical units like the usual concepts.

With the first eight of the TAE steps, people become able to say what they had been unable to say. They report telling about it everywhere, both at length and briefly. Many people report the exciting discovery: 'I can think!' What most of us learned in school was not thinking. We learned to use already-formed concepts without our whole IU.

Then, if a formal theory is needed, there are more steps, which I will discuss below. The fourteen steps and an introduction are available at www.focusing.org. Here I only want to mention a few points.

Partnership helps one say what one didn't know

Along with Focusing we teach a 'listening' which lets each thing be and be heard just as it was intended. There is room to refer to and wait for the felt sense. People soon say more than what they have already thought. In TAE we have a partner who listens in this way and writes down what we say verbatim. We need this because the precision of the new phrases that come is so quickly forgotten. ('How did I just say that?' It's written down.)

FIRST AND THIRD PERSON PROCESSES

Why 'facets' (particular events) are necessary

TAE requires recalling at least one actual instance (later four or five). Such an instance is called a 'facet', anything that actually happened and has the hue of what we are tracking. People often say, 'Oh, it happened many times', but TAE requires recalling a specific occasion.

For example, we need a facet when someone writes: 'I want my words to *match* my experience.' The word 'match' will derail any further thinking because it assumes the old representational model. When we can separate what we mean from the old way of saying it, we can refer directly to the facet, and examine what it actually consists of in that real instance. Then new phrases come and can lead to new concepts.

Why words won't do; phrases are necessary

We often think something new, but our old words bring only the old conceptual model. Then we cannot go further. Only new phrases can say new meaning. Even if people don't understand the new phrase, they notice that something new is being said.

A way to get new phrases when none come

At one stage in TAE we use a simple way to get new phrases to come. The new meaning is usually immersed in old statements and concepts. How can we separate it out? Write a sentence however insufficient. We look up a major word in it (like 'match' in the above example) in the dictionary, and vividly discover that it doesn't mean what we intended. Then we ask — very gently — 'What did you want that word to mean?'

Another word may come. Looking it up leads us to reject it as well. And so with a third. We see that every word says much that we didn't want it to mean. As we replace words one after the other, they make what I call a 'slot' in the sentence. If we say the sentence with the slot left empty (for example, if we put a hand-gesture or a '...'), then the sentence seems oddly close to saying what we mean.

Once the slot works, it can do more. Now the slot can change what the words mean, if we put them back (but only for us and only for now). Each word we tried now has a different new meaning, because it crosses with the slot. And, if we say more about these meanings, the further words that come will also have acquired new meanings.

Now, if we invite them, odd new phrases come easily. Why easily now? Because now what we are tracking no longer implies the old phrases.

Building a theory

About building a logical theory from direct reference, let me briefly state just the principle: in the early TAE Steps (1–5) we phrase many 'terms' from the felt sense. Each of them is implied by the felt sense. Therefore they imply each other. Their already existing implicit connections can yield a theory of logical connections between them.

In TAE Steps 6–8, which I don't have room here to describe, we find a new conceptual pattern and allow it to stand. It can be stated in three or four of the terms. Now we can write a precise definition for each term by stating its connections to the other terms in the pattern. Then we can also write definitions for all the others by using the already-defined terms. The pattern expands into a logical theory.

Now there are logical connections between the terms, which explicate the implicit connections they already had. The terms are now connected not only implicitly, but by logic as well.

In any context, if we want theory, a retroactive logic can always be explicated from implicit functioning. That possibility is always already implicit. (We saw that possibility when we saw that the logical consequences of each chess move were already implicit in the coming of the new move.)

The theory can develop further and further by using the pattern and the logically connected terms to define anything in its own field. The theory can also generate new statements on any other topic by crossing that topic with our pattern.[17]

Once the theory is formulated, we can use it with or without directly referring. Of course we also still have the (much carried forward) felt sense. That allows us to create a second terminology, which we may want for various reasons. Varying terminologies enable us to see different aspects of the implicit. Having more than one terminology is not a relativistic variety, but rather two explications with direct reference.

V. Two Kinds of Speech

Why don't we always speak directly from what our whole IU implies? This is because speech first forms as a cultural system of sayings and

---

[17] I call this 'reversal'. A new meaning (or the new pattern implicit in it) can cross and apply also to major topics, for example 'biology', 'evolution', 'human nature', 'nature', 'beauty', or 'value'. Instead of being subsumed under the large old topic, the new pattern provides a new way to think about biology, or evolution, human nature, etc. A new pattern can bring the large topic a new possibility which could not be seen from the usual unit model.

doings which can capture us. Please notice: I am not saying that this system *must* capture us, only that it can, and usually does. I deny most current theories which say that capture is the inherent nature of language.

I will show *why* speech captures — but need not. (We teach what makes the difference. Every segment of the population likes learning it. And once having learned, no one wants to go back to nearly automatic capture.)

Many children close the access to their IU between the ages of six and ten. Very small children have empathy with all children and animals but later most of them have none for children and animals whom the culture rejects.

Some people cannot easily feel more than the cultural situation. For example, a man's brother died. You ask him what he feels and he says 'sad'. You ask for more and he says, 'I am mourning him.' You ask him what his brother's death means to him, and he answers 'Well, what are you asking me? How would you feel if your brother died?'

Similarly, some rituals are bodily important to some people for extremely varying reasons, but if asked about it, they give the same standard account.

However, everyone has also changed or elaborated some of what the culture teaches. The deliberate part of that can be told, but direct reference to the IU is more difficult. It always includes the culture, but goes far beyond it.

The cultural system is implied by the human body. Let us first see why. Human bodies imply behaviour including speech possibilities. Most human behaviour is speech, and all human behaviour involves implicit speech. In humans the behaviour context is called the 'situation'. We have seen that the bodily-implied behaviour context — the situation — is not external nor is it internal. Situations are our bodily-implied behaviour contexts. Language is not a separated system of mere words about things. It is part of the body-process in situations.

We can see the bodily nature of language if we ask: How do the words come to us to say? I open my mouth and the words come. They come already organized in phrases and sentences that say what I want to say in this situation without my having to consider all possible words and combinations.

We see that 'a situation' is something the body has. It is not a puzzle why the words fit the situation, since a 'situation' is the bodily implied behaviour possibilities. This provides an explanation for how words come. The situation is the bodily behaviour context of possible next moves, largely speech.

Situations don't first exist and are then 'signified' by language. We don't 'symbolize' by attaching 'signifiers' to external things. The explication model we have been building explains the old seemingly artificial relation of 'signifier and signified'. Symbols (words, concepts, gestures) are not a separate system of tags pasted onto things by convention. *The symbols and the situation are internally connected because a situation is inherently the implying of a cluster of possible sayings and doings.*

Language is how cultural situations developed. Each culture consists of its typical kinds of situations and word-uses in them. Each kind of situation is a bundle of stories, scenarios, ready alternative actions and sayings.

All our doings are defined by words and by gestures like signing papers and earning money. (If you didn't sign the cheque, you didn't pay.) Situations come in kinds defined by their implicit speech and ritual.

We rarely speak directly from our own whole IU because our behaviour context implies this elaborate system of already-defined situations with already-formed sayings. I will try to show why going beyond this system has seemed impossible.

Always the same words

It can seem that we are trapped by the words. Of course we always have only the same old words of the language. We can combine words or syllables. Occasionally we add a foreign word. Otherwise we must always use the same old words.

Each word has its uses, its own meanings in certain kinds of situations. Even when we want to say something directly from our own more intricate situation, it seems we cannot. The words say their own standard meanings instead. Language is 'discursive'. The words bring their own story and carry *that story* forward. We can only hope that our words will also, indirectly, as a by-product, carry forward the situation in which we are actually living. Language seems never to say as much as our own whole situation would imply, sometimes not even anything like it.

Elsewhere I have quoted a man who said: 'Where I grew up, no matter what I really felt, it had to be one of two or three things.' Then he said 'If there is another way to talk, *I want it!*' That man keenly felt how much more his own situations implied.

Currently most philosophers say that there is no other way to speak. Words can only say what *they* mean. What *we* meant is lost, and language is blamed. They say that language can only be discursive. I deny it. There is another way:

How language can say something new; three remarkable facts about phrases

(1) A word has many uses, but a phrase may have only one.
(2) Words come to us already arranged in phrases. Phrases belong to situations; they come to the specific juncture, now.[18]
(3) In a new situation a new phrase gives the words a new use and meaning.

Usually new phrases don't come because we don't speak from direct reference to the IU of our own situation and our own thought. We move from one already-formed phrase to another. People assume they must use old phrases. Even when they sense the edge directly, they tend not to let a new phrase come. But they could.

New phrases may take a minute to form. At one moment only familiar ones may come. One needs to notice what the old ones *do not* say.

Wittgenstein demonstrated that the same word could have new meanings in new uses. He invented situations to show this (for example, many new meanings of the word 'reading'). He didn't explain it. He only wanted to show that meaning depends on use. He said he was not telling, 'only showing'. He did not explain what is involved in 'only showing'. He didn't try to make a theory from what he 'showed', because he was sure that theory must use representations, which would falsify the actual use and working of language to which he pointed.

My philosophy demonstrates that words *can* say how they are working in the saying they're doing. New phrases can let words acquire new meanings *from and about* how they work in this fresh happening of language. Wittgenstein was right that the working of

---

[18] How words come in phrases (old or new) involves four considerations at once. Syntactically the words implicitly cross along with their possible relations to each other (as adjectives, verbs, nouns, etc.). Pragmatically all their uses function implicitly to let just this one use emerge. Thirdly these two crossings must cross to be able to say just this, not something else. Fourthly, the words must belong to this particular situation, now. Philosophers have distinguished syntactic from pragmatic, but have only recently wondered how they happen in one occurring (Goldberg *et al.*, 2007). See also my 'Crossing and dipping' (1995) and 'Reply to Johnson' (1997c).

words cannot be said in representations, but words can refer to the saying they are doing.[19]

We can speak freshly because our bodily situation is always different and much more intricate than the cultural generalities. A situation is a bodily happening, not just generalities. Language doesn't consist just of standard sayings. Language is part of the human body's implying of behaviour possibilities. Our own situation always consists of more intricate implyings. Therefore new phrases can come when we refer directly to the IU.

Fresh speech from direct reference is a learned skill for most people. But once we have learned it, we can do it at any time. Then we see that our situation implies much more than the cultural kinds.[20]

The usual view is mistaken, that the individual can do no more than choose among the cultural scenarios, or add mere nuances. The 'nuances' are not mere details. Since what is culturally appropriate has only a general meaning, it is the so-called 'nuances' that tell us what we really want to know. They indicate what the standard saying really means here, this time, from this person. Of course we would know much more if the person would directly refer to that meaning, and speak from there.

Speech coming directly from IU is trans-cultural. Every individual incorporates but far transcends culture, as becomes evident from direct reference. We train people in many countries and cultures. The process is largely the same. A man briefly describes the role of Japanese fathers at some festival, just enough to take me across the culture at that one spot. Then I perfectly understand his pain from his father's neglect at that festival, and always.

Of course I understand only this individual, not the culture. During group activities I know that I don't know what is happening.

One's culture is recognizable by posture, style of movement, and much else. Culture deeply structures the body but it is never enough to live on. Communication from implicit understanding reveals that culture gives us only generalities that are largely oblivious of what it is to be a person.

---

[19] I show this in 'Words can say how they work' (1993), as well as in 'What happens when Wittgenstein asks "What happens when ...?"' (1997b).

[20] Thinking is both individual and social. The current theory of a one-way determination by society is too simple. The relation is much more complex. Individuals do require channels of information, public discourses, instruments and machines, economic support, and associations for action. The individual must also find ways to relate to the public attitudes so as to be neither captured nor isolated. In all these ways the individual is highly controlled. Nevertheless, individual thinking constantly exceeds society.

Both old and new are implied

Both the old phrases and the new situation are always functioning. In the coming of new phrases the old ones function implicitly (like old chess moves). If old phrases come, our present IU has functioned implicitly to determine which old saying came, why it came, and what it actually means in this situation here. (One can discover this with direct reference.)

But society is changing. Direct reference to IU is becoming easier and more prevalent. Individuals have been developing. The culturally defined roles have become more inadequate than ever. We innovate all day. There is more and more need to express new meanings directly from implicit understanding.

We can foresee a society in which people live more often from implicit understanding (IU) and recognize that others do. Then society won't waste so much of what a human being can be. Already we can study and measure the difference between disconnected and IU-connected talking. Many variables correlate with it. It is widely recognized that there is always novelty, and that positive new steps and healing can come from the implicit when we are in direct contact with it.

Currently most of society's efforts fail to improve schools, churches, jails, businesses, and policy planning. This is because the efforts don't reach and interact with what is implicitly happening in people. We find that if a person becomes able to refer directly to IU, then social efforts can *reach there where* they connect with implicit functioning and make something new possible. Children are excited to discover where in them fresh thinking can happen. Violent jail inmates no longer just 'act out'. Having learned Focusing they find where and how the situation 'gets to them'. 'Each time it's different!' they report (Bierman, 1999). Business meetings usually go round in circles, but with Focusing and listening people discover a kind of meeting in which they can say things they themselves have never thought before.

But with the new ways one can also go horribly wrong. New developments can make some old ways of coping impossible without supplying effective new ones. Focusing is by no means the only skill we need to learn. We need to develop along many other avenues, but Focusing does enable all other instructions to be more effective.

VI. The Changed Ground

The unit model and the explication model contrasted

In the unit model existence is thought of as just occurring–occurring–occurring. Each occurring is a discrete event. In the explication model the discrete events are also implicit intricacies with a more intricate continuity. Objects exist within the process of body–environment interaction, not just in empty space.

The unit model generates an 'external' space, a viewed space. Environmental interaction is misunderstood. The body seems to consist of views from the outside. The organism's implying seems to happen 'inside' the externally-viewed body. First person process is considered 'internal', 'subjective'.

Consciousness is cut away and seems to be a separate thing. But this thing-consciousness can never be added to logical concepts, since their inferences depend on their working alone. The concepts *require* cutting consciousness away, so an artificial 'hard problem' about consciousness is created, if consciousness is to be added to them. But consciousness cannot be understood as a separate thing.

In the old model our concepts seemed to be 'representations' which needed 'corresponding' entities in an 'external' reality. Logically connected concepts explain things and let us build new machines and technology. But something goes wrong when the concepts are taken as the overall model of reality (instead of as explications of the wider process which includes concept-formation). Then the universe seems to be the space of mere views, and we seem to exist inside a body that consists of external views. This foundation of science has long seemed absurd, and its objectivity was a puzzle.

The famously questionable ground of science has been criticized for centuries but there was no alternative. Since we are now developing the explication model, we can completely shift this shaky ground. The objectivity of concepts can be explained and established in an explication system about concept-formation and empirical testing within environmental interaction.

Which of the two models can include both? The explication model can let us think about itself as well as about the derivation of the unit model. It can show how the two models expand each other. The explication model can refer both to first person process *and* to third person views.

The third person views are products of explication within the first person process. *All concepts are explications from first person process, including the unit-concepts and the process-concepts I present.* (People will soon make better and better concepts of the new kind.)

The reciprocity of the two models

Logic depends on keeping the units the same. Therefore it can never explain how new thoughts come. In contrast, explication freshly 'carries forward' at every step. Therefore it can never have the inferential power of logical formation. We can see clearly that neither system can undercut or minimize the other.

We have to let our concepts have their own inferences. These can lead us to new places, new interactions with the environment. There we look around. What the computer did might have been too complex for our IU to follow, but we look around from the result. Then our IU may enable us to think more than the computer can follow. The implicit connections in our IU are retroactively capable of logical explication which sometimes leads to building new computers.

What we study and test in interaction must never be assumed to consist only of the conceptual units. It is a false metaphysics which has taught students to assume that a research subject is nothing but the units of the current science system.

There was always reciprocity between the two systems, but there was no way to employ it systematically. Now there is. Many advantages are gained for analysis if the wider system is available as well. New units can be generated and tried at any point.

Empirical testing is vital but we have to recognize that we cannot test the concepts themselves. We test the outcomes of *what we do*. The operations happen directly in the implicit intricacy of nature. That is why we always get more findings than our hypotheses projected, never only what confirms or disconfirms them.

Empirical testing requires replication by many independent groups. We need not believe just one. Science is a social process, but society-wide testing takes a while. Entrenched groups hold on to their views and slow things down even more.

Because of slower social process, there is always an 'established' picture of nature. Nature seems reduced to one set of concepts. What remains to be discovered seems 'not yet' reduced, as if it soon will be. But there is absolutely no chance of this. Even a single new concept or new doing can make innumerable changes in the implicit possibilities. Nature is never only the units we make and combine. Everything in nature is an implicit intricacy.

References

Bierman, Ralph (1999), 'Focusing in changing abusive fighting to constructive conflict interactions: RWV therapy groups with domestically violent men', *Paper presented at the 11th International Focusing Conference, Ontario, Canada*. Available at www.focusing.org.

Crease, Robert P. (1993), *The Play of Nature: Experimentation as Performance* (Bloomington: Indiana University Press).

Crease, Robert P. (1997), 'The philosophy of science', *The Folio*, **20**(1), pp. 32–42.

Dreyfus, Hubert L. (1992), *What Computers Still Can't Do: A Critique of Artificial Reason* (Cambridge, MA: MIT Press).

Gallagher, S. (2006), *How the Body Shapes the Mind* (Oxford: Clarendon Press).

Gendlin, E.T. (1962), *Experiencing and the Creation of Meaning. A Philosophical and Psychological Approach to the Subjective* (New York: Free Press of Glencoe). Reprinted by Macmillan, 1970.

Gendlin, E.T. (1981/1997), *A Process Model* (New York: The Focusing Institute). A corrected version (2001) is available at http://www.focusing.org/process.html.

Gendlin, E.T. (1993), 'Words can say how they work', in R.P. Crease (Ed.), *Proceedings, Heidegger Conference*, pp. 29-35 (Stony Brook: State University of New York). Also available at http://www.focusing.org/gendlin/docs/gol_2087.html.

Gendlin, E.T. (1995), 'Crossing and dipping: Some terms for approaching the interface between natural understanding and logical formation', *Mind and Machines*, **5**, pp. 547–60.
Also available at http://www.focusing.org/gendlin/docs/gol_2166.html.

Gendlin, E.T. (1997a), 'The responsive order: A new empiricism', *Man and World*, **30**(3), pp. 383–411. Also available at http://www.focusing.org/gendlin/docs/gol_2157.html.

Gendlin, E.T. (1997b), 'What happens when Wittgenstein asks "What happens when...?"', *The Philosophical Forum*. **XXVIII**(3), pp. 268–81. Also available at http://www.focusing.org/gendlin/docs/gol_2170.html.

Gendlin, E.T. (1997c), 'Reply to Johnson', in D. M. Levin (Ed.), *Language Beyond Post-Modernism: Saying and Thinking in Gendlin's Philosophy*, pp. 168–75 & 357–58 (Evanston, IL: Northwestern University Press).

Gendlin, E.T. (Forthcoming), 'We can think with the implicit, as well as with fully formed concepts' in Leidlmair, K. (Ed.) *After Cognitivism: A Reassessment of Cognitive Science and Philosophy* (n.p.: Springer).

Gendlin, E.T. & Johnson, Don H. (2004), 'Proposal for an international group for a first person science,' http://www.focusing.org/gendlin/docs/gol_2184.html.

Gibson, James J. (1966), *The Senses Considered as Perceptual Systems* (Boston, MA: Houghton Miflin).

Goldberg, A.E., Casenhiser, D. & White, T.R. (2007), 'Constructions as categories of language', *New Ideas in Psychology*, **25**(2), pp. 70–86.

O'Regan, J.K. and Noë, A., (2001), 'A sensorimotor account of vision and visual consciousness', *Behavioral and Brain Sciences*, **24**(5), pp. 939–73.

Claire Petitmengin & Michel Bitbol

The Validity of First-Person Descriptions as Authenticity and Coherence

Abstract: *In this paper we list the various criticisms that have been formulated against introspection, from Auguste Comte denying that consciousness can observe itself, to recent criticisms of the reliability of first person descriptions. We show that these criticisms rely on the one hand on poor knowledge of the introspective process, and on the other hand on a naïve conception of scientific objectivity. Two kinds of answers are offered: the first one is grounded on a refined description of the process of becoming aware of one's experience and describing it, the second one relies on a comparison with the methods of the experimental sciences. We conclude the article by providing a renewed definition of 'the truth' of a first person description.*

Keywords

Introspection, first person, description, phenomenology, consciousness, pre-reflective consciousness, awareness, epistemology, methodology, explicitation, experience, subjectivity, reliability

Introduction

The goal of this article is to show that longstanding and more recent criticisms of introspection are due to an insufficient comprehension of the introspective process. After an inventory of these criticisms, we answer them by providing a concrete description of this process, which is grounded in our practice of a first person method of verbal explicitation of experience, as well as *vipassana* meditation. Such a description leads us towards a new conception of the validity of introspective reports, conceived as authenticity and consistency instead of correspondence, a conception which is in fact the same as that which underlies the experimental sciences.

I. Criticisms of Introspection

Is introspection able to give us access to our experience? Are introspective reports trustworthy? Or on the contrary, do we have reasons to suspect that introspection — defined as the observation of one's own lived experience — is either impossible or introduces an irreducible distortion, which may be of observational, temporal, interpretative or verbal order? Doesn't an important part of our cognitive processes, of our sensorial experience and of our emotional life simply elude introspection? Furthermore, doesn't the private and singular character of experience make introspective reports impossible to verify? In this first section we draw up an inventory of these criticisms.

Stimulus error

A first argument frequently used for contesting the reliability of introspection invokes the gap often noted between the stimulus and the report on experience:

> If we compare the observer's reports with the stimuli actually exposed, we find that he may see what was not there at all, may fail to see much of what was there, and may misrepresent the little that he really perceived; introspection adds, subtracts, distorts (Titchener, 1912, p. 488).

Among the observations highlighting this gap, those demonstrating the phenomenon of 'change blindness', where a person viewing a visual scene apparently fails to detect large changes or salient stimuli in this scene (like a woman in a gorilla suit walking through a ballgame), are especially convincing (Levin & Simons, 1997; Simons & Levin, 1998; Simons & Chabris, 1999). But, as Titchener notes, this argument cannot be considered as a criticism of introspection. For introspection does not consist of observing and describing stimuli (this interpretation is the beginner's mistake, that Titchener dubbed 'stimulus error'), but of observing and describing *one's own experience* of these stimuli. The question is not whether a description corresponds to the stimuli, but to know whether it corresponds to the subject's experience: it can be false from the first point of view while being completely right from the second.

> Psychological observation is observation by each man of his own experience, of mental processes which lie open to him but to no one else. Hence while all other scientific observation may be called inspection, the looking-at things or processes, psychological observation is introspection, the looking inward into oneself (Titchener, 1898/1914, p. 27).

Impossible split

However, is such an auto-observation possible? Indeed, how can I 'cut myself into two' in order to observe myself? How can I be angry and at the same time observe myself being angry? How can I calculate differential equations and at the same time observe myself calculating differential equations?

> The thinker cannot divide himself into two, of whom one reasons whilst the other observes him reason. The organ observed and the organ observing being, in this case, identical, how could observation take place? This pretended psychological method is then radically null and void (Comte, 1945, leçon 1, p. 34).

Moreover, supposing the existence of such a split gives rise to a risk of *regressio ad infinitum*: an especially persistent introspectionist observing a mental process might wish to observe himself observing this process, and so forth 'ad infinitum and ad nauseam' (ten Hoor, 1932).

Observational distortion

A third set of criticisms concern the reliability of auto-observation. An answer to the 'impossible split' argument consists in imagining two orders or levels of experience or consciousness (Bitbol, 2008a,b), of which one would consist in observing or 'reflecting' the other, without being completely dissociated from it. Phenomenology speaks of non-reflective and reflective consciousness; a few recent authors refer to first and second order consciousness (Marcel, 2003; Overgaard & Sorensen, 2004), or of basic consciousness and meta-consciousness (Schooler, 2002). In first order consciousness the subject is immediately engaged, immersed in the flow of experience. The second order experience consists in distancing oneself from this immediate experience through an act of observation, introspection or reflection, by means of which consciousness is directed towards itself. But how can we guarantee the correspondence between first order and second order consciousness? How can we be sure that the later doesn't distort or alter the former (Zahavi, 2008)? 'If meta-consciousness requires re-representing the contents of consciousness, then, as with any recoding process, some information could get lost or become distorted in the translation (Schooler, 2002, p. 342).'

- Objectification

According to a first argument, in the act of introspection the subject considers himself as an object: what he observes then is not the original subject anymore, but an objectified and reified subject, who is lost as subject.

> One apparently never grasps the subjective, as such, in itself. On the contrary, in order to grasp it scientifically, one is forced to strip it of its subjective character. One kills subjectivity in order to dissect it, and believes that the life of the soul is on display in the result of the dissection! (Natorp, 1912, p. 103, quoted by Zahavi, 2003, p. 157).

- Immobilization

A similar argument stresses the 'freezing' character of the introspective act. To be able to observe the fluctuations of his experience, which is fundamentally in motion, and particularly the subtle movements of his thought, the subject has no other solution than to immobilize, to petrify them, which amounts to missing them.

> Now it is very difficult, introspectively, to see the transitive parts for what they really are. (...) The rush of the thought is so headlong that it almost always brings us up at the conclusion before we can rest it. Or if our purpose is nimble enough and we do arrest it, it ceases forthwith to itself. (...) The attempt at introspective analysis in these cases is in fact like seizing a spinning top to catch its motion, or trying to turn up the gas quickly enough to see how the darkness looks ... (James, 1890/1983, p. 237).

- Disruption

If it does not stop it dead, introspection disrupts the course of experience deeply: ''Tis evident this reflection ... would so disturb the operation of my natural principles as must render it impossible to form any just conclusion from the phenomenon.' (Hume, 1739-40/1969, p. 46; see T. Froese, 2009).

For Wundt (1897), this disrupting effect is felt mainly in complex thoughts, whereas for James, it is felt mainly in bodily action: 'We walk along a beam all the better if we think less of the position of our feet upon it (James, 1890/1983, p. 1128).' For Merleau-Ponty (1945), reflective consciousness hinders the natural flow of spontaneous bodily action which is irreflective, that is non reflectively self-conscious. Some experiences show that reflective consciousness alters pleasure (Schooler, 2002). 'Inner observation' could even simply destroy its object:

> If someone is in a state in which he wants to observe his own anger ranging within him, the anger must already be somewhat diminished, and so his original object of observation would have disappeared. The same impossibility is also present in all other cases. It is a universally valid psychological law that we can never focus our attention upon the object of inner perception (Brentano, 1874/1995, p. 30).

- Creation

A final criticism of observation is that it enriches or even creates experience. For example, I could invite you to turn your attention toward the tactile sensation of your feet in your shoes, or toward the noises that you can hear just now. Did these tactile and auditory sensations exist before you observed them? Did they belong to your experience, in a pre-attentive, vague and inchoate form? Or were you insensible and deaf to these sensations? Does not the very fact of turning your attention toward them simply create them?

> It is like a flashlight in a dark room to search around for something that doesn't have any light shining on it. The flashlight, since there is light in whatever direction it turns, would have to conclude that there is light everywhere. And so consciousness can seem to pervade all mentality where actually it does not (Jaynes, 1976, p. 23).

Such is the debate which opposes the supporters of the 'rich' conception and of the 'poor' conception of experience, a debate recently revived by Schwitzgebel (2007a).

> James (1890/1983) and Searle (1992) endorse the rich view of consciousness, according to which the stream of experience involves both a centre of attention and a broad periphery of consciously experienced but unattended objects and background feelings. Jaynes (1976), Dennett (1991) and Mack and Rock (1998) endorse the thin view: consciousness is limited to only one or a few objects, modalities, topics or fields at a time. The unattended hum of the traffic in the background is no part, not even a peripheral part, of your experience when you're sufficiently absorbed in other things (Schwitzgebel, 2007a, p. 7).

Temporal distortion

Therefore it seems that introspection, conceived as an observational activity unfolding simultaneously with the observed experience, is extremely problematic. But could not these problems be solved by the possibility we have of directing ourselves *retrospectively* toward our experience? In fact, it seems that most of the time we do not observe our experience at the very moment it takes place, but *a posteriori*, as Stuart Mill had noted:

> A fact may be studied through the medium of memory, not at the very moment of our perceiving it, but the moment after: and this is really the mode in which our best knowledge of our intellectual acts is generally acquired. We reflect on what we have been doing when the act is past, but when its impression in the memory is still fresh (Mill, 1882/1961, p. 64).

In point of fact, there is no introspection in the strict sense of the term, 'all introspection is retrospection' (Sully, 1881). Retrospection enables us to remedy the splitting and distorting effects of simultaneous introspection, since the subject doesn't observe himself while experiencing, but observes instead the memory of an experience — a memory which can at will be recalled, slowed down and scrutinized in its smallest details without the original experience being affected. 'You must wait to introspect until the processes that you wish to examine have passed by. Let them run their course undisturbed: then call them back by memory, and look at them. They are now dead, and cannot be changed by your observation.' (Titchener, 1898, p. 28)

The retrospective strategy, supported by James, was adopted by the school of Titchener, the school of Binet in Paris (Binet, 1903), and the school of Würzburg in Germany, notably for studying mental imagery. But another difficulty immediately arose, that of the validity of memory: how can we be sure that the memory is true to the initial experience? How can we ensure that the recalled experience is not rebuilt? Do we not in fact arrive at a retrospective falsification of conscious history, by the processes that Dennett (1991) calls 'Orwellian' and 'Stalinesque'?[1] Do we not have good reason to question the reliability of memory, whose distorting effect is well-known, by means of transformation, amplification or impoverishment of the original experience — the dimensions of experience on which attention was not focused during the initial experience being consigned to oblivion?

---

[1] Retrospective alteration of history can be obtained in two ways, according to Dennett (1991). In the Orwellian way, somebody first makes one conclusion based on partial evidence, and then changes her memory of having made this previous conclusion in order to accommodate further evidence. In the Stalinesque way, somebody does not make any intermediate conclusion but entirely reconstructs the whole sequence *ex post facto*, when all the evidence is available. However, according to Dennett, at the microtime scale of brain processes the distinction is not a real one.

Interpretative distortion

Another major difficulty of introspection results from the fact that, contrary to what Dennett sometimes misleadingly suggested by evoking our unchallengeable authority about our experience (Schwitzgebel, 2007b), an experience is not infallible: I can misinterpret the way my experience appears to me. 'One can be mistaken about one's experience just as one's experience can be mistaken' (Marcel, 2003, p. 181). My experience can be occulted by naive or theoretical preconceptions, which have two types of effect.

First, preconceptions may have a distorting effect: surreptitiously, a knowledge about the experience substitutes itself for the experience, biasing the description. Just as someone who draws a table spontaneously draws it as he knows it is: rectangular, and not as it may appear to him when every perceptive or conceptual preconception is relaxed, that is as a deformed parallelogram (Vermersch, 1997, p.7). Nisbett and Wilson's experiments show very convincingly how untrained subjects slip surreptitiously from the description of their experience toward the verbalization of explanations, generalizations, and abstract knowledge about their experience.

> Subjective reports about higher mental processes are sometimes correct, but even the instances of correct reports are not due to direct introspective awareness. Instead, they are due to the incidentally correct employment of a priori causal theories (Nisbett & Wilson, 1977).

Sometimes, it is an expectation or a motivation that substitutes for the experience.[2] 'When individuals have strong expectations about conscious experience they may access the expectation rather than the actual experience' (Schooler & Schreiber, 2004).

Second, preconceptions may have a concealing effect: when a dimension of our experience does not match up with our knowledge or our expectations, it can remain unnoticed. For example, until the publication of Nigro and Neisser's article (1983), in the field of cognitive psychology it was considered impossible that someone would be able to see himself/herself in an evoked scene, and in fact very few people described such an experience (Marcel, 2003). In the same way, the belief that thought must be expressed in images or words makes the description of unsymbolized thinking very difficult (Hurlburt & Schwitzgebel, 2007). In the medical domain, the belief that seizures are sudden, a theory which underpins the whole medical discourse on

---

[2] This could explain for example 'the placebo effect', in this case the expected effects of the medicine substituting themselves for the felt effects.

epilepsy,[3] considerably hampers the awareness and description by the patient of the preictal symptoms that could enable him to anticipate and manage his seizures (Petitmengin et al., 2007).

The distortion or screening of experience by a preconception may be even more difficult to detect if it is 'adaptive', that is if it fulfils a function,[4] the resistance of the individual or the community to the process of becoming aware being in this case proportional to the benefit received.

Verbal distortion

A last distortive effect comes from verbal description. As James wrote: 'We find ourselves in continual error and uncertainty so soon as we are called on to name and class, and not merely to feel (1890/1983, p. 191). This difficulty is partly due to the paucity of the vocabulary we have for describing our subjective experience. 'We almost completely lack the concepts and competencies that would allow us to parse, think about, talk about, and remember the complexity of experience' (Hurlburt & Schwitzgebel, 2007, p. 51). Moreover, the vocabulary we have, and the metaphors we use in order to palliate its insufficiency, transmit very powerful preconceptions and implicit theories that contribute to the distorting effect of introspection by infiltrating the description of our experience. Finally, the very effort of describing verbally some specific experiences may disturb them, introducing a 'verbal overshadowing' (Schooler, 2002). Describing amounts to decomposing and dissecting. However the experience of a perfume, the taste of a wine, an aesthetic experience, the recognition of a face, are experiences of an holistic nature, that one cannot analyze and break up into separate elements without altering them. And although it may be possible to describe a logical problem-solving task as it unfolds, by simply 'thinking aloud', describing tasks of a non discursive nature (affective decision making, analogical reasoning, insight problem solving) hampers or disrupts the process (Schooler *et al.*, 1993; Schooler & Dougal, 1999).

Blindness of introspection

Furthermore, as different researchers have noted, an important part of our experience eludes reflective consciousness and therefore introspection.

---

[3] And this is can be traced right back down to the etymology of the word 'epilepsy': the Greek term *epi-lambanein* meaning 'to surprise'.

[4] Wilson (2002) speaks of adaptive unconscious, Schooler (2002) of adaptative dissociation (of meta-consciousness).

For example, some processes of choice, of decision, are very difficult to access. We have access to the result of our thought processes, but seldom to the processes themselves, to the 'what' but not to the 'how'. As Nisbett and Wilson noted, we suffer from 'the most extreme form of inaccessibility to cognitive processes — literal lack of awareness that a process of any kind is occurring until the moment that the result appears' (Nisbett & Wilson, 1977, p. 241).

But even the 'what' often seems difficult to access. On the one hand, some subtle or ambiguous sensations (like the prodroma of an epileptic seizure or a of a stress attack) are difficult to detect. Even intense emotions — of sadness or anger for example — may remain unobserved. On the other hand, many actions are performed 'automatically', without any reflective consciousness. The most quoted example is that of absent-minded driving: we sometimes realize when arriving at a destination that throughout practically the whole journey we have been completely absorbed in our thoughts without any reflective consciousness of our perceptions — the road, the other cars, roadsigns — or of our actual driving. Studies carried out on this phenomenon of 'mind wandering' while reading show that subjects are often not aware of the fact that their mind is wandering, even when they are taking part in an experiment in which they are expressly requested to pay attention to these absences (Schooler, 2002; Schooler et al., 2005).

Non verifiabiliy of results

A last group of arguments against the use of introspection as a scientific method invokes the non verifiable character of its results. This absence of verifiability is due to two factors, the private character and the singular character of experience. On the one hand, my subjective experience is private, inaccessible to anyone else; no one therefore has the means of verifying the accurateness of my description. On the other hand, a given experience is singular, unrepeatable, neither by others nor even by myself who is experiencing it: it is therefore impossible, for me as for others, to test the accuracy of a description by reproducing the described experience.

> Introspective reports offer no means for independent checks by which they may be evaluated. Indeed, the reports are irreplicable not only by others but even by the particular introspector himself (Wundt quoted by Shanon, 1984).

In these conditions, an introspective report is neither verifiable nor falsifiable, and it is this which prevents introspection from achieving the status of a science - the verifiability of results being considered the very basis of scientific methodology. Methods for studying lived experience, called 'first person' methods, would be in principle and by nature radically different from 'third person' methods used in the natural sciences.

The following quote summarizes the situation well:

> As introspection is not a rigorous method, one must not expect any scientific results from it. By using it one cannot hope to reach results of observation and experimentation that would be repeatable and controllable, in the way public observations and experiments in physics or in chemistry are controllable - since mental phenomena that introspection observes are private, inner, non public and communicable only by the means of language, by which one expresses them (Schlanger, 2001, p. 530).

II. Response to Criticisms

This picture looks catastrophic. Behind the researcher trying to evaluate the relevance of introspection for scientific research, these criticisms question the human being in us: what do we really know about our lived experience? Since our lived experience is the most personal and intimate thing about us, we think we are familiar with it, and cannot imagine for a moment that we could fail to perceive it or be misled about it. However, if I asked the reader to describe precisely his strategies of memorization for example, or how he proceeds in writing a letter or an article, or even in spelling a simple word, it is very likely that in a first stage, I would obtain quite poor descriptions. I would probably manage to collect the description of what you *know* about processes of memorization, of what you either heard or read on this topic, but in order to know precisely the way you really proceed, it would be necessary to carry out an in-depth examination. All of us (hopefully) know how to carry out these actions, but we have only a very partial consciousness of how we go about doing them. This indigence does not only concern our intellectual processes, but also our emotional processes, or even as fundamental and pervasive experiences as our bodily and sensory experiences (Schwitzgebel, 2008).

But if we are unaware of our experience, we are especially unaware of the particular experience consisting in accessing our lived experience and describing it. This experience has very little been studied for itself. Since Titchener[5] the necessity and the very possibility of

---

[5] 'Experimental introspection is a procedure that can be formulated; the introspecting psychologist can tell what he does and how he does it' (Titchener, 1912, p. 495).

describing the introspective act have rarely been envisaged.[6] However, research by practitioners of introspection who have not only practised it but have also attempted to describe their practice, show a convergence: introspection is a particular act, a specific process consisting in achieving very precise inner gestures. But these gestures do not consist in observing one's experience, in 'in-specting' or 'retro-specting' it, in producing a description which would reflect it precisely. This conception of introspection is a naive representation that does not rely on a precise, first-person knowledge of the introspective act. Therefore criticisms which rely on this preconception (based either on theoretical ideas or on instinctive introspection) in order to contest the adequacy of introspective reports on experience, are simply irrelevant. In the continuation of this text, we will use empirical[7] descriptions of the introspective act in order to develop a new conception of the validity of an introspective report. This validity is no longer measured in terms of 'truth' — conceived as adequacy or representative accurateness, but in terms of authenticity on the one hand, and of performative consistency on the other. We do not claim to present an exhaustive description of the introspective act,[8] which would go beyond the scope of this article. But on the basis of a preliminary work of description, we intend to pinpoint some lines of epistemological reflection.

In this section we will address successively each criticism identified in the previous section.

1. Introspecting, observing and becoming aware

First let's consider the arguments of impossible split and observational distortion.

As Titchener explained when denouncing 'stimulus error', 'introspecting' is being interested in the actual experience of an object and not in the object of an experience. It is not describing the properties of an object — the shades of green of the landscape I am watching, the smooth, soft, fresh character of the surface of my notebook, the characteristics of the sound of the bell. But it is describing my visual

---

[6] Even Schwitzgebel, who supports the idea that introspection is a skill (2004), does not embark in a description of this expertise.

[7] The word 'empirical' is used here with its extended etymological meaning (*empeirikos*: who has the experience of), and not with its restricted meaning of 'falling within experimental science'.

[8] Pierre Vermersch's article (this issue) is devoted to the description of the introspective process.

experience, my tactile experience, my auditory experience, what it is like or feels like to live these experiences.

But what is my 'experience' of the objects? What else do I have at hand other than objects or contents of experience? The landscape, my notebook, and even the sound of the bell, have some stability, I can quite easily identify their characteristics and describe them. But my experience of them is evanescent, as if transparent; my first impression is that I neither know what to say nor am able to say anything about them.

> Thus in my view, Descartes got things exactly backwards. The outside world of stable objects, people, and events is what we know the most directly and certainly. The 'inner world' of conscious experience is reflected on only rarely and is known only poorly. (Hurlburt & Schwitzgebel, 2007, p. 52)

For 'transparency theorists', we cannot access our experience as such. For Searle for example (1992), as a state of consciousness can only be described in the terms of what this state represents, the consciousness of the state cannot be distinguished from the consciousness of the represented object. Similarly Dretske (1995) argues that introspection is nothing other than a sort of 'displaced perception': we only know that we are in a given mental state by being aware of the object represented by this state.

> Such experiences (if experiences they be) as seeing and feeling seem to be, as it were, diaphanous: if we were asked to pay close attention, on a given occasion, to our seeing and feeling as distinct from what was being seen or felt, we should not know how to proceed; and the attempt to describe the differences between seeing and feeling seems to dissolve into a description of what we see and what we feel. (Grice, 2002, p. 45)

However a convinced 'transparency theorist', after saying that the sensation of blue is nothing other than blue, and that it vanishes if we try to fix our attention upon it, remarks: 'Yet [this sensation] can be distinguished, if we look attentively enough, and if we know that there is something to look for (Moore, 1903, p. 450).'[9]

But what must we look for, and how do we go about it?

Let us consider the first question. Usually, the concentration of attention upon the object of experience conceals the experience itself. If I look at a landscape or a painting, I immediately recognize elements which my attention focuses on and becomes absorbed in. My gaze stretches out, projects itself toward the object, over there, I lose

---

[9] For an extensive criticism of the transparency theory, the reader may refer to (Thompson, 2007, chapter 10).

contact with the immediate visual sensation. It is a little like a person driving in a nail with a hammer, whose attention is entirely directed toward the nail, and only has a transparent or 'pre-reflective' consciousness of the contact and variations of pressure of the hammer in the palm of his hand — to refer to a well-known example. When I hear a sound, the event that is at the source of the sound (the bell), immediately recognized, masks the auditory experience. As James noted, in the experience of movement, our interest in the object toward which the movement is directed (the ball, the apple) masks the movement of the limb, which itself conceals the internal sensations of movement in the muscles and joints that actually initiate the movement of the limb (1890/1983, p. 687). All our cognitive processes are also involved: whether we are memorizing, remembering, imagining, calculating, understanding or deciding, the absorption in the object or the objective, the 'what' of the process, overrides the 'how', which stays pre-reflected. For example while writing this article, I am completely absorbed by the content of the ideas I am trying to express. But I am barely aware of the rapid succession of inner images, inner comments, slight emotions, micro-operations of comparison, appreciation, amplification, letting go, which constitute my activity of writing. I am conscious 'in action' of this micro-activity, as I am actually writing. But I am not reflectively conscious of it.

Box 1: Imagining a mountain waterfall

(See next page; NB it is very important that the footnote[10], printed on this page only to avoid splitting the box, is not read until *after* the exercise has been completed.)

---

[10] For the purpose of this written exercise, we suppose that the reader succeeds in forming an image, and our questions focus on the characteristics of this image. But a real explicitation interview, taking into account the possibility that the reader has done something different than imagining, would begin with a much more open (or 'openbiginninged', according to Hurlburt in this issue) question such as: 'When I asked you to imagine a mountain waterfall, what happened first?'. The following prompts would have been adapted to the answers of the interviewed person. Moreover, this exercise does not mean that the imagining experience must be determinate with regard to all the characteristics being asked about, as the questions posed in this box suggest.

> **Box 1: Imagining a mountain waterfall**
>
> I would like to invite you to participate in a small experiment. Take your time, here and now, to imagine a mountain waterfall. Make a pause at this point, and wait until you have completed your work of imagination before reading the next sentences.
>
> Now I propose you to answer the following questions. Did this waterfall appear in color or in black and white? Was this image clear or fuzzy? Was it stable or fleeting? Was it an imaginary waterfall, or a waterfall that you had seen before? Was the visual scene accompanied by sounds? By smells? By bodily sensations? Did you see this image as if it was a photograph or a film? Or were you 'inside the scene', in the location of the waterfall?
>
> Now if you saw a photo: where did you see it (at the top at the bottom, to the right, to the left)? How far away was this image? How big was it? If you were 'inside the scene': were you seeing it from your own eyes, from your own point of view? Or were you seeing it from the eyes of another person in the scene? Or from elsewhere in the scene? In the last case, did you see yourself looking at the waterfall?
>
> So what was the goal of my questions? It was to redirect your attention from the content of the visual experience (the waterfall), which usually absorbs our attention, toward the synchronic structural characteristics of this experience, which are usually pre-reflective: for example, the dimensions of the image, its localisation in space, or your 'perceptual position' outside or inside the scene.
>
> Now you could achieve a slightly different gesture, consisting of diverting your attention from the image once stabilized, towards the dynamics of its appearance, its genesis: was the image or scene preceded by other candidate images? Did the final image appear at once, complete, or was it progressively constituted? Which sensorial dimension appeared first, the visual, the tactile, the auditory, the olfactory, (or maybe the gustatory)? From the instant where I asked you to imagine a waterfall, did you say anything to yourself? Did you feel anything particular? When precisely did you know that you were 'imagining a mountain waterfall'?
>
> These questions help you to turn your attention from the content of the experience towards its — often pre-reflective — diachronic structure. *[See footnote 10 on previous page]*

The pre-reflective[11] part of our experience seems to include different levels of depth, which are increasingly difficult to become reflectively aware of. If all of us can easily turn our attention toward the sensation of our feet in our shoes, who among us is able to recognize the part of the body (finger, arm, shoulder, stomach or head) that initiates the movement when he or she tries to catch an object (Shusterman, 2008, p. 94)? Who among us has a clear awareness of the criteria which enable him or her to appreciate the relevance of a formulation while writing?

Let us now consider the second question: how can we go from a first order or pre-reflective to a second order, reflective or introspective[12] consciousness of experience? In an article relating a recent study, Overgaard recognizes that the distinction between first order and introspective consciousness is not only a conceptual, but also an experiential distinction. But when he asks the subjects: 'Every time you see a picture, you are not to think about it as a figure out there on the screen. Instead, you are to think of it as an experience you are having' (Overgaard & Sorensen, 2004, p. 80) what are they supposed to do? Most traditional definitions of introspection as well as recent ones imply that this act consists in observing oneself, in the same way as one would observe an object outside, but by turning one's eye inward:

> Looking inside in order to see what happens in there: this is in a nutshell the essential of introspection. (...) We look at ourselves being, thinking, acting — as if we were a sight for ourselves (Schlanger, 2001, p. 528).

In this perspective, introspection or reflection is seen as a deliberate act of objectification, separating and distancing, whose direction is simply the opposite of the usual form of objectification, which is directed towards the outside. Consciousness turns towards itself, reflecting itself. It is this kind of conception that makes the image denounced by Comte of a division of the subject himself unavoidable. 'Reflection (...) involves a kind of self-fission. (...) It makes subjective life thematic in a way that involves self-division and self-distanciation' (Gallagher & Zahavi, 2008, p. 61).

However, from the descriptions of this act which are grounded in disciplined practice quite another vision is emerging: becoming aware of one's experience does not consist in distancing oneself from it in order to observe it, considering it as an object, but on the contrary in

---

[11] To use the vocabulary of Husserl (1913), later adopted by Sartre (1936 and 1938) and Ricœur (1950). Piaget (1974) speaks of 'consciousness in action', Vermersch (2000) speaks of 'direct consciousness'. The French word for 'pre-reflective' is 'pré-réfléchi'.

[12] In the remainder of this article we will use these three terms indifferently.

reducing the distance, in coming closer to it. It is not a matter of splitting into two in order to look at one's experience, but of coming into contact with it. 'Suppose that instead of wanting to raise ourselves above our perception of things, we plunged into it to dig it out and enlarge it.'[13] It is not about stopping or fixing the course of experience, in order to observe it while immobilizing it under the beam of garish light of consciousness. In this sense James's metaphor of the light being switched on, and the visual model that underlies it, are deceptive. Rather than switching the light on suddenly to see what the room looks like in the dark, it is rather exploring it in the dark, patiently, by feel, with precision and delicacy, a little as a blind person would do. It is not a matter of 'looking at' one's experience but of 'tasting' it or 'dwelling in' it.

This exploration is encouraged by a particular attentional disposition, which is both open and receptive. Unlike focused attention, which is narrow, concentrated on a particular content, this attention is panoramic, peripheral, open on a vast area. This diffuse attention is however very fine, and sensitive to the most subtle changes. Several people have described this openness to us as a subtle shift of the area usually perceived as the centre of attention towards the back of the skull, or from the head down into the body.

This attentional disposition is also described as non intentional, receptive. This characteristic seems paradoxical because it is difficult for us to conceive of attention as being other than intentional, actively focused toward a goal and a given object. However numerous testimonies describe another type of attention that while being very alert and awake, remains loosened, detached, receptive. It does not consist in stretching toward experience to scrutinize it, recognize it, and characterize it immediately. But in being present at the singular situation, open to anything that may arise. This disposition allows us to become aware of dimensions of experience that the stretching toward a goal usually makes imperceptible. The only thing that one can do is to adopt the required attentional disposition and let consciousness come.[14] It is rather like looking at a stereogram:[15] for the motif to appear in all its depth and transparency, nothing must be forced; one

---

[13] Merleau-Ponty (1943, p. 22) quoting Bergson (1934, p. 148).

[14] This particular disposition is described in detail in (Petitmengin-Peugeot, 1999) and (Petitmengin, 2001, pp. 183-191 and 251-268). This disposition corresponds to the attitude of 'letting go' described in (Depraz et al. 2003, chapter 1.2). The reader can also refer to Charles Genoud's article in this issue.

[15] For example *Magic Eye: A New Way of Looking at the World*, Andrews and McMeel Publishing, 1993.

must simply adopt the required position of receptivity and then wait. This act is devoid of intentionality, in the two senses of the term: neither a will or particular expectancy, nor the grasping of an object.

This process does not mean either diverting one's attention from the external objects toward an inner world, to intro-spect. Because when we free ourselves from the absorption into the objects of experience to explore our experience of the objects, the separation which is usually perceived between an inner and an outer world proves to be much more permeable. This process rather enables us to come into contact with the pre-reflective dimension of experience where this scission originates (Petitmengin, 2007).

In a remarkable article (Zahavi, 2003, integrated in Zahavi, 2008, chapter 4), Dan Zahavi analyses Heidegger's answer to Natorp's criticism according to which reflection fails to account for subjective experience because it turns it into an object. Heidegger agrees with Natorp that any investigation that seeks to grasp experience as an object is bound to fail. But he argues that a true phenomenological understanding, far from implying the withdrawal and distancing from experience required if the subject is to bend backward and stare at itself, consists of gaining acquaintance, familiarity or sympathy with experience. This process 'entails neither a seizing of the life nor a stilling of its stream, but simply a going along with, or rather a being carried along with the stream of life'. (Zahavi, 2003, p. 173, quoting a 'rather unique passage' at the end of the lecture course *Grundprobleme der Phänomenologie* of 1919/1920). This remark is developed by Sartre (1934, p. 83) when he points out that 'phenomenological reduction' simply consists in relaxing *all* efforts consciousness makes to elude itself by giving itself objects, including the effort it makes to give itself an 'interior' object.

In this perspective, the process of emergence into reflective consciousness is not an observational process. It is not either a process of reflection of pre-reflective experience by a second order consciousness that would reflect, mirror or copy the first one. These are abstract representations, which are not based on real practice, they simply do not correspond to what an individual does concretely when 'introspecting.' As the etymology of the terms 'introspection' and 'reflection' reinforce these preconceptions, we consider them inappropriate and will limit their use as far as possible in the remainder of this text.

Therefore the criticisms of 'introspection' that invoke an observational distortion lose their relevance. Indeed between reflective and pre-reflective consciousness there is no relationship of correspondence, the one copying or reflecting the other one in a more or less exact way. On the contrary, during the process of becoming aware, a transformation occurs, very fortunately because this is the 'raison d'être' of this process.

> The (introspective) analysis changes the experience, and this change is not, as is sometimes supposed, an inevitable and deplorable accident, but its purpose and aim. (Bode, 1913)

It is not about minimizing or overlooking this change, but about eliciting on the one hand what it consists of, on the other hand which process induces it. The latter question — crucial because the authenticity of a description relies on a disciplined unfolding of this process — will be addressed in the following sections of this article. As for the first question, we will reformulate it in this way: 'How does reflective experience differ from pre-reflective experience?', or more simply: 'What does reflective consciousness bring to experience?' Surprisingly, this extremely important question has been little investigated. In the non observational perspective, reflective consciousness is not a second consciousness that stares at the former, at the risk of reifying, freezing, distorting or disturbing it. There is only one consciousness which, when becoming self-aware, intensifies, amplifies, lights up (Fink, 1992; Prinz, 2004). A slight form of attention to experience accompanies and accentuates this, but without focusing and without effort. This 'non observational awareness' (Marcel, 2003, p. 178) is not disturbing but liberating. Becoming aware of the pre-reflective micro-dynamics of lived experience introduces a space into it that opens up considerable possibilities of transformation. Here are some examples:

- Becoming aware of the subtle pre-reflective sensations that announce the onset of a seizure enables the epileptic patient to control his/her seizures, which improves significantly his/her quality of life (Petitmengin et al., 2007).

- Developing an early consciousness of the subtle symptoms that precede the emergence of an emotion, and of the micro-gestures that maintain and amplify it, makes it possible to learn to foil and calm the emotional process before the intensity of emotion causes possible suffering (Philippot & Segal, this issue).

- Alexander's work shows that our usual focusing on the desired goals conceals what we really do in our bodily action and posture, preventing us from seeing how what we do impedes what we want to do. Whereas being aware of our bodily experience makes us more precise and effective (Shusterman, 2008, p. 259).

- An increased mindfulness of one's bodily experience seems to play a determining role in the process of transformative learning (Mathison & Tosey, 2009, this issue).

Far from disrupting it, freezing it or shrinking it, it seems that an increased consciousness of experience makes it more efficient, more fluid and meaningful, contrary to what indeed happens in the attitude that would consist in trying to consider oneself as an object. Entering into contact with our experience does not divide us into two but gives us back our entirety, our integrity.

Finally, let's notice that the goal of *vipassana* meditation is precisely to gain such a reflective awareness of experience. A very old Buddhist sûtra express this very simply:

> When the practitioner is walking, he knows: 'I am walking'. When standing, he knows: 'I am standing'. When sitting, he knows: 'I am sitting'. When lying down, he knows: 'I am lying down'. Whatever his body does he is aware of,' (...) In eating, drinking, chewing or savouring, he does so with full awareness; in walking, in standing, in sitting, in falling asleep, in waking, in speaking or in keeping silent, he does so with full awareness. This is how he remains mindful of the body. [16]

'When walking, he knows he is walking': the *vipassana* practitioner walks while being conscious of walking, in other words he is reflectively conscious of his bodily experience — the subsequent stages of this training being mindfulness of sensations / feelings (*vedanâ*), of the mind (*citta*), and of mental contents (*dharma*). The goal is not to reach a special ('altered') state of consciousness, but to become increasingly aware of what is usually lived through but remains unnoticed, in other words it is to recognize what is there (Genoud, this issue).

2. Retrospecting and evoking

Let us now examine the argument of temporal distorsion.

How can we go from a pre-reflective to a reflective consciousness of experience? How can we come into contact with our experience? Because of the absorption of our attention into the object, the extreme rapidity of the unfolding of experience, and the richness of the pre-reflective dimension, it is usually very difficult to come into

---

[16] *Sattipatthâna-sutta (Four Foundations of Mindfulness), Dîgha-Nikâya*, 22 or *Majjhima-Nikâya*, 10.

contact with the pre-reflected dimension of experience while it is taking place. But this coming into contact may be facilitated by a specific state, the evocation state, which enables us to recall or re-enact a past experience. According to Sartre (1934, p. 30), 'Any irreflective consciousness, being a non-thetic consciousness of itself, leaves a non-thetic memory that can be consulted.'

The evocation state falls within a type of memory which has been called 'concrete memory' (Ribot, 1881; Gusdorf, 1950), and more recently 'episodic memory' (Cohen, 1989) or 'autobiographical memory' (Neisser, 1982). This type of memory is not based on a deliberate desire or project to remember; rather, the experience is memorized non-intentionally by the subject. Moreover, in concrete memory the recalling of the memory is also involuntary: it does not occur on the initiative of discursive thought, but spontaneously, usually through the intermediary of a sensorial trigger. Thus the memory cannot be deliberately set off, but it is possible to indirectly prepare for its emergence by rediscovering the sensations linked to the experience. For example, if you were asked: 'What is the first thought you had when you woke up this morning?' it is quite probable that there would be no way for recovering this memory other than returning in thought to your bed at the moment when you awoke. Therefore the trigger may be visual (in order to remember the experience, you recall the visual context of the experience, what you were seeing at that moment). The trigger may be auditory (you recall the sounds, such as the birds singing or the alarm clock going off). It may be kinaesthetic (your recall for example the position of your body). It may be olfactory or gustative (as in Proust's well known 'madeleine', the evocation of which enabled him to recall very precisely one scene, and then whole chapters, of his childhood).

The evocation state allows the emergence into reflective consciousness of dimensions of experience that were not only memorised unvoluntarily, but moreover remained unnoticed at the very moment of experience. This emergence unfolds progressively, through successive strata, each new evocation of a given experience eliciting the unfolding of a new dimension.[17]

But knowing how to elicit this evocation state is a very specific skill. This is why we consider that it is indispensable, for inexperienced subjects being asked to describe their experience, to be accompanied in this process by a skilled person. In our opinion, one of the reasons why the subjects questioned by Nisbett and Wilson (1977)

---

[17] This process is described in this issue by Vermersch who calls it 'leafing through'.

failed to describe their experience of choosing a photograph, is this lack of guidance. Because if someone describes his/her experience without evoking it precisely, relying only on a vague memory, all that he is able to do is to describe what he *believes* he has done, or *thinks* he might have done — not his experience but his beliefs, implicit theories and judgments about his experience. This is precisely what happened to Nisbett and Wilson's subjects, and this is the reason why according to us, these experiments — while being very instructive – do not invalidate at all the possibility of becoming aware of one's experience in a disciplined way. Nisbett and Wilson's subjects were simply not 'introspecting', i.e. performing the process that would have enabled them to come into contact with their experience.

'But how can we be sure that the evoked experience is true to the initial experience, and is not a rebuilt experience?' — are we often asked. This question implies that only the initial experience can be 'pure', the experience of evocation being a second order experience, an ersatz of experience likely to be distorted to various degrees. We would answer that nobody can live an experience 'in the past', there is no other experience than the present. It is therefore impossible to 're-live' a past experience, or to access it 'retrospectively', through a problematic splitting into two that would enable subjects to observe themselves. In the evocation state, the subject lives a new experience. Therefore the question of knowing in abstracto, from a 'cosmic exile' standpoint, if the experience of evocation coincides with the initial experience, or is a true copy of it, is epistemologically irrelevant. It is only from within current experience that the existence of any alleged match between experiences can be investigated. As we'll develop later on, 'being true to' does not hold between two experiences, but as an internal mark of one experience.

In point of fact the particular experience consisting of evoking a past experience, while 'slowing down' in a way the unfolding of experience, enables us to come into contact, here and now, with dimensions of experience which are usually concealed by our instantaneous absorption into objects. A certain type of memory enables us to become reflectively conscious of the structure of our experience. Therefore what is important is not that the evoked *content* is exactly identical to the content of the initial experience. What is important is not that the mountain waterfall that you are evoking now is exactly identical to the waterfall you imagined a moment ago. What is important is that, thanks to the experience of evocation, you become reflectively aware of the synchronic and diachronic *structure* of the experience of imagining.[18]

On the other hand, it is important that the process of evocation unfolds correctly. It is a very precise process, quite different from the process of constructing a description or describing a vague memory, a belief or a theory. Practiced persons have internal criteria that inform them about the intensity of their own evocation state, and know how to achieve the very precise micro-actions that enable them to elicit or to revive this state. Trained interviewers have linguistic devices able to elicit or revive this state in another person, and objective criteria for evaluating its intensity.

An example of objective indicator is the direction of the eyes: when a subject is evoking a past experience, he takes his eyes off the interviewer to look 'into space', to the horizon. At the same time, the flow of speech slows down, and the words are often cut with silences: these para-verbal clues are the sign that the subject is coming into contact with the pre-reflective dimension of his experience. Co-verbal gestures often appear, indicating that the subject is in contact — or attempting to make contact — with his experience.

Let's add that we are not condemned to be reflectively conscious of our experience only in the evocation state. Once aware of a characteristic of my experience thanks to the evocation state, I can verify its existence 'in real time'. For example, the epileptic patients we interviewed, although they became aware of their preictal symptoms while evoking a past crisis, now know how to recognize them during the preictal period. Thus evocation is a procedure whose final aim is to acquire an increasingly fine reflective awareness of one's experience in real time.[19]

3. Interpreting and bracketing presuppositions

We will now consider the argument of interpretative distortion.

If lived experience is concealed by our fascination for the objects of experience, it is also masked by our preconceptions and beliefs about experience. Can we learn to perceive our experience as it is, and not as we think or believe it is? Can we learn to 'bracket' our presup-

---

[18] 'If Melanie uses a newly (re-)created image in place of an original image, we still find something about the characteristics of Melanie's images' (Hurlburt & Schwitzgebel, 2007, p. 151).

[19] Is it possible to acquire reflective consciousness of one's experience without calling on evocation? To what extent can *vipassana* meditation for example do without evocation? An answer to this question would require a precise comparison, through first person reports, of explicitation and meditation techniques.

positions, preconceptions and implicit theories about our experience? Again, this process has been little described. Phenomenologists, who consider the 'phenomenological reduction' as the core of their method, are very discreet about the way to achieve this gesture concretely. Even in the interview methods where it is agreed that 'the main skills of the investigator's task are to bracket the investigator's own presuppositions and to help the subject bracket the subject's own presuppositions' (Hurlburt & Schwitzgebel, 2007, p. 263), these skills are little described. The practice of the interview of explicitation leads us to distinguish the *devices* that make it possible to elicit the gesture of reduction in the context of an interview, from this gesture of reduction itself.

When persons try to describe a given experiential process (whether it is cognitive, emotional or perceptual), they start spontaneously by describing what they believe they do, what they imagine they do. A particular effort is necessary to enable them to 'bracket' their representations, beliefs, judgments and commentaries, in order to access their experience itself. In the context of an interview, a set of devices enable a trained interviewer to help the person (Vermersch, 1994; Petitmengin, 2006). First of all, these devices consist in helping the subject to shift from a general description to the description of a singular experience, which is precisely situated in time and space. Then even though this experience has just been lived, the interviewer helps the subject to evoke it and stabilize this evocation (Vermersch, 1994, chapter 5; Petitmengin, 2006, p. 244–46). Afterwards, 'content empty'[20] questions help the subject to become aware of the different structural — diachronic and synchronic — dimensions of his experience, and to give a verbal description of them. It is important to note that the key question is the question 'how', the question 'why', which makes the subject irresistibly veer toward explanations and abstract considerations, being proscribed.[21] Such guidance, even when the subject first asserts: 'I am doing nothing', or 'I know how to do it, but

---

[20] 'Content-empty' questions are questions which guide the interviewee's attention towards the various moments and dimensions of his experience, which flag them without suggesting any content (Vermersch 2004). This type of 'content-empty' questioning enables the researcher to obtain a precise description without infiltrating his own presuppositions.

[21] This point is illustrated very well by Nisbett and Wilson's experiments (1977), recently confirmed by Johansson's, where verbal reports are elicited by the question 'why?'. 'To solicit the verbal reports we simply asked the participants why they chose the way they did (Johansson & al., 2006, p. 675).' When an untrained subject is asked for the reason for his choice, he slips automatically, without even noticing it, toward abstraction. It is therefore not surprising that the comparative linguistic analysis of the verbal reports of the manipulated subjects (explaining a choice that they didn't make) and of the non manipulated subjects (explaining their actual choice) shows no difference. In both cases, the subjects are

I don't know what I am doing', usually allows him to leave the level of abstract preconceptions to become aware, often with much surprise, of unnoticed processes, and to describe them very precisely.

Here again, a set of precise clues enable the interviewer/researcher to evaluate the degree of contact of the subject with his experience, and therefore the authenticity of his description (Hendricks, this issue). One of these is the concrete character of the vocabulary: the absence of abstract categories, of psychological concepts, is an indicator that the subject is not describing theoretical knowledge but is absorbed in his experience, in contact with it.[22] These concepts or categories are not present in the description. Abstracting them from the description will be the researcher's task in the aftermath of the interview.

For example, the subject does not say 'This bird song elicits in me the evocation of a spring morning' — sentence that contains a meta-knowledge (evocation) and an explanatory interpretation (elicits in me). He rather says 'I feel refreshed and cleared', 'the air is like in a spring morning'. He does not say 'I have the mental picture of an elephant', but 'I see an elephant', or even 'there is an elephant.' The more a person enters into contact with her experience, the more the vocabulary becomes simple, direct, concrete.[23]

The more the gesture of reduction is trained and refined, the more the detected and abandoned preconceptions are subtle. Because it is one thing to abandon your implicit theories about decision making to become aware of the process that led you to choose this pair of socks; and quite another to abandon your naive theories on perception to become aware of the micro-processes that led you to recognize here a pair of stockings (Schwitzgebel, 2008). Or to abandon your body image to come into contact with your concretely felt bodily experience, in other words to shift from 'the thought of the body or the body in idea' to 'the experienced body or the body in reality' (Merleau-Ponty, 1945, p. 231).

It is important to underline that the gesture of reduction is not a matter of intellectual, conceptual understanding. It does not consist in

---

not in contact with the experience associated with the process of choice, but give it a theoretical justification. A specific guidance is necessary to enable them to become aware of the 'how' of their choice and to describe it.

[22] Prinz (2004) distinguishes 'mere captioning' from 'psychological captioning' which uses psychological terms, raising the possibility that different processes could be involved.

[23] The article of Mary Hendricks in this issue provides an analysis of the somatic and linguistic criteria enabling the therapist or researcher to evaluate the 'level of experiencing', i.e. the degree of contact of a subject with his/her experience.

shifting from a naive conception to an expert conception, but in leaving the conceptual level, in agreeing to lose one's conceptual landmarks. It is a gesture of loosening, of letting go, that implies an attitude of receptiveness, humility, and in a way vulnerability. One of the clues that the subject has actually achieved this gesture is the surprise he feels when discovering an unexpected dimension, for which he cannot find any pre-existing conceptual category. It is then difficult to suspect him of being influenced by a preconception (Vermersch, 2000; Hurlburt & Schwitzgebel, 2007).

Coming into contact with experience is not therefore acquiring some new knowledge about experience, but rather striping ourselves of the knowledge that prevents us from entering into contact with experience. It is a process of simplification and distillation rather than complication and enrichment. This iterative process (Hurlburt, this issue), that enables us to free ourselves from increasingly subtle preconceptions in order to have more intimate contact with experience, seems to have a specific structure. A better understanding of this structure - the different stages of this letting go, and the succession of minute gestures that enable us to come closer and closer to experience — requires a meticulous investigation of the reverse micro-process of superimposition to experience, of its different stages and of the different mechanisms of resistance that make us impervious to it.

4. Describing experience

We will now consider the argument of verbal distortion.

If the capacity of words to describe lived experience has been questioned, the process of description itself has been little studied and described. The few descriptions that have been made show that it consists of precise inner gestures, usually concealed by the rapidity and spontaneity of verbalization: entering into contact with experience, testing the quality of this contact, intensifying this contact, letting words come, confronting words with experience to evaluate their appropriacy.[24] These gestures can be learned and perfected, or facilitated by the questions and prompts of an expert interviewer. The authenticity of a description relies on this being carried out correctly.

It has been noticed that the gestures that enable the *description* of an experience differ in subtle ways from those that enable the *expression* of this experience (Petitmengin, 2007, p. 72; Hurlburt & Schwitzgebel,

---

[24] This process is described in detail by E. Gendlin in (Gendlin, 1962) and in the context of the 'Thinking at the Edge' method (for example in 'Introduction to thinking at the edge' and 'Making concepts from experience'). See also (Petitmengin, 2007).

2007, p. 156). When I am in contact with a feeling, I can *express* it through a poem, a picture or a dance, but I can also try to *describe* as precisely as possible its sensorial characteristics, as well as the process of its emergence, transformation and disappearance. For example, I can express a given emotion by writing: 'The setting sun is lighting up the woods / Joy is opening its wings / How the sky is blue and boundless!' (Victor Hugo, 1982). But I can also make a less poetic description: 'a sensation of heat in the centre of my chest, which intensifies, becomes bigger, and then rises in my throat'. How does what someone carries out in order to enter into contact with their experience and describe it differ from what the poet does? A meticulous work of description and comparison of these two know-hows would enable us to answer this question. A possible difference might be related to the use of metaphors: whereas expression calls extensively and loosely on it, description needs precise vocabulary, which for the time being we lack. But why not create it? (Wittgenstein, 1992, § 610 p. 291) What prevents us from introducing new words that would enable us to refer to the various dimensions of our experience – for example words coming from a disciplined and collective use of metaphor or metonymy (Findlay, 1948), rather than from free metaphors as in poetic expression? Why not refine our vocabulary gradually as we become more skilful and discriminating in exploring our lived experience? Why not follow the same way by which oenologists have created a very rich vocabulary in order to describe the olfactory and gustatory experience of wine (Courtier, 2007)?

The explicitation process, with its use of verbal descriptions, has been criticised for transforming experience, and notably altering it by decomposing and dissecting it. But what do words do to experience? What does the investigation of the process of explicitation teach us about this question? One thing it teaches us is that the fact of expliciting indeed transforms experience: it does not consist in putting words on an experience that would pre-exist to them and would remain unaltered by them. But neither does it consist of dissecting experience. On the contrary, it has the effect of unfolding experience, while enriching it with new nuances. The word — whether it is 'this', or 'this strange thing' — is a sort of pointer or 'handle' that enables us to discriminate and intensify slight differences in experience. 'The snow that had just fallen had a very strange aspect, different from the usual appearance of snow. I decided to call it "micacé", and it seemed to me, as I chose this name, that this difference became more distinct and more fixed than it was before' (James, 1890/1983, p. 484). In a subsequent description, by relying on this new word ('micacé') the

THE VALIDITY OF FIRST-PERSON DESCRIPTIONS   389

subject will be able to refine his consciousness of this experience even more, to intensify his contact with it. In the same way in our study of the auditory experience (Petitmengin *et al.*, this issue), the development of an appropriate vocabulary allowed us to progressively refine our consciousness of this experience.

However, the fact of relying on words, of describing on the basis of previous descriptions, without coming back to the experience, may end up in provoking a sort of absorption into words, and in becoming cut off from experience. The freshness of contact with experience gets lost, the words become disembodied. We may have the feeling of pronouncing empty words, 'to be only in the words'. But there are some internal criteria which can inform us about this loss of contact, allowing us to revive the evocation through specific micro-operations and to enable fresh, more precise words to emerge. And the search for these internal criteria can be promoted through specific guidance by the interviewer.

Words as such don't display experience, they only point at it. As Heidegger wrote, 'phenomenological concepts cannot communicate their full content, but only indicate it' (Zahavi, 2003, p. 173). Words have the power to help the speaker to amplify, to unfold his experience. They also have the power to trigger the unfolding of an experience in the reader or listener, thanks to a specific activity of understanding, recognition, appropriation, simulation, entering the situation to feel what the other feels.[25] But words are not experience, nor do they provide it. Their whole power resides in this capacity to refine, amplify, rigidify or conceal a dimension that does not belong to the same order. In themselves, words are empty, they only become meaningful through the gesture that relates them to experience.

In this perspective, the question of knowing if a verbal report corresponds to experience exactly, reflects it precisely, loses its meaning. The validity of a description cannot be assessed according to its ability to reproduce the described *content*, but according to the quality of its own production *process*.

More generally, we are witnessing the emergence of a new conception of the validity of a description, which cannot be measured in static terms of correspondence to experience, but in dynamic terms of authenticity of the process of becoming aware and describing. Whether they are objective or subjective, the criteria of validity we

---

[25] What does the experience of 'understanding the experience of somebody else' consist of? This experience has been little studied. On this topic the reader can refer to an interesting article by Spiegelberg (1975). See also the literature on 'simulation theory of other minds' (Goldman, 1992).

have do not inform us about the adequacy of the description content, but about the subject's level of contact with experience. The validity of a description is not evaluated by comparing it with its hypothetical 'object', but according to the authenticity of the process that generated it.

5. 'Verifying' introspective reports

In order to deal more extensively with the final question of the verifiability of introspective verbal reports, we still have to differentiate carefully between three levels of abstraction: the experience itself, the description of this experience and the type of experience which is described.

Singularity, privacy and reproducibility

First of all, a given *experience* (a token of experience) is singular and non reproducible either by others or even by the person who lives it. I will never relive the instant that I am living. I will never smell again the perfume of this rose. I will never relive the present experience of imagining this mountain waterfall.

A lived experience is not only singular but private, and inaccessible to others. I do not have access to the particular quality of your experience when you are imagining a mountain waterfall, to the 'what it is like' of your experience.

The experience of *describing* a particular experience of mine (a token of description) it also singular and non reproducible. On the other hand, the result of this description is potentially accessible to anyone.

Furthermore, whereas a *token* of experience is singular, I can live a given *type* of experience several times: the experience of smelling the perfume of a rose, the experience of imagining a mountain waterfall, correspond to types of experience which are reproducible. And the experience of describing a given type of experience also corresponds to a type of experience which is reproducible: if I know the operating mode, I can reproduce at will singular descriptions of singular experiences of imagining a mountain waterfall. And all these descriptions are accessible to anybody who wants to read or hear them.

Therefore the researcher who investigates lived experience does not have access to the experience of the subjects he interviews, but he has access to the descriptions they produce.[26] And the descriptions of a given *type* of experience are reproducible (on the condition that one knows the operating mode).

Things are not different in experimental sciences. The type/token analysis apply as well. An event, whether it is astronomical, geological, or physiological, is singular and non reproducible. The measurements of a particular event are also singular and non reproducible. On the other hand, a given *type* of event is reproducible, as well as the corresponding measurements, *if the researcher knows the operating mode enabling him to make these measurements.*

Moreover, the researcher does not have access to events or processes 'in themselves', he only has access to the 'data' he can collect through the intermediary of his instruments of measurement and recording (Piccinini, 2007). The astronomer does not have access to astronomical events, but only to various ranges of (generally electromagnetic) radiations, to their spectrum, to their interferometric images, etc. The neurologist does not have access to the activity of the brain as such, but only to the neuroelectric or neurometabolic activity his tools enable him to record (to which cerebral activity cannot be reduced). Therefore the real criteria of validation of scientific descriptions cannot be their correspondence with the process 'in itself', but another criterion that a recent current of the philosophy of scientific experimentation has termed 'enlarged consistency' or 'performative consistency'.[27] Performative consistency consists of an agreement among (a) the theories, (b) the construction of devices and the understanding of their functioning, (c) the theoretical guidance of measurements, and (d) the results (Pickering, 1995). More simply, performative consistency may be limited to an agreement between the perceptive interpretation of an image and the result of actions guided by perception. Let's consider an example of this kind, discussed by Hacking (1983): the interpretation of images coming from a fluorescent microscope (or X rays). Does one need to ascertain 'correspondence' of these interpreted images with 'the real object itself' in order to consider them as valid? Not at all. On the one hand the comparison of the image with 'the object itself' is impossible (at the very most can

---

[26] But unlike Dennett, we do not think that one can access the other's experience by way of a purely theoretical and abstract reconstruction from verbal descriptions. Rather, the interviewer can only do that by relying on a process of resonance with his or her own experience (see below).

[27] Consistency is said to be 'enlarged' because it does not limit itself to a logical matching of the parts of a theory, but also concerns the active interventions of the experimenters and the answers given by their experimental devices. The fact that this system also includes experimental activity makes also qualifies it as 'performative'.

we compare several images coming from different types of microscopes). And on the other hand, the researcher can do completely without such a comparison in practice. Instead of comparing, he contents himself with *acting* under the supposition that the image is correct, and with insuring that the result of the action, controlled by a new image of the same microscope, is in conformity with what the initial image permitted him to foresee. In sum the criterion of validity of the image limits itself to an enlarged consistency between the image, the interventions that it makes possible to guide, and another image of the same type that highlights the consequences of these interventions. Validation relies on a form of consistency and not on 'correspondence' (Shanon, 1984). True, when performative coherence has been reached and stabilized in some given scientific field, it is tempting to believe that this reveals a *correspondence* between a theory and its external object. Such a shortcut may help, as a provisional incentive to use the said theory as a guide for action. But it should not be endowed with any ontological significance. Indeed, when a scientific revolution occurs and new broader cycles of performative coherence emerge, one often realizes retrospectively that former beliefs about the strict one-one correspondence between the older theory and its putative objects were unwarranted.

In the case of first person experience, two types of validation on the 'consistency' mode are possible: the validation of a singular description and the validation of a type of description.

Idiographic validation

The *public* character of a singular verbal report and of the behavioural clues that accompany it enable the researcher to evaluate its validity through a number of objective criteria. On the one hand, precise clues — linguistic clues as well as para-verbal and non verbal ones — enable the researcher to assess the level of contact of the subject with his own experience (Hendricks, this issue). These are indications of the *authenticity* of the description. On the other hand, the design of appropriate 'experiential protocols' enables the correlation of a description with objective measurements. For example, a task consisting in memorizing a matrix of numbers may be complemented by questions chosen in such a way that the response time varies according to the strategy adopted (visual or auditory). The answers to these questions bring elements of confirmation or invalidation to the description of the corresponding experieince (Vermersch, 2000). In the same vein, Hurlburt suggests creating tasks to enable correlating the description of reading strategies to measurements of the reading time (Hurlburt & Schwitzgebel, 2007, p. 274). In this case the researcher obtains indications enabling him to evaluate the degree of coherent connection of the description to the described experience.

Intersubjective validation

The public *and reproducible* character of descriptions of a same type of experience also enables intersubjective validation. In fact our lived experience, far from being a simple 'draft', is structured. Analyzing and comparing a set of descriptions of experiences of the same type makes it possible to abstract from them a structure, that is 'a network of relationships between descriptive categories, independent of the experiential content' (Delattre, 1971). Comparing the structures which have been detected in different subjects, by different research groups, for a given type of experience, may then enable the detection of generic experiential categories,[28] that is generic structures, which brings a presumptive mark of validity to the initial descriptions.[29]

The objective of this process is close to that of Husserlian phenomenological psychology, which does not consist in collecting a set of descriptions of particular subjective experiences, 'a singular and facticial sequence of lived moments' (1993, p. 99), but to identify the invariant, essential, structures of psychic life. But the methods are different: in order to identify these invariants, we do not use the Husserlian method of eidetic variation, which consists in varying in one's imagination the adumbrations of an object, in order to detect the constant, essential features, of our experience of this object. But we proceed by progressive abstraction from the description of several real experiences.[30] The identified structures are qualified as 'synchronic' when they concern the configuration of experience at a given instant. They are qualified as 'diachronic' when they concern the evolution of experience in time.

Here are a few examples of generic structures.

---

[28] Generic experiential categories are meta-knowledge. They must not be confused with the reflective consciousness (sometimes termed meta-awareness) of a singular experience, which does not require the recognition of this dimension as generic (a confusion that seems to have been made by Schooler, 2004).

[29] An example of this work of abstraction of experiential categories from a set of descriptions (of the experience of emergence of an intuition) is given in (Petitmengin-Peugeot, 1999) and (Petitmengin, 2001, chapter 2).

[30] As Merleau-Ponty wrote, 'Eidetic psychology is a reading *of invariant structures* of our experience from imaginary cases, while scientific psychology, relying on induction, is a reading *from real cases*'. (Sorbonne lectures published in *Bulletin de psychologie*, 236, XVIII, 3-6, nov. 1964, p. 147)

- Let's consider again the example of mountain waterfall. The 'what it is like' of the scene you imagined is singular and private. The content of the scene may vary indefinitely. On the other hand, whatever its content is, an imaginary scene is always perceived from a given 'viewpoint', a given perceptual — egocentric or allocentric — position. Moreover, in the experience of imagining a scene, at a given moment each sensory modality is characterised by a specific perceptual position, which may differ from one modality to the other: for example I can be in 'self' position in the visual mode, and in 'other' position in the auditory mode (Andreas & Andreas, this issue). The perceptual position is therefore a complex experiential variable belonging to the generic synchronic structure of the experience of imagining a scene.

- From the analysis and comparison of the descriptions of auditory experiences that we have collected, emerges a threefold structure of this experience, depending on whether the attention of the subject is directed towards the event which is at the source of the sound, the sound itself, considered independently from its source, or the felt sound: in other words, a generic dynamic structure of the auditory experience, or at least a sketch of such a structure (Petitmengin *et al.*, this issue).

- How does a new idea, a new understanding, or a reflective consciousness emerge? Most testimonies focus on the instantaneous and unpredictable character of this emergence, which is therefore difficult to describe and to study. But the progress of first person methods has enabled the description of this process to begin to unfold in time. While keeping an unforeseeable and instantaneous character, the emergence of an idea or understanding seems to be encouraged by a particular inner disposition, which is notably characterized by an intensification of bodily awareness and a specific attentional mode. This favourable disposition may itself be prepared by a particular inner process, which is itself likely to be induced by precise techniques. The work of collection, analysis and comparison of this process is still in progress (Gendlin, 'Introduction to thinking at the edge', 'Making concepts from experience', his article in this issue; Petitmengin- Peugeot, 1999; Petitmengin, 2001; Depraz *et al.*, 2002; Depraz, this issue; Mathison, this issue). But a succession of phases, displaying striking regularity from one experience to the other and from one subject to another, regardless of the content emerging to consciousness, is beginning to emerge from this work: in other words, a generic dynamic structure of the understanding process.

This meticulous work of detection of experiential structures from a set of descriptions is delicate and still little known, and little studied. But it is a very vast research field that is opening up.

To summarize, lived experience is private and singular. But this does not mean that the researcher is locked in his/her subjectivity. The analysis of a corpus of descriptions of a same type of experience enables the researcher to identify regularities of structure, that make an intersubjective validation possible.[31]

Does one proceed differently in experimental sciences? Under which conditions is the result of an experiment verifiable? Firstly, the type of experiment must be reproducible, which supposes that the operating mode is described with enough detail for the researcher or a colleague to be able to reiterate actions and use instruments of a same type (all other conditions being equal). Secondly, the results must be comparable either between themselves, or with a theoretical anticipation, which supposes that they are *generically* comparable. However a generic comparison cannot be made case by case but by comparing common *structures*. As the advocates of the 'structural' (or 'semantic') conception of scientific theories highlighted, what enables researchers to test theories is not their confrontation with 'raw observational data', with pure contents; it is their confrontation with structured 'data models' (Van Fraassen, 1989). The neurophysiologist for example, while interpreting electroencephalographic records, does not obtain a great deal of information from the raw, individual tracings. He is rather looking for generic signatures, typical 'waves' having a more or less constant structure. The technique of evoked potentials, which consists in accumulating records after a given stimulus, and coming to recognize typical structures (P300 wave associated with recognizing a specific stimulus, or N170 wave associated with seeing a face), or even better the time-frequency patterns (e.g., synchrony) in single-trial analysis, illustrates well the focusing of scientific method on structures.

However let's specify three methodological points.

First of all, the absence of convergence of the experiential structures detected in several individuals, several populations, or by several research teams, does not necessarily prove their invalidity. Before hastening to draw such a conclusion, it is important to look for the

---

[31] 'I suggest a distinction between, on the one hand, the particular contents of consciousness that one experiences at a given moment (i.e., specific sensations, perceptions, ideations and other mental states) and, on the other hand, the parameters that define consciousness as a cognitive system. The subject matter of a theory of consciousness is the latter, not the former.' (Shanon, 2008, p. 24) This conception is also developed in (Shanon, 1993/2008).

reasons that could explain this gap (exactly like in any meticulous experimental study).

A difference of structure may be only apparent, actually due to a divergence of interpretation. For example, a few recent authors (Monson & Hurlburt, 1993) showed that the disagreements between the Würzburg and Cornell laboratories about 'imageless thought' were due to a divergence of interpretation. The subjects of both laboratories agreed to describe 'vague and elusive processes, which carry as if in a nutshell the entire meaning of a situation' (Titchener, 1910/1980, pp. 505–506). But in the Würzburg school theoretical perspective, these 'vague and elusive processes' were imageless thoughts. In Titchener's theoretical perspective, they were not.

A difference of experiential structure may also be due to a difference of expertise. A subject who has no disciplined practice of introspection, and a subject who has been practicing vipashyana meditation regularly for twenty years for example, do not have the same perception of their experience. A subject who has been practicing an hour of daily meditation for twenty years does not perceive his experience the same way as a monk who has spent twenty years in meditative retreat. Different descriptions, different structures, only show in this case different degrees of skill, different degrees of reflective consciousness. It would be the role of a science of consciousness to characterise these degrees of skill precisely, and the experiential structure associated with each of them.

Second, let us come back to the *reproducible* character of a type of description. The reproducibility of a result is the kingpin of any scientific validation: a result or an observation must be reproducible, at least potentially, by any researcher. But in order to be reproducible, a result or observation must be accompanied by a description of its own process of production. In the context of a rigorous investigation of lived experience, this requirement means that in order to be reproducible, and therefore verifiable or falsifiable, a type of description must be accompanied by a description of the process that enables one to obtain it, in other words by a description of the very process of becoming aware and describing. Actually, this description is possible: the process of description being itself an experience, it is possible to collect its description and to detect its generic structure. This point is crucial, because it is this generic dynamic structure of the process of becoming aware and describing that enables the reproducibility of descriptions of a given type. It is this generic structure that makes a description falsifiable. It is also this structure that enables a training of this process.

THE VALIDITY OF FIRST-PERSON DESCRIPTIONS 397

In other words, the researcher is not bound to use the subjects as instruments which he would not need to know the theory nor the functioning of.[32] The researcher must take an interest in the way his data, to wit descriptions of experiences, are produced.[33] Moreover, he should himself be an expert in the process of becoming aware and describing, in order to guide the subjects in the realization of this process and to evaluate its authenticity.

Finally let's come back to the 'public' character of verbal reports. Reports on lived experience are potentially accessible to anybody. But only potentially. In the same way an EEG is accessible to anybody, but readable only by an expert who has received the required theoretical and practical training, a verbal report is not interpretable by an untrained person. The suitable skill consists for example in knowing how to detect the objective — verbal and non verbal — clues making it possible to evaluate the subject's 'level of experiencing'. But this is not all. In the case of a verbal report of experience, interpreting cannot rely only on objective clues. Whether he is evaluating the authenticity of a description or identifying the structure of the described experience, the researcher must understand the experience. However, as we noticed earlier, words do not provide experience, they only point at it. They only become meaningful through a specific gesture the skilled interpreter has to achieve in order to relate with his/her own experience. In other words, researchers in the domain of lived experience cannot avoid making a detour by their own experience. Their expertise must not limit itself to the inventory of objective signs, but must extend to the exploration of their own subjectivity.

Neuro-phenomenological intervalidation

Finally, the fact that using a given experiential structure may guide neurological analysis and help to discover original structures in the electro-encephalographic (or fMRI) data, is a strong confirmation criteria of the validity of this experiential structure. Let's take as examples two projects inspired by the research program initiated by Francisco Varela (Varela, 1996; 1997), that have paid special attention to this neuro-phenomenological circulation.

---

[32] On this point we disagree with Piccinini: 'Just as other scientists need not have a definite understanding of the processes on which they rely in collecting data, we don't need to have an exact understanding of how introspective reports are generated in order to use them as sources of data; (...) we need not know the details of the introspective process for our use of introspective reports to be legitimate'. (Piccinini, 2003, p.149)

[33] 'I suppose that no reputable scientist would venture to publish any considerable alleged discovery in the physical sciences without a careful investigation of his instruments under the precise conditions under which they were used (Dodge, 1912).'

In Lutz's protocol (Lutz, 2002; Lutz *et al.*, 2002), it is the distribution of the neuro-electric data in three classes or 'phenomenological clusters', according to the values of a generic experiential category, which made it possible to distinguish three distinct dynamic neuronal configurations or 'signatures'. In other words, it is the use of an experiential category as a criterion for neuro-electric analysis that enables the detection of an original structure on this level, which confirms in return the relevance of that category through its insertion into a coherent set of data.

In our study of epileptic seizure anticipation (Petitmengin *et al.*, 2007), the discovery of a new neuro-dynamic structure (the preictal neuro-electric desynchronisation) first allowed a refinement of the consciousness of the corresponding experiential dynamics (preictal symptoms and therapeutic countermeasures). This refined consciousness of the experiential dynamics enabled in turn the detection of an original structure in the neuronal dynamics (neuronal desynchronisation at a distance of the seizures).

These two examples illustrate a process of codetermination and mutual validation of structures, since the validation of the experiential structure does not rely on its being matched with an independent neuronal structure, but on the process of refinement and mutual constitution of the experiential and neuronal structures. In other words, the question is not to correlate on the one hand neuronal structures as they would exist 'in themselves', regardless of the activity of recording and analysis that allowed their detection, and on the other hand structures of 'pure' experience, regardless of the acts of becoming aware, of description and analysis. But it is to start and to let unfold a process of co-determination and mutual co-validation of the two processes. This is an additional illustration of the process of putting several results and research process in mutual consistency, which enables the validation of first person descriptions.

But here again, this process of guidance and validation by mutual confrontation, is not anything exceptional. It is the foundation of the whole edifice of natural sciences (Bitbol, 1996; 1998). As Quine (1974) and Piaget (1967) underlined, natural sciences cannot take advantage of any external guarantee against scepticism, and therefore of any external guarantee to validate their contents of knowledge. They only rely on the reciprocal guarantee given by the consistency of the system they form as well as by their general efficiency. This process is then at the root of the most basic methods for refining experimental data. For example, how did one check the reliability and exactness of the thermometers made of a mercury column and a calibrated glass beaker, during the first stages of the science of heat, at the end of the eighteenth century (Bachelard, 1938)? There was no absolutely reliable external standard for this, and moreover there were good reasons to suspect systematic distortions: if the glass expands with temperature in an unknown proportion in relation to mercury, indications of temperature become unreliable. But if one uses another thermometric device, which is also uncertain, to evaluate the dilation coefficient of the glass, one can correct (even imperfectly, because of the second device's uncertainty) the graduation of the first instrument. And so on.

The continuation of the process consists in converging, from mutual corrections to mutual corrections, toward one common interval of values of the temperature that is considered as 'exact'.

Nothing other than such a process of mutual validation is required to give consistency to the verbal first person reports. There is no 'correspondence' to look for with whatever else. We entirely agree on this point with Shanon's remarks (1984; 1993) about the necessity of substituting the theory of truth as consistency to the theory of truth as correspondence when evaluating the truth of first person descriptions. But we also specify at the same time the nature of the consistencies which are to be sought: consistency of descriptions and verbal/ non-verbal clues, consistency amongst the structures which have been extracted from the reports of experience, and finally broader neuro-experiential consistency.

A very basic objection may arise at this point: isn't this kind of circular procedure of validation tantamount to self-validation and unfalsifiability? Doesn't it fall prey to Popper's criticism of psychoanalysis, which was accused of being inaccessible to any possible challenge? To understand why this criticism is irrelevant, one must realize that the requirement of self-consistency is by no means a requirement of closure. For example, 'anomalies' challenging the possibility of describing experience by means of explicitation approaches may arise. But they are bound to be expressed *in terms* of these approaches, and to take the form of an *internal* discrepancy. Thus, it may be the case that several incompatible structures are extracted from reports of experience of the same type of task, and that no rationale can be found for this incompatibility by pushing the interviews further. This would trigger a process of revision of hypothesis and methods.

Here again, this does not depart from the methods of experimental research, which also accepts several levels of circularity in their very procedure of testing. One of them is that a theory is usually tested by means of instruments described and interpreted by means of this very theory. Another level of circularity is that an 'anomaly' (threatening to falsify the theory) can only be expressed in terms of this theory. For instance, Michelson & Morley's celebrated result was initially interpreted in terms of partial dragging of the ether by the Earth, and not as a relativistic effect. In this case, as in the case of explicitation reports, it is clear that circularity means neither self-validation nor complete closure.

Conclusion

To sum up, becoming reflectively conscious of one's experience and describing it is a process which does not consist in observing or reflecting upon a pre-existing experience, but in an unfolding of experience elicited by precise acts. The validity of a first person report is a validity 'in action', which cannot be measured in static terms of correspondence between the report and the experience, but in dynamic terms of performative consistency of the acts which produce it. Considerable research has to be carried out in order to specify the description of these acts and their modes and criteria of consistency. This is a research program for the years to come, which can be only performed by researchers involved in the practice of these acts. That such a research program is not only possible but also indispensible can be seen in many developments within the neurocognitive sciences themselves. For example, questions such as 'Is the experience of using of Bach-y-Rita's TVSS visual,tactile, a mixture, or a new sensory modality?' imperatively require first-person inquiry (Froese & Spiers 2007).

Acknowledgments

The authors thank Benny Shanon, Evan Thompson, Tom Froese and Dorothée Legrand for their very helpful comments on an earlier version of this article.

References

Andreas C. and Andreas T. (2009), 'Aligning perceptual positions: A new distinction in NLP', *Journal of Consciousness Studies*, this issue.
Bachelard, G. (1938), *La formation de l'esprit scientifique* (Paris: Vrin).
Bergson, H. (1934/1975), *La Pensée et le Mouvant* (Paris: Presses Universitaires de France).
Bitbol M. (1996), *Mécanique quantique, une introduction philosophique* (Paris: Flammarion).
Bitbol M. (1998), 'Some steps towards a transcendental deduction of quantum mechanics', *Philosophia naturalis*, **35**, pp. 253–80.
Bitbol M. (2008a), 'Is consciousness primary?', *NeuroQuantology*, **6**, pp. 53–71.

Bitbol M. (2008b), 'Consciousness, situations, and the measurement problem of quantum mechanics', *NeuroQuantology,* **6**, pp. 203–13.
Block, N. (1995), 'On a confusion about a function of consciousness', *Behavioral and Brain Sciences,* **18**, pp. 227–47.
Bode, B.H. (1913), 'The method of introspection', *The Journal of Philosophy, Psychology and Scientific Methods,* **10**, pp. 85–91.
Brentano F. (1874/1995), *Psychology from an Empirical Viewpoint* (London: Routledge).
Cohen G. (1989), *Memory in the Real World* (Psychology Press).
Comte, A. (1945), *Cours de philosophie positive. Leçons 1 à 45* (Paris: Hermann).
Courtier, M. (2007), *Le dictionnaire de la langue du vin* (Paris: CNRS éditions).
Depraz N. (2009), 'The failure of meaning', *Journal of Consciousness Studies*, this issue.
Depraz, N., Varela, F., Vermersch, P. (2003), *On Becoming Aware: The Pragmatics of Exepriencing* (Amsterdam: John Benjamins).
Delattre, P. (1971), *Système, structure, function, evolution* (Paris: Maloine).
Dennett, D.C. (1991), *Consciousness Explained* (Boston, MA: Little, Brown).
Dodge, R. (1912), 'The theory and limitations of introspection', *The American journal of Psychology,* **23**, pp. 214–29.
Dretske, F. (1995), *Naturalizing the Mind* (Cambridge, MA: MIT).
Findlay J. N. (1948), 'Recommendations regarding the language of introspection', *Philosophy and Phenomenological Research,* **9**, pp. 212–36.
Froese, T. (2009), 'Hume and the enactive approach to mind', *Phenomenology and the Cognitive Sciences,* **8**(1), pp. 95–133.
Froese, T. & Spiers, A. (2007), 'Toward a phenomenological pragmatics of enactive perception', *Proc. of the 4th Int. Conf. on Enactive Interfaces,* Grenoble, France: Association ACROE, pp. 105–108.
Fink, E. (1992), *Natur, Freiheit, Welt* (Würzburg: Königshausen & Neumann).
Gallagher, S. and Zahavi, D. (2008), *The Phenomenological Mind* (London: Routledge).
Gendlin E. (1962/1997), *Experiencing and the Creation of Meaning* (Evanston, IL: Northwestern University Press).
Gendlin E., 'Introduction to thinking at the edge', http://www.focusing.org
Gendlin E., 'Making concepts from experience', http://www.focusing.org
Genoud C. (2009), 'On the cultivation of presence in meditation', *Journal of Consciousness Studies*, this issue.
Goldman, A.I. (1992), 'In defense of the simulation theory', *Mind and Language,* **7**, pp. 104–19.
Grice, H.P. (2002), 'Some remarks about the senses', in A. Noë and E. Thompson (Ed.), *Vision and Mind*, pp. 35–54 (Cambridge, MA: MIT Press).
Gusdorf G. (1950/1993), *Mémoire et personne* (Paris: Presses Universitaires de France).
Hacking, I. (1983), *Representing and Intervening* (Cambridge: Cambridge University Press).
Hendricks, M. (2009), 'Experiencing Level: An instance of developing a variable from a first person process so it can be reliably measured and taught', *Journal of Consciousness Studies*, this issue.
Hugo, V. (1982), 'Fuite en Sologne', *Les chansons des rues et des bois* (Paris: Gallimard).
Hume D. (1739–40/1969), *A Treatise of Human Nature*, ed. E.C. Mossner (London: Penguin Books).
Hurlburt R.T. (2009), 'Iteratively apprehending pristine experience', *Journal of Consciousness Studies*, this issue

Hurlburt, R. and Schwitzgebel, E. (2007), *Describing Inner Experience? Proponent Meets Skeptic* (Cambridge, MA: MIT Press).
Husserl E. (1913/1950), *Idées directrices pour une phénoménologie* (Paris: Gallimard).
Husserl E., 'La Phénoménologie', article pour l'*Encyclopedia Britannica* traduit de l'allemand par J.F. Courtine et J.L. Fidel (1993), *Notes sur Heidegger* (Paris: Éditions de Minuit), version 2, pp. 93–114.
James W. (1890/1983), *Principles of Psychology* (Cambridge, MA: Harvard University Press).
Jaynes, J. (1976), *The Origin of Consciousness In the Breakdown of the Bicameral Mind* (Boston, MA: Houghton Mifflin).
Johansson, P., Hall, L., Sikström, S., Tärning, B., Lind A. (2006), 'How something can be said about telling more than we can know: On choice blindness and introspection', *Consciousness and Cognition*, **15**, pp. 673–92.
Levin, D.T. & Simons, D.J. (1997), 'Failure to detect changes to attended objects in motion pictures', *Psychonomic Bulletin and Review*, **4**, pp. 501-506.
Lutz, A. (2002), 'Toward a neurophenomenology of generative passages: a first empirical case study', *Phenomenology and the Cognitive Sciences*, **1**, pp. 133–67.
Lutz, A., Lachaux, J.P., Martinerie, J., Varela, J. (2002), 'Guiding the study of brain dynamics using first person data: synchrony patterns correlate with on-going conscious states during a simple visual task', *Proceedings of the National Academy of Sciences* (USA), **99**, pp. 1586–91.
Mack, A. & Rock, I. (1998), *Inattentional Blindness* (Cambridge, MA: Harvard University Press).
Marcel, A.J. (2003), 'Introspective report', *Journal of Consciousness Studies*, **10** (9–10), pp. 167–86.
Mathison J. and Tosey P. (2009), 'Exploring moments of knowing; neuro-linguistic programming and enquiry into inner landscapes', *Journal of Consciousness Studies*, this issue
Merleau-Ponty, M. (1943), *Éloge de la Philosophie* (Paris: Gallimard).
Merleau-Ponty, M. (1945), *Phénoménologie de la Perception* (Paris: Gallimard).
Monson, C.K. and Hurlburt, R.T. (1993), 'A comment to suspend the introspection controversy: Introspecting subjects did agree', in R.T. Hurburt (ed.), *Sampling Inner Experience in Disturbed Affect*, pp. 15–26 (Plenum Press).
Mill, J. S. (1882/1961), *Auguste Comte and Positivism* (Ann Arbor, MI: University of Michigan).
Moore, G.E. (1903), 'The refutation of idealism', *Mind*, **12**, pp. 433–53.
Natorp, P. (1912), *Allgemeine Psychologie nach kritischer Methode* (Tübingen: J.C.B. Mohr), French translation by E. Dufour & J. Servois (2007), *Psychologie générale selon la méthode critique* (Paris: Vrin).
Neisser, U. (1982/1999), *Memory Observed, Second Edition. Remembering in Natural Contexts* (Worth Publishers).
Nigro, G. and Neisser, U. (1983), 'Point of view in personal memories', *Cognitive Psychology*, **15**, pp. 467–82.
Nisbett, R.E & Wilson T.D. (1977), 'Telling more than we know: Verbal reports on mental processes', *Psychological Review*, **84**, pp. 231–59.
Overgaard, M. & Sorensen, T.A. (2004), 'Introspection distinct from first order experiences', *Journal of Consciousness Studies*, **11** (7–8), pp. 76–95.
Petitmengin C. (2001), *L'expérience intuitive* (Paris: L'Harmattan).
Petitmengin C. (2006), 'Describing one's subjective experience in the second person. An interview method for a science of consciousness', *Phenomenology and the Cognitive Sciences*, **5**, pp. 229–69.

Petitmengin, C. (2007), 'Towards the source of thoughts: The gestural and transmodal dimension of lived experience', *Journal of Consciousness Studies*, **14** (3), pp. 54–82.

Petitmengin, C., Navarro V., Le Van Quyen, M. (2007), 'Anticipating seizure: Pre-reflective experience at the center of neuro-phenomenology', *Consciousness and Cognition*, **16**, pp. 746–64 .

Petitmengin C., Bitbol M., Nissou J.M., Pachoud B., Curallucci H., Cermolacce M., Vion-Dury J.(2009), 'Listening from within', *Journal of Consciousness Studies*, this issue

Petitmengin-Peugeot C. (1999), 'The intuitive experience', in F. Varela and J. Shear (Eds), *The View from Within*, pp. 43–77 (Exeter: Imprint Academic).

Philippot P. and Segal Z. (2009), 'Mindfulness based psychological interventions: developing emotional awareness for better being', *Journal of Consciousness Studies*, this issue

Piaget J. (ed. 1967), *Logique et connaissance scientifique* (Paris: Gallimard).

Piaget J. (1974), *La prise de conscience* (Paris: Presses Universitaires de France).

Piccinini, G. (2003), 'Data from introspective reports', *Journal of Consciousness Studies*, **10**, (9–10), pp. 141–56.

Piccinini, G. (2007), 'First-person data, publicity, and self-measurement' <http://www.umsl.edu/~piccininig/First-person%20Data%20short%202.htm>

Pickering, A. (1995), *The Mangle of Practice* (Chicago: University of Chicago Press).

Prinz, J. (2004), 'The Fractionation of Introspection', *Journal of Consciousness Studies*, **11** (7-8), pp. 40–57.

Quine, W.V. (1974), *The Roots of Reference* (Chicago: Open Court).

Ribot T. (1881), *Les maladies de la mémoire* (Paris: Alcan).

Ricœur P. (1950), *Philosophie de la volonté* (Paris: Aubier).

Sartre J.P. (1934), *La transcendance de l'ego* (Paris: Vrin, 1978).

Sartre J.P. (1936), *L'imagination* (Paris: PUF).

Sartre J.P. (1938), *Esquisse d'une théorie des émotions* (Paris: Hermann).

Shanon, B. (1984), 'The case for introspection', *Cognition and Brain Theory*, 7, pp. 167–80.

Shanon, B. (1993/2008), *The Representational and the Presentational: An Essay on Cognition and the Study of Mind* (London: Harvester-Wheatsheaf; second edition Exeter: ImprintAcademic, 2008).

Shanon, B. (2008), 'A psychological theory of consciousness', *Journal of Consciousness Studies*, **15** (5), pp. 5–47.

Schlanger, J. (2001), 'Introspection, rétrospection, prospection', *Revue de Métaphysique et de Morale* 2001/4, 32, pp. 527-541.

Schooler, J.W. (2002), 'Re-representing consciousness: dissociations between experience and meta-consciousness', *Trends in Cognitive Science*, **6** (8), pp. 339–44.

Schooler, J.W., Dougal, S. (1999), 'The symbiosis of subjective and experimental approaches to intuition', *Journal of Consciousness Studies*, 6 (2–3), pp. 280–87.

Schooler, J.W., Ohlsson, S., Brooks, K. (1993), 'Thoughts beyond words: When language overshadows insight', *Journal of Experimental Psychology: General*, **122**, pp. 166–83.

Schooler, J.W., Schreiber C.A. (2004), 'Experience, meta-consciousness, and the paradox of introspection', *Journal of Consciousness Studies*, 11(7-8), pp. 17–39.

Schooler, J.W., Reichle, E.D. & Halpern, D.V. (2005), 'Zoning-out during reading; Evidence for dissociations between experience and meta-consciousness', in D.T. Levin (Ed), *Thinking and Seeing* (Cambridge, MA: MIT Press).

Schwitzgebel, E. (2004), 'Introspective training apprehensively defended: Reflections on Titchener's Lab Manual', *Journal of Consciousness Studies*, 11(7–8), pp. 58–76.

Schwitzgebel, E. (2007a), 'Do you have constant tactile experience of your feet in your shoes? Or is experience limited to what's in attention?', *Journal of Consciousness Studies*, **14** (3), pp. 5–35.
Schwitzgebel, E. (2007b), 'No unchallengeable epistemic authority, of any sort, regarding our own conscious experience – Contra Dennett?', *Phenomenology and the Cognitive Science*, **6**, pp. 107–13.
Schwitzgebel, E. (2008), 'The unreliability of naïve introspection', *Philosophical Review*, **117** (2), pp. 245–73.
Searle, J.R. (1992), *The Rediscovery of the Mind* (Cambridge, MA: MIT Press).
Shusterman, R. (2008), *Body Consciousness: A Philosophy of Mindfulness and Somaesthetics* (Cambridge: Cambridge University Press).
Simons, D.J. & Levin, D.T. (1998), 'Failure to detect changes to people during a real-world interaction', *Psychonomic Bulletin and Review*, **5**, pp. 644–49.
Simons, D.J. & Chalbris, C.F. (1999), 'Gorillas in our midst: Sustained inattentional blindness for dynamic events', *Perception*, **28**, pp. 1059–74.
Spiegelberg, H. (1975), 'Phenomenology through vicarious experience', in *Doing Phenomenology. Essays on and in phenomenology*, pp. 35–56 (The Hague: Martinus Nijhoff).
Stern D.N. (2009), 'Pre-reflexive experience and its passage to reflexive experience: A developmental view', *Journal of Consciousness Studies*, this issue
Sully, J. (1881), 'Illusions of introspection', *Mind*, **6** (21), pp. 1–18.
Ten Hoor M., (1932), 'A critical analysis of the concept of introspection', *The Journal of Philosophy*, **29** (12), pp. 322–31.
Titchener, E.B. (1898/1914), *A Primer of Psychology* (New-York: Macmillan).
Titchener, E.B. (1910/1980), *A Textbook of Psychology* (New-York: Scholars' Facsimiles and Reprints).
Titchener E.B. (1912), 'The schema of introspection', *American Journal of Psychology*, **23**, pp. 485–508.
Thompson E. (2007), *Mind in Life. Biology, Phenomenology, and the Sciences of Mind* (Cambridge, MA: The Belknap Press of Harvard University Press).
Van Fraassen, B. (1989), *Laws and Symmetries* (Oxford: Oxford University Press).
Varela, F. (1996), 'Neurophenomenology: A methodological remedy for the hard problem', *Journal of Consciousness Studies*, **3** (4), pp. 330–35.
Varela, F. (1997), 'The naturalization of phenomenology as the transcendance of nature: Searching for generative mutual constraints', *Alter: Revue de Phénoménologie*, **5**, pp. 355–85.
Vermersch P. (1994/2003), *L'entretien d'explicitation* (Paris: Éditions ESF).
Vermersch P. (1997), 'Questions de méthode. La référence à l'expérience subjective', *Alter: Revue de Phénoménologie*, **5**, pp. 121–36.
Vermersch P. (2000), 'Conscience directe et conscience réfléchie', *Intellectica*, **31**, pp. 269–311.
Vermersch P. (2009), 'Describing the practice of introspection', *Journal of Consciousness Studies*, this issue
Wilson T. (2002), *Strangers to Ourselves: Discovering the Adaptative Unconscious* (Cambridge, MA: Harvard University Press).
Wittgenstein L. (1992), *Investigations philosophiques* (Paris: Gallimard).
Wundt W. (1897), *Outlines of Psychology* (Leipzig: Wilhelm Engelmann).
Zahavi, D. (2003), 'How to investigate subjectivity: Natorp and Heidegger on reflection', *Continental Philosophy Review*, **36** (2), pp. 155–76.
Zahavi, D. (2008), *Subjectivity and Selfhood: Investigating the First-Person Perspective* (Cambridge, MA: MIT Press).

www.ingramcontent.com/pod-product-compliance
Lightning Source LLC
Chambersburg PA
CBHW021133230426
43667CB00005B/102